Retention and Productivity Strategies for Nurse Managers

Retention and Productivity Strategies for Nurse Managers

Carol Jorgensen Huston, R.N., M.S.N.

Associate Professor of Nursing
California State University
Chico, California

Bessie L. Marquis, R.N., C.N.A.A., M.S.N.

Professor of Nursing
California State University
Chico, California

Philadelphia **J. B. LIPPINCOTT COMPANY**

Cambridge   New York   St. Louis   San Francisco

London   Singapore   Sydney   Tokyo

Production: Editorial Services of New England, Inc.
Composition: Publication Services, Inc.
Printing/Binding: R. R. Donnelley & Sons

6 5 4 3 2 1

Library of Congress Cataloging-in-Publication Data

Huston, Carol Jorgensen.
  Retention and productivity strategies for nurse managers.

  Bibliography: p.
  Includes index.
  1. Nursing services – Personnel management.
2. Nursing services – Administration. I. Marquis,
Bessie L. II. Title.
RT89.3.H87 1989   362.1'73'0683   88-27304
ISBN 0-397-54739-0

Any procedure or practice described in this book should be applied by the health-care practitioner under appropriate supervision in accordance with professional standards of care used with regard to the unique circumstances that apply in each practice situation. Care has been taken to confirm the accuracy of information presented and to describe generally accepted practices. However, the authors, editors and publisher cannot accept any responsibility for errors or omissions or for consequences from application of the information in this book and make no warranty, express or implied, with respect to the contents of the book.

I would like to dedicate this book to my beautiful children, Kristin and Shauna, and to my wonderful and supportive husband, Tom. I would like to thank my husband for encouraging me to actively pursue the other great loves of my life: nursing, teaching, and writing.

CJH

I would like to dedicate this book to my husband, in thanks for the multitude of household chores he performed willingly and without request so that I could write this book. I also want to thank Ahna for the use of her computer and the word-processing lessons, which had the unexpected outcome of making me computer proficient. Lastly, I would like to thank my longtime friend and model nursing CEO, Jeanne Madison, for her encouragement and support.

BLM

Preface

This book developed as an outcome of a ten-year study on retention that indicated that most organizations view high attrition rates as inevitable. The results of that study, which were published in the March 1988 issue of *Journal of Nursing Administration*, prompted us to begin examining what proactive roles organizations could take to increase not only retention, but also productivity. What we discovered was a wealth of classical and current research in support of our observations, and the observations of many of our managerial colleagues, that people do respond to appropriate managerial strategies; that is, that managers and thus organizations can be proactive in implementing strategies that focus on the growth and development of human resources.

We have made a conscientious effort to present realistic human resource strategies in this book. Both financial accountability and cost-effectiveness were considered. We believe that contemporary principles of managing human resources are cost-effective, and we have attempted to show that neglect of human resource needs leads to a high cost to organizations in terms of attrition and loss of productivity.

Although this book focuses primarily on personnel management for nurses, the content is applicable to any staffing mix. Likewise, although the hospital is frequently used as a point of reference, the human resource strategies suggested are applicable in a variety of health care settings.

In addition to the retention study, several other factors shaped the book's development. First is our extensive experience in management as practicing administrators, educators, and authors. Second is our personal belief that the current practice of frenzied recruitment is not an acceptable solution to the nursing shortage if the underlying human resource management problems of the organization are not corrected. Last is our strong personal belief about the potential of human beings; we believe that people try to live up to high expectations if they are supported financially, psychologically, and intellectually while doing so.

This book was designed primarily for use by middle-level nursing managers, although many of the topics it covers are also applicable to first-level managers. The book is also designed for personnel managers, nurse recruiters, and heads of non-nursing departments. Although most top-level nursing executives have a broad-based sophistication about nursing management, they may find the book useful as a teaching tool or may be able to adapt the tools for implementation in their organizations. Lastly, the book is appropriate for graduate students in various fields of health care administration and as a supplemental text for senior students studying leadership or management.

We feel this book offers several salient features that distinguish it from other nursing human resource management books. First, the book includes topics that are traditionally absent or are covered only superficially in most books on human resource management for nurses; the chapters on coaching, the impaired employee, grievances and arbitration, employee socialization and resocialization, career development, and management ethics are examples. Second, the strategies suggested in each chapter are supported by current non-nursing as well as nursing research in personnel management. Lastly, in order to assist managers in implementing many of these strategies, each chapter includes specific tools for implementation. These tools are applicable to almost any health care organization, and readers are encouraged to adapt them for use in their organizations whenever possible.

However, the value of this book is limited if readers and organizations are not willing to honestly examine how they manage human resources and consider how they might improve their management strategies. It is our hope that managers will use this book to (1) look at themselves and their organizations' beliefs about human resource management, (2) determine how they can improve the management of human resources to increase productivity and retention, (3) implement programs, and (4) realize positive outcomes from changes they implement.

Carol Jorgensen Huston
Bessie L. Marquis

Acknowledgments

We wish to thank our numerous faculty colleagues at California State University, Chico, for their encouragement and support during the writing of this book. We are also indebted to the milieu in which we work. The academic system itself encourages its members not only to be productive, but to excel. Although we have been employed in various organizations throughout our nursing careers, we have never before found that so much was expected of us. And we have never been so productive, so well supported during our endeavors, or so handsomely rewarded, as we have in academia.

We also wish to acknowledge our nursing management colleagues, who have taught us so much. We are especially indebted to those managers who have shared their ideas and suggestions in our numerous workshops, talks, and seminars. Our undergraduate students have also been a constant source of encouragement, and our graduate students have made a special contribution to this book.

Contents

List of Tools for Implementation

Retention and Productivity Strategies for Nurse Managers

·UNIT ONE
Introduction to Human Resource Management

THE HEALTH care industry is continuing to undergo a major redefinition of roles and responsibilities. Recent patterns of supply and demand, as well as current economic realities, have led to the development of a regional physician surplus, the implementation of diagnostic-related groupings as a means of reimbursement for government-supported patients, and a severe nursing shortage. This in turn has altered the way health care organizations view employees, especially nurses. There is an increased focus on the value of the individual employee and a growing movement toward humanism within organizations. This refocusing on the needs of the individual employee is not a result of altruistic philosophies, but a recognition that optimal management of human resources can result in not only a more stable workforce, but increased productivity as well.

This new emphasis on meeting employee needs as well as organizational needs has resulted in proactive (in contrast to reactive) reorganizational changes. Health care organizations and their managers must be willing to examine their values honestly and seek congruence between stated values and actions. Organizational, nursing service, and unit philosophies must be examined and rewritten to reflect the value of the nurse to the organization. Only then can congruent organizational and management philosophies become the cornerstone for all future planning.

This future planning is proactive. Nurse administrators can no longer passively wait to see whether their staff will remain loyal to them and their organization. They must create a motivating work environment that provides for employee needs such as recognition, achievement, opportunity for advancement, satisfying work, participative management, and fair compensation. The inadequacy of both a current and a future nurse employee pool has changed the focus from recruitment to retention. Increasing nurse retention in a severe nursing shortage is not an option; it has become an economic necessity.

The renewed interest in humanism as a way to retain more nurses and increase productivity has resulted in unique management challenges. Changing the focus from organizational needs to a combination of organizational and employee needs has often resulted in changes in the way human resource management is organized. It is rarely possible or even desirable for one department to meet the individual needs of many employees. As a result, the responsibility for personnel management in many institutions has been expanded to every manager within the organization. This role overlap carries a great risk; communication within the organization is now more complex, and there is always a potential for conflict. However, there has never been a time when the need for wise and effective supervision has been greater. A new breed of nursing managers is emerging that can balance employee and organizational needs while also maintaining a high level of productivity. This truly is optimal human resource management.

1
The Art and Science of
Managing Human Resources

HUMAN RESOURCE management can be broadly defined as maximization of human resources for optimal personal and organizational growth. The goals of management and the needs of the people who work in an organization are met jointly through the mutual planning of objectives. In the past, the term *human resource management* was often used synonymously with *personnel management*, although personnel management traditionally placed organizational needs above human needs. In this book, however, the two terms will be used interchangeably.

Because the health care industry is labor intensive, it is vital for nurse managers to understand human resource management and to maximize the recruitment, selection, and retention of a highly skilled professional staff. An adequate supply of professional nurses must be assured to meet the ever-changing and increasingly complex needs of the health care system. Nurse managers must understand how to identify and select employees who will be motivated to meet organizational goals; they must also be able to use retention strategies to create a stable and economical work force.

Chapter 1 briefly describes the prominent theorists of the human relations era and discusses components of the personnel process such as recruitment and retention. The impact of the current nursing shortage on the need for optimal human resource management and the intensity of the nursing shortage in regards to the current as well as future nurse applicant pool are examined.

In addition, the challenge of nursing as a labor-intensive profession is presented. The importance of retaining nurses as a valuable resource for nursing managers is outlined, as are stressors unique to professional nursing. Tools for implementation include checklists for measuring employee satisfaction and tools that assess the cost of turnover in institutions.

THEORISTS OF THE HUMAN RELATIONS ERA

Human resource management places the emphasis on the "human" resource, rather than on capital or physical resources. Historically, personnel management focused primarily on technical means of production, viewing worker satisfaction as relatively insignificant. However, in the last 50 or 60 years, industrial psychologists and sociologists in the United States have begun focusing on the "human element" as a critical factor in productivity. In a *"human relations era,"* people rather than machines are emphasized, and the focus is on participatory management.

Among the catalysts leading to the shift toward humanism were studies done by Elton Mayo at the Hawthorne works of the Western Electric Company near Chicago, Illinois, between 1927 and 1932. Initially, the studies began as an investigation of the relationship between light illumination in the factory and productivity. However, they revealed that, regardless of changes in the environment, workers responded positively to the attention paid to them by management as subjects in the study. This so-called Hawthorne effect indicated that people respond to being studied and will alter their behavior in whatever way they feel will continue to gain them attention.

Douglas McGregor reinforced the findings of the Hawthorne studies in his work entitled *Theory X* and *Theory Y.* According to McGregor, managerial attitudes about employees (and hence how they treat those employees) can be directly correlated with employee satisfaction. Theory X managers believe that employees are basically lazy, need constant supervision and direction, and are indifferent to organizational needs. Theory Y managers believe their employees enjoy work, are self-motivated, and willingly contribute to organizational goals.

Chris Argyris theorized that counterproductive employee behavior indicates a failure on the part of the organization to meet worker needs, rather than a failure of the employee. According to Argyris, managerial domination causes discouragement and passivity among employees. Thus, employee failure or termination is a direct result of management's not meeting employee self-esteem and independence needs.

Abraham Maslow continued this work by looking at human needs and motivation. Maslow identified a hierarchy of five important needs and stressed that human resource development should focus on helping individuals achieve the fourth and fifth stages of self-esteem and self-actualization. Maslow emphasized the need for managers to recognize that all employees are motivated by different things at different times in their lives.

Ouchi proposed the egalitarian organization, in which employees participate fully in the management of the organization. This approach, known as *Theory Z* and *Japanese management*, expanded McGregor's Theory Y and supported democratic leadership. Components of Theory Z include consensus decision-making, the fitting of employees to their jobs, job security, the movement of employees slowly through the ranks to assure competence and success, quality circles (formal employee/management problem-solving work groups), and holistic concern for the workers.

In the 1980s there continues to be a great deal of emphasis on productivity, with unprecedented attention to the importance of human resource management. Managers must be attuned to the new social values of workers in the 1980s and 1990s, including a general decline in the belief in the work ethic, a shifting balance between technical and professional workers, the increasing frequency of mid-life career changes, a trend toward education as a lifelong pursuit, and declining motivation to manage among the younger generation (Schuster, 1985). Nurse executives today are expected to possess a business mindset with regard to delivering patient care, financial acumen, and knowledge of economic trends and health policy, *and* they are expected to be expert managers of human resources (Miller, 1987). In addition, human resource management not only must result in employee motivation and greater retention, it also must result in greater productivity.

Nurse managers in the 1980s and 1990s must be proactive in making organizational changes that recognize the value of the nurse employee as a valuable member of the health care team. Scherer (1988) identified human resource management strategies that have allowed visionary nurse managers to attract and keep nurses. One of the managers described utilizes a combination of primary nursing and decentralized nursing administration. A second nursing manager has centralized all departments participating in patient care under nursing service so as to better focus on the patient. A third manager assists staff in developing contractual agreements between patients and nurses so that patients assume great responsibility for their own recovery. A fourth manager is reorganizing the structure so that nursing units become franchises.

Kramer (1988) studied 16 magnet hospitals that possessed characteristics similar to the best run companies in the corporate community. Most of these magnet hospitals were moving toward all registered nurse (RN) staffs and had fluidity and informality that allowed for quick and easy communication and exchange of information at all levels. In addition, employees were trained to feel empowered and were rewarded for productivity, and the hospitals consistently acted in accordance with their desire to deliver quality care for the consumer. Leaders were highly visible and accessible, and enthusiasm was common in the management team.

Fifield (1988) examined "productivity excellent" hospitals and found that lean management and good morale were characteristics of successful hospitals. Employee morale generally was high because of proactive management strategies that recognized employee growth and development, participative management, the need for recognition, and the intrinsic value of the employee. Good working conditions and a higher than average nonmanagement compensation package also contributed to worker satisfaction and productivity. Regardless of the strategy used, it becomes clear that nurse managers must be attuned to the wants and needs of their employees and be proactive in making organizational changes that result in retention and increased productivity.

THE IMPACT OF THE NURSING SHORTAGE ON HUMAN RESOURCE MANAGEMENT

There has always been a need for skillful human resource management, but this need has intensified with the current nursing shortage, which will reach epidemic proportions in the 1990s. Trends indicate that by the year 2000 there will be about one-half as many nurses as needed (Styles and Holzemer, 1986).

Although nursing has experienced periodic shortages before, many experts argue that the current nursing shortage is different and far more severe than any experienced thus far. Prior shortages consisted of inadequate numbers of working nurses in specialized areas and in specific parts of the country. Since the nurse pool itself was adequate to meet the need, the solution centered around recruiting inactive nurses and drawing from the new graduate nurse pool. Many nursing administrators today are erroneously continuing to focus solely on increasing their supply of new nurses. Nurse administrators must recognize that the "revolving door syndrome" will probably occur again as the nursing shortage worsens (Prescott and Bowen, 1987). This syndrome is characterized by nurses becoming more easily dissatisfied as they become aware that jobs are plentiful, thus making it more difficult for hospitals to retain them.

Today, both the future and current nurse employee pool is inadequate. One half of the nation's baccalaureate nursing programs reported a loss of 19% of total full-time undergraduate enrollments in the past two academic years. Nursing candidates have turned to other career options in search of increased financial reward and career mobility. In addition, reduced availability of scholarships and financial aid as a result of government cutbacks deter potential candidates from entering baccalaureate nursing education. A 1986 survey of entering male and female freshman college students found that only 2.7% of 204,491 students intended to pursue nursing careers, the smallest number in the past 20 years. Between 1974 and 1986, the aspiring nurse population enrolled in universities fell by nearly three fourths, from 9.1% to 2.6% (Green, 1987).

Because nursing continues to be primarily a female occupation, the impact of the women's movement on the future nursing pool is significant. Women have been encouraged to enter occupations traditionally held by males, and altruistic professions have been devalued. Forty-three thousand freshman college women planned to become nurses in the fall of 1983. That number had dropped to 20,000 by the fall of 1986 (Green, 1987). In contrast, the number of freshman women interested in medical school now exceeds the number interested in nursing, and the number of women in the business sector has skyrocketed. This can be attributed, at least in part, to a negative and largely inaccurate image of nursing by the public (Sullivan et al., 1988). Prospective students are being advised, "You're too bright to be a nurse, go into medicine." The public image of the nursing profession continues to be that of a low-salaried, female occupation, instead of a valued health care profession.

In examining the current nursing pool, eight out of ten hospitals studied nationwide in 1986 reported unfilled RN positions. Hospitals plan to hire 14% more registered nurses this year than last year (NAHC Recruitment Survey, 1987), and vacancies for registered nurses in hospitals have doubled since 1985. Critical care and medical surgical positions remain the hardest positions to fill. A commonly held, but erroneous, belief about the current nursing shortage is that many nurses have left health care and have become inactive or have pursued careers outside the health care field. In actuality, nurses have one of the highest rates of employment among predominantly female occupations. Almost 80% of registered nurses are actively employed, whether full-time or part-time, as compared with 54% of American women, and only 6% of nurses are employed in other occupations and are not seeking a nursing position. Thus, it is unlikely that unemployed nurses represent a large potential resource to the applicant pool (Aiken et al., 1987). If nurse administrators are to maximize limited resources, the need for optimal human resource management is apparent.

NURSING AS A LABOR-INTENSIVE PROFESSION

The health care industry is the third largest industry in the United States after government and retailing, with eight million people employed in the health sector (Ginzberg, 1987). Figures for 1986 indicate there are approximately 1.5 million nurses employed in the profession. Nursing is a labor-intensive profession; in other words, a high percentage of the operating costs must be devoted to labor costs. An average hospital must allocate approximately 50% of its budget for payroll, and more than three quarters of this figure is for nursing salaries.

Between two thirds and three quarters of working nurses are employed in hospitals. Despite the fact that national demand for inpatient hospital care has hit an all-time low, hospitals have dramatically increased the nurse/patient ratio. In fact, in the last 14 years there has been an 82% increase in the ratio of nurses to patients, from about 50 registered nurses per 100 patients to over 90 per 100 (Aiken, 1987). Registered nurses have replaced ancillary personnel. In 1968, about one third of nursing service personnel were registered nurses; by 1986, this proportion approached 60% (Aiken, 1987).

These changes in the staffing mix are directly related to newer modes of implementing patient care, such as primary nursing and total patient care. These modes have been implemented in an effort to improve the quality of patient care as well as to increase the motivation and retention of registered nurses. It is important to recognize that the strategy of altering the mode of care as a means of increasing retention is in danger of being eliminated. As hospitals face both economic constraints and a nursing shortage, modes of patient care delivery that *appear* to carry a high price tag, or require a high number of skilled registered nurses, are a frequent target for reactive decisions (Marquis, 1988).

It becomes obvious then that because nursing is a labor-intensive profession, the costs of recruitment and turnover add a staggering component to the manpower budget. Recruitment bonuses of $1000 to $5000 have become commonplace, and recruiting abroad is quickly diminishing as a resource. Economically, the cost of hiring a new employee is reported as being from $1280 to $8000, and the cost of new graduate hires exceeds that figure (Hicks and White, 1981; Hinshaw, Smeltzer, and Atwood, 1987). Quoted turnover rates range from about 13% to 200%, depending on the hospital and its location. A 50% turnover rate of approximately 1.5 million nurses means that approximately 750,000 nurses are changing jobs every year. An often-quoted value for turnover cost is $2500 per nurse. Multiplying this figure by the turnover rate gives a staggering turnover cost of almost two billion dollars (Vogt et al., 1983). Tool 1-1 demonstrates the economic cost of turnover for a given agency.

Thus, the emphasis must begin to focus on retention. Human resource managers must look for causes of turnover, even in the entry process. Are new employees sabotaged early in their career? Are they hired for appropriate positions? Is orientation of new employees nonfunctional? Is recruitment success judged by volume or by the quality of the match between employee and position? Patterson and Goad (1987) found that 57% of the nurses interviewed who had recently changed their jobs stated their former employers could have induced them to stay if certain needs had been met.

Nursing administrators must begin to look at the work force they currently employ as unique individuals and must begin to identify those work factors that improve worker satisfaction and motivation.

UNIQUE STRESSORS IN THE NURSING PROFESSION

In understanding and meeting needs unique to nurses, one must first identify the physical, intellectual, and emotional stressors that are inherent to nursing practice.

Physically, nursing is hard work, involving long hours, weekend and night shifts, a constant reorientation to circadian rhythm, and exposure to disease processes.

Intellectually, nursing requires a broad base of knowledge and nursing skills. Yet despite increasing responsibilities, nurses are given limited autonomy in clinical situations and little involvement in management decision-making in setting standards for care. The American Hospital Association (1987) said in a recent publication that "nurses want and need both recognition and respect for their hard won knowledge and skills. Nurses need to know that others in the health care system value their contributions."

Emotionally, nurses are subject to unrelenting, intense human emotions. Nurses must be sensitive and caring if they are to be attuned to their client's needs, yet continuous, close, and emotional contact with patients is draining. Nurses, by their nature and what they believe they should be able to accomplish

---

Tool 1-1   Measuring the Economic Cost of Turnover

Step 1
Size of the facility × occupancy rate × days per year of care = *patient care days per year.*

Step 2
Number of nurses employed × turnover rate each year (%) = *number of nurses to be replaced.*

Step 3
Number of nurses to be replaced × turnover cost per nurse = *total turnover cost per year.*

Step 4
Total turnover cost per year ÷ patient care days per year = *increase/ decrease in costs per patient care day as a result of turnover.*

Sample problem
300 beds × 70% occupancy rate × 365 days per year = 76,650 patient care days per year.

250 nurses employed × 30% turnover rate each year = 75 nurses to be replaced annually.

75 nurses to be replaced × $2500 replacement cost = $187,500.

187,500 ÷ 76,650 = ~ $2.50 increase in costs per patient day.

---

in the work setting, often have feelings of inadequacy and frustration as they try to balance institutional demands with patient care needs (Vogt et al., 1983).

Commitment to caring as a humanistic and scientific concept is essential in the practice of nursing at all levels, yet unfortunately this caring role frequently seems to conflict with organizational goals. "It is crucial that nurses in administrative roles support the caring values of the nurses they manage. An intellectual accommodation must be made between the pressures to conform to the traditional business philosophy of administration and the humanistic philosophy inherent in professional nursing" (Miller, 1987).

A nurse manager's ability to create a positive work environment through his or her own management expertise will have a direct effect on worker satisfaction and thus on retention. Table 1-1 identifies the results of a 1980 survey that describes job factors of importance to nurses (Wandelt et al., 1981). It is interesting to note that salary is the highest ranked factor. In a 1988 survey, salary ranked only fifth among the top ten dissatisfiers in nursing (Huey and Hartley, 1988). Factors that influence nursing satisfaction, and thus retention, are changing. Tool 1-2 is a checklist that should be helpful for agencies evaluating possible areas of employee dissatisfaction.

Price and Mueller, in a 1981 study, stated that most nurses, regardless of their age and the amount of time worked, are similar. They want an increased variety of work, greater participation in work-related decisions, improved communication about work, and greater advancement opportunities. Pfaff (1987) stated that nurses in long-term care facilities want increased responsibility, potential for advancement, and increased autonomy in decision-making. Huey and Hartley (1988) stated that staff nurses want better RN/patient ratios, administrative support, adequate salaries, and a sense of being an important member of the health care team. They also want greater flexibility in work scheduling, child care, and more autonomy in nursing judgment. Tool 1-3 can be used by employees as a measure of job satisfaction.

Table 1-1. Top Ten Dissatisfactions of Employed Nurses

---

1. Salary
2. Amount of paperwork
3. Support given by administrators of the facility
4. Opportunity for furthering professional education
5. Adequacy of laws regulating the practice of nursing
6. Support given by nursing administration
7. Acceptable child care facilities available
8. Inservice education available
9. Fringe benefits available
10. Competence of non-RN staff

Data from Wandelt, M.A., et al., "Why Nurses Leave Nursing and What Can Be Done About It." *American Journal of Nursing*, 81(1): 72–77, 1981.

Tool 1-2   Check List for Evaluating the Quality of Worklife in an Organization

---

1. Adequate and fair compensation   yes   no

2. Safe and healthful working conditions   yes   no

3. Immediate opportunity to use and develop   yes   no
   human capacities

4. Future opportunity for continued growth and   yes   no
   security

5. Social integration in the work organization   yes   no
   (membership in supportive work groups
   marked by patterns of reciprocal help,
   social-emotional support, and affirmation of
   the uniqueness of the individual)

6. Constitutionalism in the work organization   yes   no
   (privacy, free speech, equity, and due process)

7. Work and total life space (the balanced role of   yes   no
   work defined by work schedules, career
   demands, and travel requirements that do not
   take up leisure and family time on a regular
   basis)

Adapted from Walton, R., "Quality of Working Life: What Is It?" *Sloan Management Review*, Fall, 1973, p. 11, by permission of the publisher. Copyright © 1973 by the Sloan Management Review Association. All rights reserved.

The organization that attempts to meet the unique needs and wants of nurses will have a motivated and productive staff, which in turn promotes retention. Such an organization must place the patient at the pinnacle of the institution's hierarchy and, in that scheme of things, must place the person most directly responsible for the patient's 24-hour care, the staff nurse, at the top of the organizational pyramid—with administration existing to support the nurse's activities (Huey and Hartley, 1988).

The current nursing shortage has prompted nursing administrators to re-examine the personnel process in an effort to promote worker satisfaction while attaining organizational goals. This shifting of focus from recruitment to retention renews the emphasis on humanism in nursing management.

KEY CONCEPTS CHAPTER 1

1. The philosophy of human resource management is that organizational goals can be met without negating the needs of the workers within that organization.

2. In human resource management people are given priority over machines and participatory management is strongly encouraged.

3. The current severe nursing shortage is different from prior shortages in that it is a national shortage, with an inadequate current and future applicant pool.

4. The economic cost of turnover to health care organizations and the inadequate applicant pool reinforce the need for management to change their focus from recruitment to retention strategies in personnel management.

5. Nursing as a profession presents physical, intellectual, and emotional stressors. In shifting their focus toward humanism, management must begin to identify stressors that lead to job dissatisfaction among nurses.

Tool 1-3   Are You Satisfied with Your Job?

To find out how satisfied you are with your job, take this test. Check the "S" line beside each aspect of your job that satisfies you. Check the "N/A" line if the item doesn't apply to your situation. Leave the lines blank if you're dissatisfied with that aspect of your work.

	S	N/A
1. Earnings	_____	_____
2. Financial security	_____	_____
3. Prospects for a comfortable retirement	_____	_____
4. Prospects for future earnings	_____	_____
5. Time for recreation and family activities	_____	_____
6. Opportunities for travel	_____	_____
7. Time for travel	_____	_____
8. Community in which you live	_____	_____
9. Prestige on the job	_____	_____
10. Advancement potential	_____	_____
11. Professional prestige	_____	_____
12. Administrative details of the job	_____	_____
13. Committee work required	_____	_____
14. Written reports necessary	_____	_____
15. Nonprofessional aspects of the job	_____	_____
16. Routine job activities	_____	_____
17. Time for study in your field	_____	_____
18. Opportunity to advance professionally	_____	_____
19. Chance to talk shop	_____	_____
20. Opportunity to direct others' work	_____	_____
21. Opportunity to help in policymaking	_____	_____
22. Opportunity to be your own boss	_____	_____
23. Interesting coworkers	_____	_____
24. Intelligent, competent coworkers	_____	_____

	S	N/A
25. Fun and relaxation with coworkers	_____	_____
26. Competition	_____	_____
27. Demands of patients	_____	_____
28. Demands of supervisors	_____	_____
29. Intellectual challenge	_____	_____
30. Variety of activities required	_____	_____
31. Chance to improve skills	_____	_____
32. Chance to do research	_____	_____
33. Physical fatigue	_____	_____
34. Pressure on the job	_____	_____
35. Hours	_____	_____
36. Opportunity to use learned skills	_____	_____
37. Opportunity to use aptitudes and abilities	_____	_____
38. Opportunity to use education	_____	_____
39. Fulfillment of personal needs	_____	_____
40. Feeling of achievement	_____	_____
41. Feeling of being needed	_____	_____
42. Feeling of accomplishment	_____	_____
43. Credit for work done	_____	_____
44. Thanks from those you benefit	_____	_____
45. Recognition from your supervisors	_____	_____
46. Peer recognition	_____	_____
47. Personal satisfaction of job well done	_____	_____
48. Chance to see results of work	_____	_____
49. Chance to follow job through to its conclusion	_____	_____
50. Chance to evaluate own work	_____	_____
51. Chance to evaluate others' work	_____	_____
52. Opportunity to use initiative	_____	_____
53. Freedom to make decisions	_____	_____
54. Personal autonomy	_____	_____
55. Freedom to use own judgment	_____	_____

	S	N/A

56. Opportunity to do socially significant tasks _____ _____

57. Opportunity to improve others' health _____ _____

58. Opportunity to improve others' appearance or comfort _____ _____

59. Opportunity to help others find success or happiness _____ _____

60. Opportunities for varied work experience _____ _____

SCORING

To determine your score, follow these steps:

1. Count the number of "S" responses and write the total in the box below:

   S ☐

2. Count the number of "N/A" responses and subtract that number from 60. This gives you the total number of relevant items on the test.

   60 − N/A ☐ = No. of relevant items ☐

3. To determine your percentage of "satisfied" responses, divide your answer in Step 1 by your answer in Step 2:

   S ☐ ÷ No. of relevant items ☐ = Percentage of satisfied responses ☐

4. To determine your final score, multiply your answer in Step 3 by 100:

   Percentage of satisfied responses ☐ × 100 = Final score ☐

ANALYSIS

High score—above 75

You are very satisfied with your job. You are probably committed to your work and devote most of your energy to your job. You also may associate much of your personal identity with your work.

Medium score—75 to 25

You're generally satisfied with your job, although you would like to change certain aspects—perhaps enjoy a higher salary, a fuller use of your abilities, or less stress.

Low score—below 25

This range shows a general dissatisfaction with your job.

Review your answers to the test to figure out which aspects you find
unsatisfactory. You could be in the wrong job for your interests and
abilities; perhaps some minor changes in your present job (for example,
new colleagues or a department transfer) could lead to greater
satisfaction; or you may just want to look for a job that provides more
satisfaction in the areas that are most important to you.

REFERENCES

Aiken, L., "Nurses for the Future: Breaking the Shortage Cycles,"
AJN, 87(12):1616–1620, 1987.

Aiken, L., and Mullinix, C., "Special Report – The Nurse Shortage:
Myth or Reality?" *N Engl J Med*, 317 (10):641–646, 1987.

American Hospital Association, *The Nursing Shortage: Facts,
Figures, and Feelings: Research Report*, American Hospital
Association, Chicago, Illinois, 1987.

Fifield, F.F., "What is a Productivity-Excellent Hospital?" *Nursing
Management*, 19(4):32–40, 1988.

Ginzberg, E., "Nurses for the Future: Facing the Facts and Figures,"
AJN, 87(12):1596–1600, 1987.

Green, K., "Nurses for the Future: What the Freshmen Tell Us,"
AJN, 87(12):1610–1613, 1987.

Hicks, G., and White, C.H., "The Costs of Orienting and Training
New Nurses," *CNA Insight*, 5(27):2, 1981.

Hinshaw, A.S., Smeltzer, C.H., and Atwood, J.R., "Innovative
Retention Strategies for Nursing Staff," *JONA*, 17(6):8, 1987.

Huey, F.L., and Hartley, S., "What Keeps Nurses in Nursing – 3500
Nurses Tell Their Stories," *AJN*, 88(2):181–188, 1988.

Kramer, M., "Magnet Hospitals: Part I. Institutions of Excellence,"
JONA, 18(1):13–24, 1988.

Kramer, M., "Magnet Hospitals: Part II. Institutions of Excellence,"
JONA, 18(2):11–19, 1988.

Link, C., "Nurses for the Future: What Does a BS Degree Buy? An
Economist's View," *AJN*, 87(12):1621–1627, 1987.

Marquis, B., "Attrition: The Effectiveness of Retention Activities,"
JONA, 18(3):25–29, 1988.

Miller, K., "The Human Care Perspective in Nursing Administration," *JONA*, 17(2):10–12, 1987.

National Association for Health Care Recruitment Survey, June,
1987.

Patterson, S.W., and Goad, S., "Incentives for Retention: The
Psychological Dimension," *Nursing Management*, 18(2):69–70,
1987.

Pfaff, J., "Factors Related to Job Satisfaction/Dissatisfaction of Registered Nurses in Long-Term Care Facilities," *Nursing Management*, 18(8):51–55, 1987.

Prescott, P.A., and Bowen, S.A., "Controlling Nursing Turnover," *Nursing Management*, 18(6):60–66, 1987.

Price, J., and Mueller, C., *Professional Turnover: The Case for Nurses*, Spectrum Publications, New York, 1981.

Scherer, P., "Hospitals That Attract and Keep Nurses," *AJN* 88(1):34–40, 1988.

Schuster, F.E., *Human Resource Management*, Second Edition, Reston Publishing Company, Reston, Virginia, 1985.

Styles, M.M. and Holzemer, W.L., "Educational Remapping for a Responsible Future," *Journal of Professional Nursing*, 2(1):64–68, 1986.

Sullivan, E.J., Printz, J.R., Shafer, M.R., and Schultz, B.K., "Strategies for Recruiting Students," *Nurse Educator*, 13(2):37–40, 1988.

Vogt, J., Cox, J.L., Velthouse, B., Thames, B., *Retaining Professional Nurses—A Planned Process*, C.V. Mosby Company, St. Louis, 1983.

Walton, R., "Quality of Working Life: What Is It?" *Sloan Management Review*, Fall, 1973.

Wandelt, M.A., et al., "Why Nurses Leave Nursing and What Can Be Done About It," *American Journal of Nursing*, 81(1):72–77, 1981.

ADDITIONAL READINGS

Astin, A.W., and Green, K.D., *The American Freshman: Twenty Year Trends; 1966–1985*, American Council on Education, Los Angeles, 1986.

Benham, L., "Manpower Policy and the Supply of Nurses," *Industrial Relations*, 12:86–94, 1973.

Scherer, P., When Every Day Is Saturday; The Shortage," *AJN*, 87(10):1285–1290, 1987.

Seybolt, J.W., "Dealing with Premature Employee Turnover", *JONA*, 16(2):26–32, 1986.

Tobin, B.K., "Would You Encourage Your Child to Be a Nurse?" *Nursing Life*, 7(3):42–45, 1987.

White, C.H., "The Nursing Shortage: There Is No Solution," *CHA Insight*, 5(20):2, 1981.

White, C.H., and Arstein-Kerslake, C., "The Market-Driven Hospital Workforce," *CHA Insight*, 10(6):822–826, 1986.

2

The Impact of Philosophy on Human Resource Management

THE ASPECT of organizational management having the greatest impact on how an organization manages people is the set of beliefs and values that the organization holds. Both individuals and organizations have a basic philosophy that is derived from their values and beliefs, and it serves as the basis for all actions and decisions that individuals and organizations make. This entire book rests on the assumption that managers and their organizations are willing to examine their personal and current beliefs and determine how those beliefs affect retention and productivity. If individuals and organizations want to improve the productivity and retention of their employees, it may be necessary for them to alter how they view human resources.

Since it is possible that the philosophy of an individual may differ greatly from that of an organization, it is important for nurse managers to be cognizant of their own personal philosophies, as well as the set of beliefs that guide organizational actions. Cherniss (1980) claims that one of the factors that contributes to burnout is incongruence between the values of the individual and those of the organization. This chapter, therefore, will be devoted to an examination of how values are derived, how an organization's philosophy influences the internal environment of the organization, and the impact of both organizational and personal philosophies on human resource management. Examples are given of an organization mission statement and an organizational philosophy, including an interpretation of each. This chapter should enable the nurse manager to write unit and departmental philosophy effectively. Additionally, this chapter teaches how to determine and interpret an organization's operational, written, and implemented philosophies. A tool to evaluate organizational and personal value congruency is also included.

VALUES VERSUS POSITIVE ATTITUDES

Many people mistake positive attitudes for values. The difference between having a positive attitude regarding something and holding it as a true value is both major and important. For example, one might have a positive attitude regarding the American Nurses' Association (ANA) but not belong to this organization. However, the individual who belongs to the ANA, pays dues, and works in the organization can be said to value the ANA. The difference in the two examples is that in the second case the individual is willing to give up something (e.g., time, money, resources) in order to maintain the value. Values, therefore, are something that result in individuals taking action; however, a positive attitude often may not result in action. Most organizations and most individuals have few real values but may have many positive attitudes. McNally (1980) identified the following four characteristics that determine a true value:

1. It must be freely chosen from among alternatives.
2. It must be prized and cherished.
3. It must be consciously and consistently repeated.
4. It must be positively affirmed and acted on.

Unless all four criteria are met, the individual or organization does not hold the philosophical statement as a true value, although the attitude toward it may be positive. Many organizations dealing in health care profess to value nursing and often have a philosophy that states this value. However, if that organization's actions are closely observed, it might be discovered that those in charge only have a positive attitude about nursing care and do not hold it as a true value. If, for example, an organization states in its philosophy that quality patient care is valued, then the nursing staffing hours should reflect that value; that is, there should be adequate nursing staffing hours to provide quality patient care.

Beach (1980) maintains that those who establish and manage organizations set the tone for that enterprise through their pattern of beliefs, values, and attitudes. Furthermore, he believes that the philosophy of an organization is made evident by its relationship with its customers, employees, and the public at large. One should be able to determine the philosophy of a hospital by the way that institution treats its employees, patients, and the community.

CHANGING AND DEVELOPING VALUES

If one examines both personal and organizational values over time, it becomes evident that values do not remain constant but change and evolve as society progresses. Both individuals and organizations need to periodically examine their philosophies to determine how their values have changed. Examples of how management values have changed over time is evidenced by the change in child labor laws, the opening of many formerly closed occupations to women, and changes in maternity leave.

Ouchi (1981) reflected that one of the reasons Theory Z management techniques were often not successful in this country is because organizations neglected to seriously examine their philosophies and missions before implementing such techniques. Ouchi maintained that before an organization can change, it must first spend considerable time exploring its mission, purpose, and philosophy and, if necessary, adjust the philosophy so that it supports the changes to be made (Ouchi, 1981). Individuals also need to be aware of their changing personal values. Marquis and Huston (1987) stated that there is periodic need for value clarification. Both individuals and organizations with unclear values have difficulty setting priorities, dealing with conflict constructively, and developing goals and objectives.

VALUES OF INDIVIDUALS AND ORGANIZATIONS

Nearly all decisions that deal with human resource management are based on moral principles derived from our personal and organizational value system. Should salary be based on merit or seniority? Should an employer reject qualified nonminorities who compete for jobs in order to provide jobs for minorities who were formerly discriminated against? Should you give a poor recommendation to inadequate nurses, which may result in their not being able to get other jobs? These are some important issues that face both individual nurse managers and health care institutions today.

In order to reduce intrapersonal conflict due to differing values of the organization and the individual nurse manager, the nurse manager must first consciously examine his or her own personal set of beliefs. To assist individuals in clarifying personal values, Hamilton and Kiefer (1986) identified seven steps necessary for value clarification. Use of these steps is especially helpful when nurse managers find they are experiencing some conflict about personnel decisions. When policies of the organization and personal values are not congruent, the following suggestions offered by Hamilton and Kiefer may be helpful in cases of value conflict:

1. Listen to your responses, including social, physical, intellectual, emotional, and spiritual feelings. Before you can recognize your values, you must become consciously aware of all your feelings.

2. Differentiate internal sources from external sources. As we learn new things, the new knowledge may have an effect on our values, but it is important for us to determine if the new information has changed our values. Individuals are frequently influenced by the values of others, not realizing that they are internalizing others' values as their own. An example of adopting another's value as our own is the ability of young people to value whatever their "significant other" values.

3. Take time to experience full awareness of your internal responses. Pay special attention to your reaction. Are you satisfied with your behavior, and is it consistent with your values?

4. Act on your internal responses. This is the time for you to decide if you want to change your values. You must be accountable for behavior that conflicts with your values.

5. Evaluate your alternatives. What alternatives exist for you that would allow you to act in a manner that would still be consistent with your values? There is always more than one way for a situation to be solved, even if your values are clearly defined and internalized.

6. Establish patterns of behavior that are consistent with your values. Seek out behaviors that reflect your internal values.

7. Trust your beliefs, preferences, likes, and dislikes. Gain confidence in the decisions you make, and learn to believe in yourself (Hamilton and Kiefer, 1986).

It is important to note the difference between being rigid and unchanging in our attitudes and values, and being so unclear about our values that we adopt anyone's values without hesitation. These are two opposites of a continuum. Individuals with strong value systems and open minds who are willing to learn new information that could change their values will be successful as managers in a changing world. Successful nurse managers stand up for what is right and trust their own instincts. This allows them to take risks, even when what they are risking are their own positions. At the same time, they are willing to learn, to compromise, and to examine the values of organizations that might have different values than they hold themselves.

HOW TO DETERMINE AN ORGANIZATION'S PHILOSOPHY

Since the values of an organization may differ from those of the individuals who work there, suggestions have been given to assist individuals in determining the true values of the organization. Let's assume there is an individual with a great deal of awareness about his or her own values and beliefs, and although the values and beliefs have changed somewhat since youth, this has not occurred without much thought and consideration. This individual is promoted to a management position, or takes a management position as a new employee. What means can be used to determine the values of the organization?

It is hoped that no one would take a position in an organization without first determining something about its philosophy, and especially not a position of management and leadership. All goals and objectives, fiscal planning, and human resource management decisions are derived from the institution's mission and purpose.

Therefore, it is impossible for individuals to carry out their duties without experiencing conflict, unless there is an acceptable congruence between the institution's values and that individual's own values. Cherniss (1980) cites numerous studies that show a causal relationship between burnout in human service organizations and inconsistency among members of the team in relation to their goals. These goals are formed from the values of the organization, and these values, Cherniss believes, have a particularly strong influence on the adjustment of the novice. This makes it critical for the novice nurse manager to examine the values of an institution prior to accepting a position. The following suggestions will assist individuals in obtaining an understanding of an organization's philosophy:

1. *Prior to accepting a position, ask to see a copy of the institution's mission statement.* This is sometimes referred to as the statement of purpose and is a simple statement of why the institution exists. A sample mission statement can be seen in Table 2-1, including an explanation of the meaning of the statement.

2. *Examine the philosophy of the organization carefully.* A statement of philosophy can usually be found in the policy manuals available to the staff at the institution or, on request, from top-level administration. Langford (1981) states that the philosophy should speak to (a) the mission of the organization,

---

Table 2-1. Sample of a Hospital Mission Statement

The primary purpose of Community Hospital is to provide a professionally organized, up-to-date, and comprehensive health care program to the communities it serves.

It is also Community Hospital's purpose to serve as an effective component of the socioeconomic system of the area, providing support to its commerce as a health resource, and contributing to the social and cultural life of the area. The hospital strives to serve as a responsible and concerned employer providing a suitable work environment. As a corporate member of the community, it seeks to contribute its appropriate share to proper community development and maintenance of a viable environment consonant with its resources and in keeping with its mission.

Interpretation: It is obvious from reading the mission statement that this is a community-oriented facility. There is no mention in the mission statement of research, education, or advancing medical science. The nurse manager working in this environment would be expected to become involved in the community. The mission statement also mentions a commitment to providing a good working environment, so it would be expected that the nurse manager in this organization would be supported and compensated adequately.

(b) the level of responsiveness to the community, (c) any special approaches to care, and (d) any particular beliefs regarding employees and patients. A sample of a hospital philosophy and its interpretation is included in Table 2-2.

3. *Observe the environment of the institution.* Sometimes the real values of an organization can be depicted by how space

---

Table 2-2.   Sample of a Hospital Philosophy

The original intent of our communities in establishing this hospital was to provide quality health care at the local level. It was felt that a local hospital would offer patients an increased proximity to their homes, families, and familiar surroundings, which is supportive to the healing process. Today, as in 1929, we feel that this assumption is still valid. In addition, the need for local services is also reinforced by the increasing burden of transportation expense on patients and families who must travel to other areas for medical care.

The hospital shall always strive to be self-supporting and independent. Its guiding principle has been, "What we attempt—we do well. What we cannot do well—we do not attempt." It recognizes fully the economic necessity of centralizing specialized treatment systems in surrounding communities and encourages their use as referral agencies. However, it also feels strongly that every effort should be made to provide the majority of patients with a continuum of care—from critical onset through convalescence—within the confines of the community.

Providing this type of service presents constant challenges to the hospital. It is essential, for example, that continuing efforts be made to recruit sufficient physicians of appropriate specialties, both local as well as visiting consultants, to provide a well-rounded program of primary care within the hospital and/or the community. In addition, the hospital must continue to maintain a level of technology and staffing that is supportive of its medical staff and responsive to the needs of its patients.

In order to provide this type of high-quality patient care, adequate financial resources are essential. The Board of Directors and the medical and management staff must ensure that the hospital is economically sound and that its resources are used efficiently. Since income from patient and third-party insurers comprise the bulk of revenue, it is mandatory that reimbursements for services be proper and reasonable.

The hospital also recognizes that philanthropy is an important supplement to hospital income. Voluntary donations may, in fact, be essential to the success of certain worthwhile hospital projects or programs. Continuing efforts will be made to inform the community of the evolution of the hospital, not only as an inducement to giving, but also as a public communication and education service.

Recognizing that advances in medical science, the continuing increase in federal and state programs, the interest of the public in cost containment, and other factors are resulting in major changes in the course of health care delivery, Community Hospital addresses itself to the need to prepare for these changes. The hospital is aware of its role both as a catalyst for desirable change and as a positive influence in the field of health care and in the general life of the community.

Interpretation: The philosophy has been drawn from the mission statement in Table 2-1. This philosophy is much longer than most hospital philosophies. It states in specific terms what the philosophy is, rather than leaving the reader with vague and ambiguous statements. Additionally, the philosophy incorporates all four of Langford's criteria for a clearly written philosophy. To gain practice in assessment of philosophy, readers are encouraged to use the organization value assessment, found in Tool 2-1, to assess this philosophy.

---

is allotted or how resources are managed. If the top nurse administrator has an unappealing office that is much smaller and more austere than that of the personnel director, it might be an indication of the value the institution places on nursing. Other observable examples of institutional values are the way the buildings are maintained and the friendliness of the staff.

4. *Talk with many different levels of individuals connected with the health care organization.* Talk with other nurses, both staff nurses and nurses in management positions. Many times the written philosophy of an institution appears congruent with an individual's values, but the actual implementation of that philosophy is not. Be sure also to obtain the view of the organization from non-nurse members of the health care organization, especially physicians and employees from other departments.

5. *Attempt to determine how the health care facility is viewed by members of the community.* It is often very revealing to talk with former consumers. Ask patients and families how they were treated. Attempt to discover what the reputation of the facility is in the community.

It is unfortunate that many nurse managers accept positions in an organization and suffer conflict and frustration because they failed to adequately research the organization's values. Individuals often spend more time and energy researching auto purchases than they do investigating the organizations where they work. Marquis and Huston (1987) maintain that, "it is unrealistic for a manager to accept a position under the assumption that she can work to change the organization's philosophy to more closely align with her personal philosophy." This view is supported by McFarland, who states that such a change would require an extraordinary amount of energy and would produce inevitable conflict, since any organization's philosophy reflects a long historical development and is tied closely to the individuals who played a role in its development (McFarland, Leonard, and Harris, 1984).

THE ROLE OF VALUES IN IMPLEMENTING PERSONNEL POLICIES

The way managers deal with individuals is based on the two underlying philosophies that have been discussed, the philosophy of the organization and the philosophy of the individual manager. The personnel policies that guide managers in their decision-making regarding human resources are developed using the philosophy of the organization as a guide. However, the interpretation of those personnel policies and their subsequent implementation are directly affected by the individual manager's value system. It is possible, therefore, for two different managers in an organization to reach very different conclusions and arrive at different actions, even though the personnel situation is the same. The fundamental assumptions that individuals hold will influence their actions. For example, do they believe that people can be trusted? Do they believe that people are basically good and industrious? Do they believe that people need explicit rules and regulations in order to perform well? Let us examine two very different philosophies of managing people. The first philosophy is what McGregor (1960) termed *Theory X*, which is a pessimistic view of human behavior. This management philosophy has also been termed *authoritative* or the *traditional* approach to managing people at work. The extreme opposite philosophy of management is frequently termed *Theory Y* but is also referred to as a *modern* or *humanistic* approach to management, as was discussed in Chapter 1. It is obvious that these terms represent two contrasting views. In actual practice, however, most managers have beliefs about people that incorporate parts of each of these philosophies. It is rare to find a manager who is wholly authoritative or wholly humanistic in the implementation of personnel policies. In Chapter 5 we will examine how assumptions of the manager influence the motivation of the worker, but this chapter examines only the two different belief systems in their purest form.

TRADITIONAL MANAGEMENT PHILOSOPHY

An early view of humans, held by both workers and management, was that humans are selfish and rebellious, and need tight reins to control their naturally occurring baseness. This view of mankind is perhaps best described by the political philosopher Machiavelli. Later philosophers expressed other themes that supported this view, such as social Darwinism, or survival of the fittest. Adam Smith in 1776 argued that the nation was best served when individuals pursue their own self-interest. Even much of the nation's early fiction was woven around the theme that hard work and self-denial is all that is necessary to be successful, and that lack of success is due simply to laziness or unimaginativeness. It must be emphasized that this view was held by workers and managers alike. Indeed, the concept of hard work and self-denial resulting in rewards is still a very strong belief in the United States, and much of our society believes that being poor or unsuccessful is the result of a lack of initiative on the part of the individual.

This philosophy produces a supervisor or manager who strongly believes that the average worker avoids responsibility, lacks ambition, and needs to be closely supervised. Managers feel their job is to obtain obedience for the orders passed down from above, and they tend to be production centered rather than people oriented. Although at first glance this philosophy of the nature of humans sounds rather negative, it has many positive aspects. For example, this belief system creates a climate in which workers have a clear understanding of role expectations as rules are clearly spelled out. It produces maximum efficiency and frequently achieves satisfactory results up to a certain level. This type of bureaucratic management is standard in most military forces and is common in private industry and government-operated businesses.

The negative aspects of this philosophy regarding the behavior of humans is evidenced by the lack of real enthusiasm it elicits in workers. Creativity and feelings of responsibility and autonomy are sacrificed in favor of a predictable, but moderate, level of performance. The type of paternalism that is fostered by this type of belief is frequently welcomed by workers, since they need exchange only high productivity, loyalty, and cooperation for employer-guaranteed job security, adequate pay, and decent working conditions. The worker willingly gives up autonomy and shared decision-making for the obvious benefits of this traditional management philosophy.

MODERN OR HUMAN RESOURCE PHILOSOPHY

The behavioral scientists have had a great deal of influence on the more recent view of human nature. As sociologists began to investigate the individual in the workplace during the late 1950s and early 1960s, a completely different set of beliefs about the worker became known. This set of beliefs about human nature has become the basis for the philosophy held by many present-day managers. This philosophy is characterized by an optimistic view of humans. Humans are seen as having potential for growth and achievement. They are potentially creative, trustworthy, and cooperative.

Managers holding this set of beliefs feel their job is to nurture workers and tap into their productive drives. The manager's goal is to build a team effort and to be the representative of the team to top-level management. The manager is both people and production oriented. Emphasis is placed on the higher motives of increasing production through activating the employees' motives of achievement and creativity. External controls are seen as less important than responsibility and self-control.

Many critics of this style of management feel this philosophy fosters ineffective management that results in a relinquishment on the part of the managers to run the business of the organization. Critics maintain that the modern approach to management dilutes the legitimate authority necessary in a chain of command. Another difficulty with this philosophical approach is that it requires a greater spectrum of talents from managers than the traditional approach.

The benefits for workers in having managers with this set of values seem obvious. Workers are nurtured and encouraged to achieve. The manager shares decision-making and responsibility with the employees, who in turn feel they are trusted and have some control over their work environment.

AN EXAMINATION OF THE MANAGER'S VALUES

So much has been written about humankind and its work that one would think that current managers would generally hold a philosophy that would support the modern theory of management. However, Beach (1980) reports that according to current research, present-day managers continue to hold both types of beliefs. For example, Beach maintains that most managers believe in some parts of humanistic management, such as shared goals, participative management, and the worker having shared control. However, researchers reveal that these same managers had grave doubts about the ability of the average worker to demonstrate initiative, individual action, and leadership. Beach feels that the vast majority of executives throughout the world lean closer to the traditional values and beliefs than to a philosophy that supports modern management theory. However, he does see hope that the future will produce a greater number of well-educated managers who philosophically trust the worker more, grant more discretion to their subordinates, and allow employees to share in decision-making. Tannenbaum and Davis (1969) support this view and feel the future of personnel management will see managers move (a) away from negative evaluations of employees and toward actions that confirm them as human beings, (b) away from being fearful of differences in people and toward utilizing and accepting those differences, (c) away from game playing and toward a more healthful, authentic behavior, (d) away from nontrust and toward a more trusting relationship with employees, and (e) away from competition and toward a greater emphasis on collaboration. Tool 2-1 for this chapter is a sample checklist to assist managers in assessing organizational and personal values.

It is evident that in recent years the sciences of management, sociology, and psychology have had a significant impact on organizational philosophy, and subsequently on how people are managed at work; but it is also evident that many managers retain a distrust and nonacceptance of subordinates. This belief system leads to human resource management decisions that often result in reduced productivity and increased attrition. If organizations and managers wish to make continued progress toward a more humanistic approach to managing people, they must be willing to examine their personal and organizational values and initiate change where necessary.

KEY CONCEPTS CHAPTER 2

1. All personnel management decisions are influenced by personal and organizational philosophy.
2. Both personal and organizational values are capable of changing over time.
3. Unless the belief system of the manager and organization are reasonably congruent, there will be value conflict.

Tool 2-1   Value Assessment Tool

Assessment of organizational values

1. What are the specific values mentioned in the organizational mission and philosophy statement?

2. What specific commitment to nursing care is made?

3. Is there a reference to the type of care provided, i.e., quality care, adequate care, safe care?

4. What references are made regarding education and/or research?

5. What specific commitment to medical care is made?

6. Does the organization stress quality of work life?

7. What are the three major beliefs or values of the organization that are specifically mentioned in the philosophy?

Assessment of personal values

1. What are your values regarding health care?

2. What values would you be willing to sacrifice your job for?

3. Does the organization mission statement reflect your philosophy?

4. What value do you place on work?

5. Prioritize your values of work, family, personal life, and personal health.

6. What value do you place on the work that you do?

7. Do you have strong values about health care, teaching, research, or nursing that are not mentioned in the organizational philosophy?

8. Do you feel you can work in this organization and be true to your own values?

---

4. Personnel policies are derived from the organization's philosophy but are implemented using the manager's management philosophy about how individuals should be managed.

5. There are two very different sets of beliefs held by managers; one is traditional, and one is modern.

6. Most managers have a set of beliefs that include values from each type of management philosophy.

REFERENCES

Beach, D., *Personnel: Management of People At Work*, Fourth edition, Macmillan Publishing Co., New York, 1980.

Cherniss, C., *Professional Burnout in Human Service Organizations*, Praeger Publishers, New York, 1980.

Hamilton, J., Kiefer, M., *Survival Skills for the New Nurse*, J.B. Lippincott Company, Philadelphia, 1986.

Langford, T., *Managing and Being Managed*, Prentice-Hall, Englewood Cliffs, NJ, 1981.

McFarland, G., Leonard, H., Morris, M., *Nursing Leadership and Management: Contemporary Strategies*, John Wiley and Sons, New York, 1984.

McGregor, D., *The Human Side of Enterprise*, McGraw-Hill Company, New York, 1960.

McNally, M., "Values. Part I: Supervisor nurse," *Journal of Nursing Leadership and Management*, 11:27, 1980.

Marquis, B., Huston, C., *Management Decision Making for Nurses: 101 Case Studies*. J.B. Lippincott Company, Philadelphia, 1987.

Ouchi, W. G., *Theory Z: How American Business Can Meet The Japanese Challenge*, Addison-Wesley, Reading, MA, 1981.

Tannenbaum, R., Davis, S., "Values, Man and Organizations," *Industrial Management Review*, 10(2):67–86, 1969.

ADDITIONAL READINGS

Argyris, C., *Integrating the Individual and the Organization*. John Wiley, New York, 1964.

Cantor, M., "Philosophy, purpose and objectives: Why do we have them?" *J Nurs Admin* 3:21, 1973.

Drucker, P., *The Practice of Management*. Harper and Row, New York, 1954.

Mayo, E., *The Human Problems of an Industrialized Civilization*. Macmillan, New York, 1953.

White R.K., Lippert, R., *Autocracy and Democracy: An Experimental Inquiry*. Harper and Row, New York, 1960.

3
The Responsibility for Human Resource Management

HEALTH CARE facilities utilize many organizational structures in meeting personnel management needs. Human resource management may be coordinated from a specific personnel department that is centralized within the institution, or it may be decentralized to all management levels within the organization. Even if human resource management is coordinated from within a specific office in an institution, the responsibility for this management extends to all first-level, middle-level, and top-level managers in the health care setting.

The implementation of human resource management is complex and requires special skills and abilities of managers at all levels of the organization. Each manager or level within the organization may have a different perception of what his or her role should be in human resource management and how the human resource plan should be implemented. Some individual variation in how different managers implement the plan is expected and should actually be encouraged. However, the management team must be careful not to lose sight of the overall organizational goal in human resource management: the creation of a work environment that results in increased productivity and worker satisfaction. If this goal is internalized as the basis for all human resource management planning, the individual implementation or actual organizational structure used to implement the plan becomes less critical.

Chapter 3 will discuss the relationship between the type of personnel department in the organization and the responsibility and autonomy required at each level of nursing management. Specific responsibilities for first-, middle-, and top-level managers will be defined. The need for good communication between the different levels of nursing management and other departments in the organization will be emphasized. In addition, since the quality of supervision has such an impact on productivity and retention, characteristics of effective supervision will be discussed. Tools for implementation include sample business letter and memo formats for communication between interdepartmental nursing personnel, between different levels of the nursing hierarchy, and outside the organization.

STRUCTURING HUMAN RESOURCE MANAGEMENT

Managers seem to be constantly re-evaluating where, in the organizational chart, the responsibility for the design and administration of personnel activities should be located; therefore, the organizational structure for personnel management varies widely. Initially, human resource management was often the sole responsibility of personnel departments within an organization, and operating managers played only a secondary and advisory role. Gradually, a shift in responsibility has occurred, and it is generally recognized that human resource management is and must be a responsibility of both the traditional personnel department and operating managers (Milkovich and Glueck, 1985).

Personnel management may be centralized, decentralized, or fall on a continuum anywhere in between. In centralized personnel management, the responsibility for planning and implementing human resource management is given to a single department within the organization. This results in a greater consistency in personnel planning and generally is more cost effective as personnel managers become more experienced at what they do.

In decentralized personnel management, the responsibility to design and implement human resource management strategies is placed at the unit level. Allowing personnel management decisions to be made at the level at which they will be implemented has many advantages. These include the increased probability that personnel decisions made will be more closely related to department objectives and needs. In addition, there is the possibility of increased flexibility in meeting employee needs. There may be some difficulty, however, in the decentralized personnel plan with consistent treatment of employees. In addition, inadequately trained or incompetent managers may perform this task at a less-than-optimal level, and there is greater potential for unit conflict with the overall goals or philosophy of the organization. Many organizations claim to have decentralized their personnel processes but withhold fiscal authority at the unit level, which is necessary to implement the plan.

Because centralization of personnel decision-making must be viewed on a continuum, it is important to recognize that many organizations utilize a combination approach. An example might be a personnel department that advertises and does the initial screening of new employees, but gives the operating manager at the department level the authority to actually interview and select new employees.

It is important in such a mixed approach that roles and authority be clearly defined. There is great potential for conflict between the personnel manager and the operating manager at the unit level if the authority and responsibility for personnel decisions is blurred. In fact, there are often great differences in the objectives or orientation of the two managers. For example, the personnel manager may have an overall goal of filling vacant positions at the minimum wage necessary to attain a minimum competency level. The operating manager may feel that a specific level of expertise or skills is required in meeting the requirements of the position, although this may require a long and expensive search for prospective employees.

Table 3-1 identifies the results of a survey administered to 27 personnel managers and 55 operating managers in which they identified which personnel activities they believe belonged within the personnel department itself. Clearly, the potential for conflict is apparent and the need for clear communication imperative.

Table 3-1. Personnel Activities Wanted in Personnel Departments by 27 Personnel Executives (E) and 55 Operating Managers (M)

Activities	Policy		Advice		Service		Control	
	E	M	E	M	E	M	E	M
Collective bargaining	30	44	30	29	22	35	11	25
Complaints/grievances	37	51	68	69	52	51	26	27
Counseling	37	40	37	69	48	55	19	27
Discipline	41	49	57	71	33	27	4	29
Employee communication	37	44	52	51	59	60	19	27
Job descriptions	48	42	30	54	48	38	63	31
Job design	15	25	37	38	19	24	19	15
Recruiting	59	69	37	31	59	44	44	44
Performance appraisal	52	46	56	58	22	24	30	42
Pay raises	37	58	56	62	33	31	22	40
Hiring decisions	30	44	59	69	30	47	30	33
Lay offs and discharges	48	42	41	66	37	35	22	29
Average responses	41.0	49.6	43.9	50.8	37.6	40.9	28	31.3

Adapted from White, H., and Boynton, R., "The Role of Personnel: A Management View," *Arizona Business* 21, 1974.

RESPONSIBILITIES ASSOCIATED WITH DIFFERENT LEVELS OF NURSING MANAGEMENT

In examining personnel management, Heneman and Schwab (1978) stated that there are four primary components that are best handled at different places by different people. These components are:

1. Formulation of personnel policy

2. Implementation of policies

3. Audit and control—the establishment of standards and procedures to see that organizational policies are maintained

4. Innovation—research and development of new practices, procedures, and programs

Before looking at which individuals within the organization should be responsible for each component of human resource management, it is essential to understand the terminology used in classifying managers. Managers are typically classified into one of three categories: top-, middle-, or first-level managers.

The top-level manager looks at the organization as a whole, coordinating both internal and external influences on the organization and generally making decisions regarding the staffing mix and organizational needs. Frequently, the top-level manager focuses on forecasting the demand for labor replacement needs (employment planning) and formulating general personnel policy. It is very important that the top-level manager recognize the importance of proactive personnel planning so as to avoid crisis or problematic personnel policy setting.

Although the determination of personnel policy requires input from many members at different levels of the organizational structure, top-level managers generally are responsible for personnel policy, as they are unique in having an understanding of the legal, ethical, legislative, regulatory, community, fiscal, and human resource ramifications in setting policy. In addition, top-level managers have a clear understanding of overall organizational goals and objectives, and can ascertain that personnel policy represents a compatible extension of the organization's overall philosophy. Examples of top-level managers may include the Chief Executive Officer, the Chief Nursing Executive, and other administrators.

Middle-level managers are usually responsible for the implementation of personnel policy that has been determined by top-level managers. Well-written personnel policies are useless if they are not implemented appropriately. These managers coordinate the efforts of lower levels and act as the channel between employees and top-level managers. Middle-level managers are more involved in day-to-day operations than top-level managers but still provide some input into long-term planning and the establishment of staffing policy on their units. Frequently middle-level managers are actively involved in the recruitment, selection, induction, orientation, evaluation, transfer, counseling, promotion, and termination of employees. Examples of middle-level managers include nursing supervisors, head nurses, department heads, and unit managers.

First-level managers are concerned primarily with the work flow through their specific units of the organization. They deal with immediate problems encountered in the day-to-day operations of the unit and deal with both organizational and personal needs. First-level managers may deal with personnel issues such as work schedules, making patient assignments, and minor employee problems. Examples of first-level managers might be a primary care nurse, a team leader, and a charge nurse.

As discussed earlier in this chapter, many health care organizations today have decentralized the responsibility for personnel management among a personnel department and the three levels of the management hierarchy. Traditionally organizations with personnel departments have given the responsibility for audit and control to the personnel department. This occurs because the coherence and integrity of the personnel process depends on good personnel policies that, in turn, require follow-up to be sure they are being properly practiced. This requires a strong and centralized audit of actual practice (Heneman and Schwab, 1978).

Likewise, the personnel department can play a vital role in innovation, providing up-to-date information on current human resource trends and new methods of solving problems. This information, in turn, is shared with top-level managers for inclusion in future policy setting. Table 3-2 gives an example of how an organization might divide personnel management responsibilities between the traditional personnel department and the nursing management hierarchy.

EFFECTIVE AND EFFICIENT COMMUNICATION IN HUMAN RESOURCE MANAGEMENT

Meeting human resource management needs of employees is a tremendous responsibility that requires clear, effective, and efficient communication among all members of the organization. Handbooks on organizational policies are usually found in each department in the form of a compact, looseleaf publication. However, this may be only a symbol of organizational communication. Organizational communication must be systematic, have continuity, be fully integrated into the organizational structure, and encourage an exchange of views and attitudes.

Jay Jackson (1957) identified characteristics of large-scale organizations that make communication particularly difficult:

1. Spatial distance within an organization can be a barrier to communication.
2. Different subgroups or subcultures within the organization have their own value systems and identities, and members form allegiances to their own subgroups. This results in

Table 3-2. Division of Personnel Management Responsibilities Between Nursing Management and the Personnel Department: A Sample Approach

Personnel Management

- Recruitment, testing, and job analysis
- Establishment of position descriptions
- Wage and salary compensation
- Employee benefits and services
- Development of employee handbook
- Grievances and arbitration
- Audit and research of policies and programs
- Innovation—forecasting manpower needs
- Employee relations
- Maintenance of personnel records
- Coordination of training and staff development programs

Top-Level Managers

- Determination of organizational personnel policies, goals, and strategies
- Complying with public manpower policy
- Determination of wage and salary controls

Middle-Level Managers

- Recruitment, interviewing, selection, induction, personal appraisal, employee inventory, counseling, transfer, promotion, and termination of employees
- Employee counseling

First-Level Managers

- Job orientation and training
- Staff development
- Staffing
- Assignment of workload

different translations of messages from management, depending on the significance of the messages in relation to the subgroup's values and what the subgroups are striving to accomplish.

3. People are structured into different systems or relationships in organizations. A work structure exists in which certain people are expected to complete tasks with other people. An authority structure exists in which some workers are in charge of supervising other workers. A status structure determines which individuals have rights and privileges, and a prestige structure allows some individuals to expect differential treatment. The friendship structure encourages interpersonal trust. All of these systems influence who should communicate to whom and in what manner.

4. Organizations are in a constant state of flux. Relationships, subgroups or subcultures, and geographical location constantly change, and because of this it is difficult to communicate decisions to all the people who are affected by them.

Organizations with both centralized and decentralized personnel management require effective communication if human resource needs are to be met for optimum productivity. *Effective* refers to "doing the right job." *Efficiency*, in contrast, refers to the optimal use of resources and may be simply defined as "doing the job right" (Laliberty and Christopher, 1984). Effective communication must be translated into efficient communication. This means that the communication should result in the right work being done, at the right time, by the most qualified individual, at the least cost.

WRITTEN COMMUNICATION WITHIN THE ORGANIZATION

Communication may take many forms in the organization. Written communication is utilized most often in a large-scale organization, as it is virtually impossible to see that all individuals needing to have knowledge of an event in a large-scale organization could be contacted verbally. Written communication, by virtue of its very nature, suggests attention and deliberation on the part of the sender and gives receivers a record for reference and review (Palmer and Deck, 1987). In personnel management, this written communication may take the form of hiring and recruitment ads, performance appraisals, and letters of reference. It may also announce changes in policy, procedures, events, and organizational change.

The written communication issued by the nursing manager reflects greatly on both the manager and the organization. Thus, the nurse manager needs to be able to write clearly and professionally, and use language that is understood. There is great danger in written communication because there is usually no feedback mechanism available for the sender of the message to clarify the intent of the message (Marquis and Huston, 1987). One way to minimize the inherent difficulties in written communication is by having other supervisory personnel read and imterpet memos prior to their distribution.

HealthCare Education Associates (1988) suggest the following guidelines for writing good letters and memos:

1. Know what you want to say before you start writing; this means that you must think clearly before you can write clearly.

2. Put people into your writing; when you write about a subject, discuss it in terms of the people affected by it. Avoid words such as *administration, authorization,* and *implementation,* which are abstract and impersonal.

3. Use action words; action verbs have a stronger impact.

4. Write plainly; use familiar, specific, and concrete words. Plain writing is more easily understood and thus more apt to be read.

5. Use as few words as possible; find one good way to make a point and trust that your reader will understand it.

6. Use simple, direct sentences; keep sentences under 20 words and include only one idea in a sentence. Make positive statements that clearly delineate your position on an issue. Tell the pertinent facts first.

7. Give the reader direction; be consistent in the tone of the message to establish a clear point of view.

8. Arrange the material logically; a logical presentation of facts increases the reliability that the reader will place in the writer. The material may be organized deductively, inductively, by order of importance, from the familiar to the unfamiliar, in chronological order, by close relationship, or by physical location.

9. Use paragraphs to lead readers; a paragraph should not exceed eight to ten lines in a memo, or be more than five to six lines in a letter.

10. Connect your thoughts; to connect your thoughts, you must add enough details, use repetition to tie thoughts together, and use transitional words to tell the reader when you are moving to a new thought.

11. Be clear; be certain your pronouns are clearly defined.

12. Express similar thoughts in similar ways.

Personnel managers are required to write a great deal in performing their job. Much of this writing is in the form of letters. Tool 3-1 shows the preferred basic format for any formal business letter.

Tool 3-1   Business Letter Format

SKIP FOUR TO EIGHT LINES, DEPENDING ON THE LENGTH OF
THE LETTER

DATE

    SKIP FOUR TO EIGHT LINES

INSIDE ADDRESS—Check the spelling and address for accuracy.

    DOUBLE SPACE

RE: (pronounced ray or ree, means regarding)—This optional device
alerts the reader to the subject of your letter.

    DOUBLE SPACE

SALUTATION— Write "Dear . . ." Abbreviate titles such as "Mr.,"
"Mrs.," and "Dr."; spell out titles such as "Reverend" and "Senator."

Use a comma (,) for informal letters and a colon (:) for formal letters—if
you are on a first name basis, use a comma; otherwise, use a colon.

If you are uncertain as to the sex of the person you are writing to,
address by title—"Dear Hospital Administrator"—or try "Dear Sir or
Madam."

    DOUBLE SPACE

BODY OF LETTER—Single space within the paragraph and double
space between paragraphs. (If you use the indented form, you do not
need to double space between paragraphs.)

    DOUBLE SPACE

COMPLIMENTARY CLOSING—Capitalize the first letter of the first
word and put a comma at the end—"Sincerely,".

    SKIP FOUR LINES IF THE LETTER IS TYPED

SIGNATURE (typed)—Place your written signature above your typed
name.

    DOUBLE SPACE

ENCLOSURES—If you are enclosing anything, indicate here, typically
with "Enc." or "Encs."

You may, if you choose, begin the complimentary closing and signature
at the center of the page; this is called the semiblock form.

Reproduced by permission from HealthCare Education Associates, *Professional Writing Skills For Health Care Managers*, p. 46. St. Louis, 1988, The C.V. Mosby Co.

Memos, unlike letters, are distributed internally within the organization. Human resource management requires tremendous intradepartment and interdepartment communication, and much of this communication occurs in the form of memos. The primary purpose of most memos is to inform, instruct, recommend, or document. HealthCare Education Associates (1988) suggest the following guidelines for writing effective memos:

1. Write memos that make the main point at the beginning.
2. Give only essential information in the memo.
3. The memo should be written simply, without inflated or authoritarian language.
4. Headings should be used in the memo to direct the reader to specific issues.

Most organizations have an established form for memos. This form is generally in a block format, with no indentations from the left-hand margin. Tool 3-2 gives an example of the standard format for an organizational memo.

CHARACTERISTICS OF EFFECTIVE SUPERVISION

Having good written communication skills is only one attribute required of effective supervisors. Supervisors are the members of the management team who are most accessible and who have the greatest immediate impact on the worker; thus, their importance in promoting optimal human resource management cannot be underestimated.

> To the worker, the supervisor is the organization. The supervisor is tangible, immediate management, not a 32-page booklet describing company benefits and worker obligations, not a notice on the bulletin board, and not a lay-off or a recall telegram. The supervisor is a leader, coach, and teacher who has the authority of knowledge and leads through persuasion. Capable of creating a work climate that motivates people and maximizes their human assets, the supervisor can often get extraordinary results from ordinary people by helping them recognize and develop their abilities. The supervisor is immediately accessible from above and below. Few suffer from as much pressure. And few are so inadequately prepared for it.*

---

*From Koger, W.E., "Supervisory Employees," in Famularo, J. (ed.), *Handbook of Human Resources Administration*, Second Edition, McGraw-Hill, New York, 1986.

Tool 3-2   Memo Format

Date:

    DOUBLE SPACE

To: If the memo is to be distributed to more than one person, alphabetical order is the easiest method of listing. You may list by rank if you prefer.

    DOUBLE SPACE

From:

    DOUBLE SPACE

Subject: In a few words, state the reason you are writing the memo. This lets the reader know at a glance what you will be talking about.

    TRIPLE SPACE

Signature:

    TRIPLE SPACE

Copies: You may need to send copies of your memo to different
cc: people. You should indicate this here, using the abbreviation cc: followed by the names of those persons receiving copies of the memo.

Reproduced by permission from HealthCare Education Associates, *Professional Writing Skills for Health Care Managers*, p. 68. St. Louis, 1988, The C.V. Mosby Co.

This quote gives the reader an idea of the responsibilities and expectations placed on supervisors. The ability of the supervisor to successfully meet these expectations has a direct impact on productivity and retention in the organization. In fact, it is fair to say that employee motivation and increased productivity are not possible if supervision is not effective. Stevens (1987) identified the following characteristics necessary in an effective management team:

1. *Clinical expertise*. Managers must have clinical expertise at or above the level of their employees if they are to gain the power and authority associated with expertise.

2. *Sound judgment*. Managers must demonstrate basic common sense in their problem solving. Common sense and a willingness to make decisions is all that is required of many management decisions.

3. *Objectivity*. It is very important that managers be able to look at the "big picture" over the needs of any one individual.

4. *Commitment*. Managers must have a strong commitment to departmental and organizational goals.

5. *Perseverance*. Managers must realize that success and needed change only occur with hard work and perseverance. This closely correlates with their commitment to the department and the organization.

6. *Self-confidence*. Managers must balance the need to be somewhat immune to idle criticism with the need to be open to suggestions on how to improve their performance. In addition, managers must have enough self-confidence to separate performance criticism from personal criticism.

7. *Initiative*. Having both the ability and the willingness to solve problems are a necessity for managers.

8. *Good interpersonal skills*. Conflict management and the ability to appropriately counsel employees for the purpose of self-growth are essential skills in human relations.

9. *Realistic expectations*. It is very easy to accomplish great things if resources are unlimited. Learning how to be productive and setting realistic goals in the face of inadequate resources provides a different challenge.

Lyles and Joiner (1986) have also identified seven personal characteristics that contribute to supervisory effectiveness in the health care field:

1. *Solid foundation of technical knowledge.* Supervisors must have a well-developed knowledge base to serve as a resource to their employees and to appropriately analyze and evaluate their employees' performances.

2. *Ability to complete work through other people.* Supervisors must have "people power" in that they must be able to guide the work of others through their own personal powers and abilities. This entails delegation at the right time and to the right individual.

3. *Desire to achieve at high levels.* Supervisors' motivations often set the tone for the motivational levels of their workers. Supervisors who are motivated to achieve motivate all their employees to reach their optimal levels. All the ability in the world is useless if individuals are not willing to take risks.

4. *High expectations of achievement from others.* Workers generally succeed at the level that is expected from them. Supervisors who believe their employees can function at high yet realistic levels motivate them to do so.

5. *Confidence in one's own ability and the ability of the workers.* Supervisors must have not only self-confidence, but also confidence in the ability of their workers. Because the two are inextricably linked, the work performance of both parties is affected.

6. *Ability to instill a sense of value in others.* Employees who place a high value on what they are doing perform at a higher level. Effective supervisors have the potential to greatly affect the value system of their employees.

7. *Ability to communicate.* The essence of supervision is completing work through other people, which requires effective communication. This includes excellent sending and receiving skills.

Other supervisory skills that the authors feel should be added to these lists include:

1. *Management skills and knowledge.* It has erroneously been assumed by many top- and middle-level managers that because an individual has excellent clinical skills he or she also knows how to manage. Management skills must be taught to managers at all levels of the hierarchy in an effort to avoid setting them up for failure.

2. *Honesty and fairness.* Employee trust and respect are impossible if supervisors are not honest and fair in dealing with their subordinates.

3. *Future thinking.* Effective supervisors look ahead in planning so as to avoid crisis management.

4. *Empathy.* Supervisors must be able to understand and identify with the feelings or ideas of their employees. This does not mean that they cater to every demand or wish of their employees, but that they do recognize and attempt to understand the position of their employees.

It is fair to say that an organization can be only as good as the quality of managers it employs at all levels within the organizational hierarchy. It is imperative to build a management team that understands the components of human resource management and that implements them in the supervision of employees. This requires a clarity and congruence of organizational and managerial goals regarding human resource management. It also requires conscientious and carefully orchestrated communication of those goals and how they are being implemented. Because human resource management is a dynamic process, each organization must continually reassess its internal environment to assure that the environment is one that promotes retention and productivity.

KEY CONCEPTS CHAPTER 3

1. The responsibility for personnel management extends to all first-, middle-, and top-level managers in an organization.

2. Centralized personnel management results in greater consistency in personnel planning and is generally more cost effective. Decentralized personnel management allows personnel decisions to be made at the unit level, which more closely meets unit needs and objectives.

3. Because of the potential for conflict, the roles and responsibility for personnel management must be clearly defined in organizations that give the responsibility for personnel management to both traditional personnel departments and to operating managers.

4. There are many barriers to communication in large-scale organizations, with written communication generally being the most frequently utilized form of communication.

5. Written communication carries great risk because it does not allow for feedback from the receiver regarding the intent of the message. Nursing managers must learn how to write professional letters and memos that reduce the likelihood of confusion and conflict.

6. It is essential that the management team understand the characteristics of effective supervision and that they implement these in order for optimal human resource management to be obtained.

REFERENCES

HealthCare Education Associates, *Professional Writing Skills for Health Care Managers; A Practical Guide*, C.V. Mosby, St. Louis, 1988.

Heneman, H.G., III, and Schwab, D.P., *Perspectives on Personnel/Human Resource Management*, Richard D. Irwin, Homewood, IL, 1978.

Jackson, J.M., "The Organization and its Communication Problems," *Society of Public Health Education*, Communication Monograph 1:10, 1957 (also reprinted in Stone, S., Firisch, S., Jordan, S., et al. (eds.), *Management for Nurses*, C.V. Mosby, St. Louis, 1984).

Koger, W.E., "Supervisory Employees," in Famularo, J. (ed.), *Handbook of Human Resources Administration*, Second Edition, McGraw-Hill, New York, 1986.

Laliberty, R., and Christopher, W.I., *Enhancing Productivity in Health Care Facilities*, National Health Publishing, Owings Mills, MD, 1984.

Lyles, R.I., and Joiner, C., *Supervision in Health Care Organizations*, John Wiley and Sons, New York, 1986.

Marquis, B., and Huston, C., *Management Decision Making for Nurses: 101 Case Studies*, J.B. Lippincott, 1987.

Milkovich, G.T., and Glueck, W.F., *Personnel/Human Resource Management: A Diagnostic Approach*, Fourth Edition, Business Publications, Plano, TX, 1985.

Palmer, M.E., and Deck, E.S., "Assertiveness: Phone Calls, Memos and I Messages," *Nursing Management* 18(1): 39–42, 1987.

Stevens, S.L., "Operationalizing a Departmental Manager Role," in Lewis, E.M., and Spicer, J.G. (eds.) *Human Resource Management Handbook*, Aspen Publications, Germantown, MD, 1987, Chapter 31.

White, H., and Boynton, R., "The Role of Personnel: A Management View," *Arizona Business*, 21, 1974.

ADDITIONAL READINGS

DiVincenti, M., *Administering Nursing Service*, Little, Brown and Company, Boston, 1972.

Elfrey, P., *The Hidden Agenda—Recognizing What Really Matters at Work*, John Wiley and Sons, New York, 1982.

Hamilton, J.M., and Kiefer, M.E., *Survival Skills for the New Nurse*, J.B. Lippincott, Philadelphia, 1986.

Kirsch, J., *The Middle Manager and The Nursing Organization: Human Resources/Fiscal Resources*, Appleton and Lange, Norwalk, CT, 1988.

Schutz, C., Decker, P., and Sullivan, E.J., *Nursing Management: An Experiential/Skill Building Workbook*, Addison-Wesley, Menlo Park, CA, 1986.

Simms, L.M., Price, S.A., and Ervin, N.E., *The Professional Practice of Nursing Administration*, John Wiley and Sons, New York, 1985.

Sullivan, E.J., and Decker, P.J., *Effective Management in Nursing*, Second Edition, Addison-Wesley, Menlo Park, CA, 1988.

· UNIT TWO
Planning for Effective Human Resource Management

TOO OFTEN managers in present-day health care organizations spend less time in planning than they do tending to crises. Yet, it is primarily due to poor planning that crises occur. Planning may be defined as deciding in advance what to do, who is to do it, when it is to be done, and where it is to be accomplished. Planning is not only the most critical phase of both the management and the personnel process, but it is also the process that must occur first.

Planning is essential for various reasons but, most important, because it eliminates uncertainty and chance. It focuses attention on goals and consequently assists in building a team effort to accomplish those goals. It gives direction to everyone in the organization regarding priorities and resource allocation. Good planning also establishes a method for control, thereby making an economical operation possible and establishing a means for determining accountability.

There are many different types of planning, but all planning in an organization should form two types of hierarchies or pyramids. The first hierarchy involves the flow of planning; that is, all plans formulated at levels below the highest level of administration must be compatible with those developed at a higher level. Therefore, unit philosophy, goals, and objectives must be compatible with departmental goals, which in turn must be compatible with organizational goals. The second hierarchy of planning is in the type of planning that is carried out in an organization. The first level must be accomplished prior to subsequent levels. The following types of hierarchical planning are used by organizations:

1. *Purpose or mission.* This type of planning is the reason the organization exists or was formed. It explains the aim of the organization.

2. *Philosophy* (sometimes included with the mission statement). This is the set of values and beliefs that guides all actions and decisions of the organization. The philosophy is the foundation of all subsequent planning.

3. *Assessment planning.* This planning must be accomplished prior to the setting of goals and objectives and includes an assessment of both the internal and external environment of the organization. There are many ways an organization can accomplish its purpose, but if the organization has not taken a complete assessment of the economical and community constraints, objectives may be selected that are not possible to accomplish. Conversely, the organization may overlook opportunities because it has not recognized available resources, either within the organization itself or in the community. Assessment planning is frequently the most neglected area of planning.

4. *Goals and objectives.* These plans are the end points toward which the organization is working. It might be said that if the philosophy is the cornerstone on which the organization is based, then the goals and objectives are the blueprints for that organization.

5. *Strategic planning.* These plans may involve (1) strategies for introducing planned change, (2) strategies to obtain resources, or (3) futuristic strategies of a long-term nature. Long-term strategic planning is particularly important in large complex organizations.

6. *Policies.* Policies consist of plans reduced to statements that guide the organization in its decisions. Policies are much more flexible than rules.

7. *Procedures.* These are plans that have very specific steps to be used to carry out policies.

8. *Rules.* These are plans that define a specific type of action or nonaction. Rules allow no room for discretion and should, therefore, be used with caution.

9. *Budgets.* These are fiscal plans that are expressed in numerical terms.

10. *Job design.* These are plans that are designed for specific personnel classifications. Although job design includes job descriptions, it is much more encompassing than job descriptions.

This unit will address the various types of planning in relationship to the management of human resources. The need for planning at the top, middle, and unit levels of the organization will be discussed.

Certain principles and guidelines apply regardless of the level or type of planning that is being carried out. In addition to plans requiring a hierarchy and being in compliance with other higher level plans, Marquis and Huston (1987) list four additional principles of effective planning:

1. Regardless of the time span involved, planning will always utilize the same process.

2. The length of each plan is determined by the amount of time required to accomplish all the tasks that are necessary to ensure successful implementation of the plan.

3. All plans must be flexible.

4. All plans must include some method of evaluation and a regular review process so that progress can be measured and, if necessary, mid-course corrections made.

REFERENCES

Marquis, B., Huston C., *Management Decision Making for Nurses: 101 Case Studies.* J.B. Lippincott, Philadelphia, 1987.

4
Nursing Department Planning: Impact on Human Resource Management

MANY PROBLEMS occurring in management that subsequently affect retention and productivity are the result of poor planning. This is particularly true in the first stages of planning, i.e., writing an appropriate philosophy and goals.

Managers of human resources should be able to write a unit philosophy that correlates with that of the organization and then develop goals and objectives that reflect this philosophy. Figure 4-1 depicts the relationship of the institutional philosophy to other departments within the institution. In this figure the term *goal* refers to the global mission statement rather than the goals that are developed from the philosophy.

Once the nursing service philosophy has been developed, but prior to the setting of specific goals and objectives, prudent managers will assess the constraints and the assets of the external and internal environment of their organizations. For example, a manager's philosophy may espouse a belief that each patient has the basic right to receive quality nursing care. The manager might define this as, "a personal service based on needs as they relate to an individual and to a clinical disease or condition." Nurse managers need to develop goals and objectives

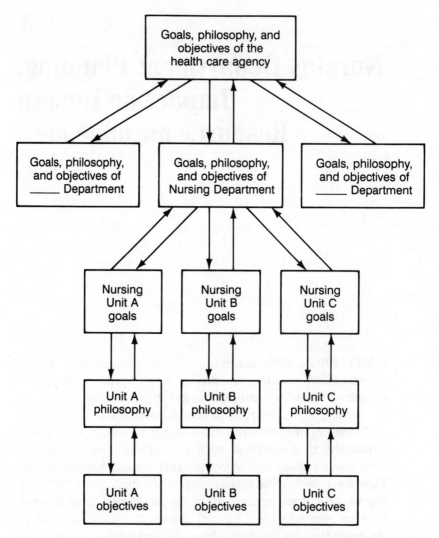

FIGURE 4-1. *Hierarchy of philosophy.* (From Schweiger, J.L., *The Nurse As Manager*, p.6, John Wiley & Sons, New York, 1980. Copyright © 1980 by John Wiley & Sons, Inc.)

that reflect the adopted philosophy, but there are various means for doing this. Managers could carry out their philosophy by any or all of the following goals: (1) individualized patient care, (2) use of care plans and care conferences, and/or (3) implementing primary nursing care management. However, before they set any specific goals and objectives, they need to determine the following: (1) Does this entail a change from past practice? (2)

What are the resources available to carry out their goals? (3) What constraints might be present? and (4) Can they put their philosophy into practice by methods other than those they have envisioned?

This chapter will assist managers in writing a nursing department philosophy that is congruent with the organizational philosophy. Managers will also be assisted in assessing both the internal and external environment of the organization. Goals and objectives for the nursing service will be developed, and the nursing service department's relationship to other departments in the organization will be examined. Tables and tools for implementation include a sample nursing philosophy, nursing service goals and objectives, an organizational chart, and check lists for assessing the internal and external environment.

DEVELOPMENT OF PHILOSOPHICAL CONGRUENCE

To avoid writing a nursing service philosophy that is not supported by the larger organization, top-level nursing managers need to examine the philosophy carefully. After reading the nursing service philosophy given in Table 4-1, the reader should return to the organizational philosophy that is shown in Table 2-1 in Chapter 2. It soon becomes obvious that the two philosophies have several inconsistencies. The first inconsistency occurs in the third paragraph of the nursing service philosophy, where there is mention of the importance of research and teaching. These two concepts are never mentioned in the mission or philosophy of the parent organization. Second, the organizational philosophy stressed community involvement, and the nursing service philosophy does not address this issue. There are, however, many likenesses in the two philosophies, as both speak to the needs of patients and to the responsibility of the organization to its employees. Both philosophies also reflect an agreement on the acceptance of accountability by employees.

One method of avoiding incongruent philosophies and goals between the organization and its departments is for all departments to be involved in periodic review of the larger organization's philosophy. Likewise, top-level nursing service management should involve personnel from many levels in reviewing

---

Table 4-1. Philosophy of Nursing Service

Our philosophy of nursing is based on respect for the dignity and worth of the individual. We believe each patient has the basic right to receive effective nursing care, which is a personal service based on the patient's needs as they relate to the patient as an individual and to his or her clinical disease or condition.

Recognizing the obligation of nursing to help restore the patient to the best possible state of physical, mental, and emotional health and to maintain the patient's sense of spiritual and social well-being, we pledge intelligent cooperation in coordinating the nursing service with the medical and allied professional practitioners.

Understanding the importance of research and teaching for the improvement of patient care, the Nursing Department will support, promote, and participate in these activities.

Using knowledge of human behavior, we shall strive toward mutual trust and understanding between the nursing service and the nursing employees to provide an atmosphere for developing the fullest possible potential of each individual member of the nursing team.

It is our belief that the nursing personnel are individually accountable to the patient and his or her family for the quality and compassion of the patient care rendered and for upholding the standards of care as delineated by the nursing staff.

---

and rewriting nursing philosophy. Understanding the beliefs and ideals of the organization is one way to build a team spirit and inspire employees. This type of employee participation increases loyalty and, thereby, increases retention. Involving employees in writing and developing the philosophy and purpose of the organization has been an effective tool used by many excellent companies and magnet hospitals (Kramer and Schmalenberg, 1988).

INTERNAL AND EXTERNAL ORGANIZATIONAL ENVIRONMENT

Although the term *organizational environment* has been around for some time, there still exists some confusion regarding its meaning. Smith and associates (1980) have defined the organizational environment as "the factors or events that have a marked impact upon the organization's performance and are beyond the immediate or complete control of the organization."

Synonyms for *internal environment* are *working climate, organizational culture*, and, simply, *working conditions*. The internal environment of the organization is essentially those things that are officially within the jurisdiction of the organization and that have an impact on the work to be done. It may include the social atmosphere, noise levels, or work stations. It includes employees' perceptions of the general working conditions within the organization. It is possible for there to be many different perceptions of the working environment among employees of the same organization.

The internal environment may be assessed in various ways. The most obvious way is to observe the environment. Managers who spend time with employees in their working environment, reviewing the work stations and observing types of social interaction among employees, will be able to more closely match organizational goals to what it is possible to accomplish. Top-level managers should also request input from lower level managers in assessing the internal environment of the organization. Lastly, but not of least importance, is the need to include employees in any assessment of the internal environment. Managers may feel that employees' perceptions are incorrect, but as long as they remain they must be dealt with.

For example, the organization may adopt a philosophy that it embraces modern technology and desires to be a leader in automation. Before the nursing service can decide on their goals and objectives for putting the philosophy into practice, they need to assess the internal environment. Perhaps the ward secretaries feel that the nursing stations are not large enough to accommodate a computer or that the noise level would be too high. Therefore, the goals of the nursing service might be modified, and, instead of adding a computerized system to nursing stations, they might begin by using computerization for staffing and for operating room scheduling until the perceptions of the ward secretaries can be altered. The goals and objectives would still reflect the philosophy of the organization but would have a greater probability of success. Tool 4-1 may be used for assessing the internal organizational environment.

The *external environment* is those things that lie outside the complete control of the organization but that have an impact on the realization of goals. The external environment includes such things as unions, competitors, the consumer, the community, government regulations, technology, the organization's assets, availability of resources, and the economic and fiscal climate. The nurse manager will fail to meet goals and objectives if he or she does not adequately assess the external environment prior to setting goals. For example, the nurse manager could

Tool 4-1 Assessing the Internal Environment

Physical environment

1. Is the environment attractive?
2. Does it appear that there is adequate maintenance?
3. Are nursing stations crowded? Noisy?
4. Is there an appropriate-sized lobby? Are there quiet areas?
5. Is there sufficient seating for families in the dining room?
6. Are there enough conference rooms?

Social environment

1. Are many friendships maintained beyond the workplace?
2. Is there an annual picnic and/or Christmas party that is well attended by the employees?
3. Do employees seem to generally like each other?
4. Do all shifts and all departments get along fairly well?
5. Are there certain departments that are disliked or resented?
6. Are employees on a first name basis with coworkers? Doctors? Charge nurses? Supervisors?

Supportive environment

1. Are there educational reimbursement funds available?
2. Are good low-cost meals available to employees?
3. Are there adequate lounges for employees?
4. Are there funds available to send employees to workshops?
5. Do employees receive recognition for extra effort?
6. Does the organization help pay for the Christmas party or other social functions?

Power structure

1. Who holds the most power in the organization?
2. Which departments are viewed as powerful? As powerless?
3. Who gets free meals? Special parking places?
4. Who carries a beeper? Wears a lab coat? Has overhead pages?

5. Who has the biggest office?

6. Who is never called by his or her first name?

Safety environment

1. Is there a well-lighted parking place for employees arriving or departing after dark?

2. Is there an active and involved safety committee?

3. Is it necessary to have security guards?

Communicative environment

1. Is upward communication usually written or verbal?

2. Is there much informal communication?

3. Is there an active "grapevine"? Is it reliable?

4. Where is important information exchanged? The parking lot? The doctors' surgical dressing room? The nurses' station? The coffee shop? In surgery? In the delivery room?

Organizational taboos and heroes

1. Are there special rules and policies that can never be broken?

2. Are there subjects or ideas that are forbidden?

3. Are there relationships that cannot be threatened?

---

accomplish the first philosophical statement in Table 4-1 by having as a goal primary nursing with an all-RN staff. But, if there are not adequate numbers of registered nurses in the area, the nurse manager will fail to meet this goal. Perhaps a more appropriate goal, which would also support this philosophical statement, would be to assign the same nursing personnel to patients as often as possible and to have individualized care plans on every patient, which are followed by all members of the staff.

Smith and co-workers (1980) maintain that planning is a mental process that begins with a philosophy but incorporates the process of thinking before any action is taken. They elaborate by stating that the thinking process should include an

Tool 4-2   Assessing the External Environment

Financial environment

1. Are there forces in the payment structure that could impact upon the organization's finances, such as changes in reimbursement?
2. Are there outstanding high-interest loans?
3. Is it likely that the number of patient days will decrease in the near future? Increase?
4. Is the organization fiscally sound?

Consumer environment

1. How does the average consumer view the organization?
2. Is the hospital recognized and supported by the community?
3. What do family members feel about the nursing care?
4. How are the physicians viewed by patients?
5. What are the age group and needs of the patient population?

Competitors

1. Who is the major competitor?
2. What is your organization's image compared with that of your leading competitor?
3. Are your competitors planning on expanding services?
4. What unique services do you offer that other facilities do not offer?
5. How do salaries and benefits in your organization compare to those of other local organizations?

Collective bargaining

1. Is there likely to be a change in collective bargaining? From nonunion to unionization or from unionization to nonunion?
2. If presently unionized, how are relationships between the union and management?
3. Are present relationships likely to change in the near future?

Community

1. Is the community growing in population?
2. What changes are taking place in the community?

3. Does the organization receive favorable publicity in newspapers, radio, and television?

4. Is the hospital supported by the community in an active manner as evidenced by a large volunteer group and an involved board of trustees?

Medical staff

1. Does the hospital have difficulty in attracting and retaining a qualified medical staff?

2. Is the medical staff supportive of the total organization? Of administration? Of the nursing staff?

3. What role does the medical staff have in decision-making?

4. Are there too few or too many physicians in the community?

Government regulations

1. What proposed state or federal regulations will affect the organization?

---

assessment of the business environment, that assessment to be used as a backdrop for future planning. We should *desire* the future, but in order to make the future happen we must use thinking in our planning so that we *shape* the future (Smith et al., 1980). The nurse manager who shapes the future and makes that future happen is a proactive nurse, rather than a reactive nurse. Increased retention and productivity of nursing staff will occur if the nurse manager uses thinking in the planning process. Tool 4-2 can assist in assessing the external environment of the organization.

WRITING GOALS AND OBJECTIVES

There are differing opinions among business writers regarding the definition of the terms *goals* and *objectives*. Some view the goal as a more global, less specific, statement and the term *objective* as a more definitive procedure on how the goal is to be accomplished. Others view the objective as the beginning or starting point of planning and the goal as the end result of meeting objectives. Two examples of written goals and objectives are included in Tables 4-2 and 4-3. The goals and objectives in Table 4-2 are more global than those in Table 4-3.

However, even the written objectives in the second set of goals do not meet the requirements of most planning theorists, because they do not have time frames for accomplishment, nor is there a specified way to evaluate whether the objectives have been met. Morrisey (1977) also feels objectives should be accompanied by the maximum cost in dollars that will be incurred to achieve the objective. For the purposes of this book, we will use the term *goal* to mean a global, less specific statement than the

---

Table 4-2. Goals and Objectives of Nursing Service

To develop recognition of the patient's need for independence, and right for privacy, and to assess the patient's level of readiness to learn and accept facts that relate to his or her illness.

To provide effective patient care relative to the patient's needs, insofar as the hospital and community facilities permit, through the use of nursing care plans, individual patient care, and discharge planning, including follow-up contact.

To encourage therapeutic interaction with the patient in order to assist the patient in acceptance of, and adjustment to, his or her condition.

To carry out the regime of care as ordered by the doctor with intelligent application to the individual needs of the patient.

To develop and adhere to standards of care for each disease entity.

To create an atmosphere conducive to favorable patient and employee morale and to personnel growth.

To appreciate and acknowledge the contribution and worth of all personnel in assuring improved patient care.

To continually evaluate the competency and attitude of all employees in the Nursing Department in a manner that produces growth in the employee and upgrades nursing standards.

To provide an inservice program for orientation of new employees and for the continued staff development of all personnel in the Nursing Department.

To develop an awareness and understanding of the legal responsibilities in nursing.

To study and evaluate the quality of nursing care and implement improvements through the use of patient care audit.

To interpret, implement, and uphold hospital policy.

To support the financial plan of the hospital by the use of an annual nursing budget.

To cooperate with all departments within the hospital in furthering the purposes of the institution.

To foster and maintain good public relations.

To uphold the policy of cost containment by eliminating waste of supplies and assisting in product evaluation.

To recognize the nursing responsibility to provide patient education, both pre- and post-operative, for specific chronic diseases, and maternal child health.

To support patients and their families through emotional crises caused by hospitalization, death, and terminal illness.

Table 4-3.   Goals and Objectives of Nursing Care for Unit A

---

1. To maintain a safe environment for the patient by:
   a. Utilizing the guidelines as outlined in the safety manual
   b. Having an effective infection control by use of an infection committee and by using the guidelines of the isolation manual
2. To coordinate both nursing and non-nursing services by:
   a. Explaining and scheduling procedures
   b. Interpreting services to the patient
3. To carry out a therapeutic medical plan of care as ordered by the physician by:
   a. Having an understanding and knowledge of accepted medical practice
   b. Noting and following through with the physician's plan of care
4. To assess, plan, implement, and evaluate a nursing plan of care by:
   a. Use of short- and long-term nursing goals
   b. Cooperation of all shifts in the use of nursing care plans
   c. Evaluating the nursing care through use of (1) a charting audit, (2) a patient questionnaire form, and (3) team conferences
5. To help the patient grow from his or her illness experience by:
   a. Teaching aspects of health and illness
   b. Assisting the patient with problem-solving
   c. Allowing the patient as much autonomy as is feasible in regards to his or her illness
6. To do for the patient what he or she is unable to do by:
   a. Using skilled bedside techniques in procedures and treatments
7. To act as a family member surrogate and to relieve the anxiety of illness by:
   a. Showing compassion and interest in the patient
   b. Using therapeutic and listening techniques of communication
   c. Answering questions and giving reassurance
8. To think of the patient as a member of an open system by:
   a. Including members of the patient's family in aspects of teaching

---

term *objective*, unless the two terms are used together. When the term *objective* is used alone without the more global term *goal*, it should be written in the following manner:

1. The objective should be explicit.
2. The objective should be measurable.
3. Information needed to evaluate the objective should be retrievable.
4. Time frames or target dates for completion should be included.
5. When appropriate, the cost to achieve the objective is included.

Clearly written goals are very important tools for achieving effective management, but many managers find them difficult to write. Morrisey (1977) suggests the following format be used to assist in writing clear objectives:

1. Write the word *to* followed by an action verb.
2. Write a single key result to be achieved.
3. Write the word *by* and state the target date for accomplishment.
4. State the maximum cost in terms of dollars and/or time.

Writing good objectives requires time and practice. The sample goals and objectives for Unit A, Table 4-3, include three objectives for the goal of helping the patient grow as a result of his or her illness (goal 5). None of the three objectives are written in measurable terms or with other criteria as listed above. If rewritten appropriately, in measurable objectives, they may appear like this:

1. All patients are to have evidence of appropriate teaching, relative to their nursing diagnosis, recorded on the nurses' progress notes prior to discharge.
2. All patients and/or their families are to be included in formulating a problem list, and documentation of their inclusion will be found in the admission nursing history.
3. All patients are to be given choices regarding time of, and method of, treatments and procedures, and this will be documented on their nursing care plans and will be updated daily.

It soon becomes apparent that the rewritten objectives are much more definitive and measurable. Marquis and Huston (1987) maintain that objectives must be clearly communicated to the personnel responsible for carrying them out. It is important, therefore, that they be written in a manner that reduces chances for ambiguity.

If goals and objectives are to be meaningful to the nursing staff, and if the staff are to be committed in carrying them out, they must be involved in the process of developing and reviewing them. This is especially true on the unit level, and Chapter 5 will further explore how unit managers can involve personnel in planning at the unit level.

All objectives should be reviewed annually. At that time, the global goals should be revised as necessary and all objectives measured and evaluated for compliance. Those objectives that have not been met need to be analyzed to determine why they were not met. Often the evaluation process will tell the nurse manager much about his or her unit or department. Knowledge is gained as much by examining what was not accomplished as by examining what was; therefore, noncompletion of an objective should never be viewed as a failure, but as a chance for the manager to gain important knowledge about the personnel and department.

COMPONENTS OF PERSONNEL PLANNING

As was discussed in Chapter 2, the top-level nursing administrator has responsibility to be involved in the planning and development of all policies that affect personnel in the organization. The stage of planning that follows the development of objectives is the formulation of policies that will assist the manager in making decisions. Beach (1980) defines a policy as a plan of action that commits the organization to a specific course of action. If the manager does not have a voice in policy development, it is very likely that policies will be formulated that will make the management of his or her human resources more difficult.

Policies do not include details of implementation. That is the role of a procedure. Lower level managers should be allowed some discretion in carrying out organizational policy, and that is why policies should serve as guidelines, not absolutes. Just as it is necessary for the philosophy, goals, and objectives to be congruent, it is necessary that policies of various departments be congruent; that is, nursing service should not have a policy that is radically different from that of other departments, unless the difference is articulated in an overriding policy. An example is the policy of some organizations prohibiting nepotism, often accompanied by the statement that in "hard-to-hire" positions managers can seek waivers to this policy. In most organizations, there are general policies that affect all departments, as well as specific organizational policies that may affect only one department.

In order for personnel policies to not adversely affect retention and productivity, the employees must understand them and must view them as being consistently applied throughout all departments. It is important, therefore, for nurse managers to understand how the nursing service and their units or departments fit into the total picture of the organization.

IMPACT OF INTERDEPARTMENTAL RELATIONSHIPS ON PLANNING

In addition to understanding organizational policies, managers should acquaint themselves with the overall formal structure of the organization. This includes the chain of command and the span of control. Even at the first level of nursing management, nurses will need to deal with other departments, so it is imperative that they understand the organizational chart. They need to know if a problem should be taken to the personnel department or to their immediate superiors. The written personnel policies and the organizational chart should guide managers in such decisions. Managers who understand the structure and relationships in an organization will be able to expedite decision-making and will also have a greater understanding of the organizational environment.

The organizational structure, as depicted on a chart, can assist individuals with role identity and with the expectations of a given role (Figure 4-2). The organizational chart defines formal relationships by the use of horizontal lines. If the lines are unbroken, positions are deemed to have formal superior/subordinate relationships, with the chain of command flowing from the top of the chart downward. The longer the chain of command, the more centralized the organization is, and the shorter the chain of command, the more decentralized it is. The broken lines denote staff positions, which are positions that are advisory. Advisory positions do not have, inherent in them, legitimate authority. Inservice education positions are usually advisory or staff positions. Inservice educators do not have the authority to hire or fire nurses who appear below them on the organizational chart.

Status and formal power are represented on the chart by the position level on the chart. Individuals holding positions depicted at the top of an organizational chart have more formal status and power than do those on the bottom. The number of positions directly under a position on the organization chart is said to be the span of control of the person occupying the

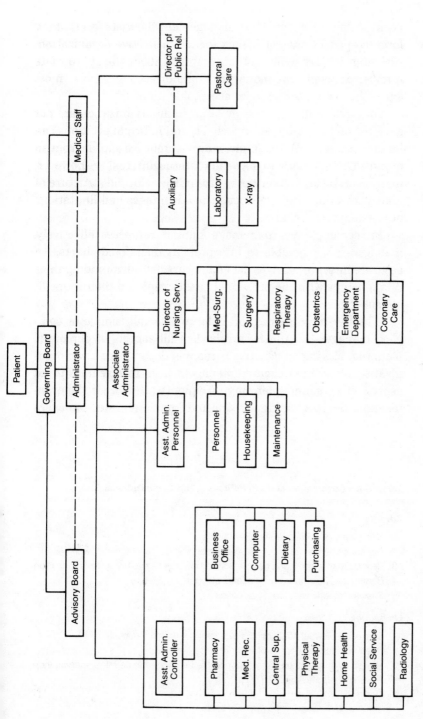

FIGURE 4-2. *Organizational chart*

position directly above. Most management theorists feel that too large a span of control makes for an ineffective organization. Although writers differ in their opinions about the appropriate number of people one manager should directly supervise, most agree that seven to ten is an acceptable number.

Of course, informal relationships in an organization are not depicted on an organizational chart, and informal positions can be very powerful. For example, many secretaries appear from an organizational chart to have low status. In reality, however, many secretaries are very powerful in the informal structure of an organization. Table 4-4 lists the advantages and limitations of organizational charts.

In learning how to manage human resources effectively, managers must be able to interpret organizational charts. An accurate interpretation assists managers in understanding their relationships with the personnel department and their immediate superiors.

Whether the organization is large or small, simple or complex, managers should be involved in all aspects of personnel planning. Having an effective personnel department in an organization should not exclude managers from involvement in all aspects of personnel planning. Frequently, the larger the organization, the less the input requested from lower level managers

---

Table 4-4.   Advantages and Limitations of the Organizational Chart

---

Advantages

1. Maps lines of decision-making authority
2. Helps people understand their assignments and those of their coworkers
3. Reveals to managers and new personnel how they tie into the entire organization
4. Contributes to sound organizational structure
5. Shows formal lines of communication

Limitations

1. Shows only formal relationships (not informal or informational)
2. Does not indicate degree of authority
3. May show things as they are supposed to be or used to be rather than as they are (becomes obsolete fairly quickly)
4. Possibility of confusing authority with status

---

regarding personnel policy decisions. Yet it is particularly essential in large organizations that all nurse managers be involved with personnel policy development.

Planning is an essential part of the process of human resource management. Managers must have a clear understanding of the goals and mission of the organization so they can communicate those goals and values to their subordinates. When everyone working in the organization has a commitment to the mission of that organization, the end result will be a team effort. It is this sense of team work and commitment that builds the type of loyalty that will ultimately increase retention and productivity.

KEY CONCEPTS CHAPTER 4

1. The philosophy, goals, and objectives of an organization flow from the top of the organizational hierarchy to the bottom.
2. There is a hierarchy in planning development.
3. A major part of the "thinking" of planning is in the assessment of the internal and external environment.
4. The more specifically objectives can be written, the more effectively they will be communicated to others.
5. In order to increase their effectiveness, nurse managers should understand their positions in relation to both the organization and other departments.
6. All nurse managers have a responsibility to be involved with personnel planning.

REFERENCES

Beach, D., *Personnel: The Management of People at Work*. Fourth Edition, Macmillan, New York, 1980.

Kramer, M., and Schmalenberg, C., "Magnet Hospitals, Part I: Institutions of Excellence," *JONA*, 18(1):13–24, 1988.

Marquis, B.L., Huston, C.J., *Management Decision Making For Nurses: 101 Case Studies*, J.B. Lippincott, Philadelphia, 1987.

Morrisey, G.L., *Management by Objectives and Results for Business and Industry*, Second Edition, Addison-Wesley, Reading, MA, 1977.

Smith, H.R., Carroll, A.B., Kefelas, A.G., Watson, H.F., *Management: Making Organizations Perform*, Macmillan, New York, 1980.

ADDITIONAL READINGS

Cantor, M., "Philosophy, Purpose and Objectives: Why Do We Have Them?" *JONA* 3:21, 1973.

Fry, S.T., "The Ethic of Caring: Can It Survive Nursing?" *Nursing Outlook* 36(1):48, 1988.

Lasagna, J.B., "Translating Distant Goals into Immediate Objectives," *Supervisor Nurse* 4:32, 1973.

Levenstein, A., "Philosophy for Nurses?" *Nursing Management* 13:49, 1982.

McNally, M., "Values. Part I: Supervisor Nurse," *J Nurs Leadership and Management* 11:27, 1980.

Strasen, L., *Key Business Skills for Nurse Managers*, J.B. Lippincott, Philadelphia, 1987.

Sullivan, E.J., and Decker, P.J., *Effective Management in Nursing*, Addison-Wesley, Menlo Park, CA, 1985.

Swansburg, R.C., "Planning: A Function of Nursing Administration, Part II," *Supervisor Nurse* 9:76, 1978.

Vestal, K.W., *Management Concepts for the New Nurse*, J.B. Lippincott, Philadelphia, 1987.

5
Human Resource Planning at the Unit Level

ALL UNITS within the organization are involved in the planning process and play an important role in human resource management. Unit level planning is separate and distinct from planning by nursing service and the organization, although all must be congruent.

One example of planning at the unit level is determining the most appropriate type of patient care delivery system for that particular unit. This requires analyzing available and appropriate staffing mixes. In addition, job design and analysis and standards for work performance must be defined. In this example, the ramifications of planning at the unit level are significant in that the mode of patient care delivery chosen will have a direct impact on worker satisfaction and thus on productivity.

Chapter 5 will discuss various types of patient care delivery systems and the criteria that should be used in selecting a patient care delivery system for a particular unit. In addition, the determination of work standards and job analysis will be addressed. Tools for implementation include a sample job analysis form and several position (job) description formats.

PATIENT CARE DELIVERY SYSTEMS

There are four primary means of organizing patient care delivery on the unit level: (1) case method or total patient care, (2) functional or task-oriented nursing, (3) team or modular nursing, and (4) primary care nursing (Marquis and Huston, 1987). Case method nursing, one of the earliest forms of organizing nursing care, was the primary method of patient care delivery prior to World War II. In case method nursing, the registered nurse assumes total responsibility for the care of a given group of patients during the time that he or she is with those patients. This requires self-direction and a fairly broad expertise on the part of the nurse. Case nursing usually results in high employee and patient satisfaction, as patient care is more holistic in focus and staff feel that the lines of responsibility and accountability are clear. Case nursing is inappropriate, however, if not all caregivers are adequately trained or prepared to care for their patients. Case method nursing may be considered more expensive than other delivery systems, as professionally trained individuals are doing tasks that might be accomplished equally as well by less trained, and thus less highly paid, members of the health care team.

Case method nursing lost popularity with the advent of World War II, which required an increase in the number of health care workers needed to provide care both at home and abroad. Because so many registered nurses had left hospitals to care for the wounded at the battlefront, high numbers of ancillary personnel with little formal training were drawn into the hospital setting to assist in caring for patients. This lack of adequate professional staff required hospitals to maximally utilize the capability and training of each of the personnel they did have. This mode of nursing, called *functional* or *task-oriented nursing*, involves assigning certain personnel to accomplish certain tasks, rather than assigning them to care for a specific patient. For example, functional nursing delivery might include a medication nurse, a treatment nurse, a bathing aide, a linen changer, and an employee to feed patients. This type of patient care delivery mode can be economical in that it allows for the use of many ancillary, relatively unskilled workers. These workers gain expertise from repetitively doing relatively simple tasks and become very efficient at their particular task. There is little confusion regarding job responsibilities and lines of accountability. Patient and employee satisfaction, however, may be very low in functional nursing. The potential for employee boredom and demotivation is high. Likewise, the probability of fragmented patient care and incomplete meeting of patient needs is also high.

This fragmentation of patient care was the impetus for the development of the next major mode of nursing care delivery in the 1950s. In this mode, known as *team* or *modular nursing*, auxiliary or professional staff work together to provide care to a group of patients under the direction of a registered nurse. In modular nursing, the team is generally limited to two individuals. In traditional team nursing, generally there are more than three individuals on each team. The registered nurse who directs the team is called the *team leader* or *modular leader* and is responsible for knowing about and planning the care for each patient on the team, regardless of whether he or she provides any direct care to them.

The team leader also coordinates intrateam communication through individual team members or through regularly scheduled team conferences for patient care planning. Team nursing allows the team leader to assign team members to complete tasks that utilize their unique skills and abilities. Individual patient needs can be met by the staff member who has the greatest expertise in that area. Likewise, team nursing can be economical in that it allows for patient care to be accomplished with a relatively high proportion of ancillary staff.

Team nursing can, however, result in low employee and patient satisfaction if there is inadequate intrateam communication or if staffing changes so frequently that team members do not have the opportunity to get to know each other's strengths and weaknesses. In addition, patient care can become fragmented in team nursing. Lines of responsibility and accountability may be poorly defined, and team members may feel they are making no significant contribution to the care planning of patients.

The concept of primary nursing as a patient care delivery mode was pioneered at the Loeb Center by Lydia Hall and Marie Manthey in the 1960s. Primary nursing is a patient care delivery mode that combines the concepts of total patient care and an all-professional nursing staff. In primary nursing, the registered nurse ("primary nurse") assumes 24-hour responsibility for the care planning of one or more patients from the time of admission to the facility to the day of discharge. Primary nurses provide total patient care to those patients during the time they are actually present in the facility. During the time they are not working, physical care is provided by "associate nurses," who implement the care plan developed by the primary nurses.

Primary nurses are responsible for establishing and maintaining clear communication among the patient, physician, associate nurses, other members of the health care team, and themselves. All these individuals provide feedback into care planning, which is reviewed on a regular basis. This type of patient care delivery system should result in holistic, high-quality patient care, and staff satisfaction is generally high after the staff has become accustomed to it, given adequate staffing levels. This satisfaction is probably related to the high autonomy and responsibility given to the primary nurses. As in total patient care, however, an inadequately prepared or trained primary nurse will probably be incapable of making the decisions necessary to coordinate a multidisciplinary team or may lack the clinical expertise to identify changing patient needs and conditions. Economically, primary nursing, when implemented correctly, has proven to be a cost-effective patient care delivery mode, although it may be difficult to recruit and retain an all-professional nursing staff.

SELECTING THE OPTIMUM PATIENT CARE DELIVERY SYSTEM FOR A SPECIFIC UNIT

There is no "one best" patient care delivery system for all institutions or, for that matter, for all individuals. At times, the greatest productivity occurs when work is completed by individuals. At other times, work should be structured so that it is accomplished by groups of employees working together (Hackman, 1977).

Wise managers should examine various criteria in order to select the optimal patient care delivery system for their specific units. Unfortunately, many units select their patient care delivery system based on the latest fad or the most "popular" delivery mode at that time (Marquis and Huston, 1987). In fact, some units change patient care delivery systems frequently, assuming that if someone else is achieving high patient and staff satisfaction, something must be inherently wrong with the system they are currently using. Such changes in the mode of patient care delivery should be undertaken only if a change is actually needed; that is, if patient and employee satisfaction are low, quality of work is low, or work is inefficient. All patient care delivery systems should meet the following criteria (Marquis and Huston, 1987):

1. The delivery system should provide the level of care that has been determined in the health care facility's philosophy (i.e., quality, adequate, or safe patient care).
2. The mode of delivery of patient care must be cost effective.
3. The patient care delivery system should provide satisfaction to the patient and his or her family (satisfaction and quality of care differ, and either may be provided without the other being present).
4. The mode of delivery must provide some degree of fulfillment and role satisfaction to the nursing personnel.
5. The patient care delivery system must allow for the utilization of the nursing process.

When a change in the pattern of patient care management is required, it is necessary to involve others in the change (Beyers and Phillips, 1979). Administrative personnel must be knowledgeable about the goals, methods, benefits, and needs that the new patient care mode will require, and a commitment must be made by top-level management to support the change in patient care delivery mode throughout the process.

In order for management to select the optimal patient care delivery system for a unit, it is important they they recognize and consider the unique role and needs of each unit. Some of these factors include:

1. *The staffing mix.* What is the mix of educational and experience levels among the staff? Is there an adequate number of highly trained professional nurses available to assume a delivery mode such as total patient care or primary nursing? Is there or has there been stability in retention? How successful have prior efforts been to recruit an all RN staff?
2. *Cost.* Although any of the patient care delivery systems should be cost effective if implemented correctly, the unit must look at market salaries for their area. Is the administration willing to support economic costs required to

change to a different type of patient care delivery system? Can a higher level of nursing care result in a reduction of length of hospital stay?

3. *Patient population needs.* Are patient needs such that they require a high level of nursing care? Can ancillary personnel be used to meet basic patient needs? Would another patient care delivery system continue to meet patient needs at the same or a higher level? What is the average length of a patient stay?

4. *Level of technology.* What level of technology is utilized within the facility? What level of expertise and training is required of your staff in meeting these technological needs?

5. *Importance of staff satisfaction.* How important is it that staff needs of self-esteem and self-actualization are being met? Are there other employers in the area that can draw employees away from your unit? Do employees have a strong sense of loyalty to your unit and your organization?

6. *The philosophy of the organization.* Does the organizational philosophy stress quality of care or the need for holistic care? Are patient teaching and family counseling emphasized? Is economical health care a top priority? Would the institution support the change from one patient care delivery system to another? Is the organization willing to decentralize authority and responsibility such as that which would be needed in primary nursing? Is collaborative practice encouraged between the medical and the nursing staff? Does the philosophy encourage interdepartmental cooperation?

7. *Philosophy of the unit.* Is the delivery system currently utilized or planned congruent with the unit philosophy?

8. *Motivation of the employees.* Do staff members want increased autonomy and decision-making? Are staff members self-directed?

JOB ANALYSIS

After nursing administrators have selected the optimal mode of patient care delivery system for their unit, the manager must determine exactly what jobs or work need to be completed and by whom. This is done through job analysis and job design.

Job analysis means determining the exact requirements and standards necessary for each job to be completed. Job analysis usually collects information about specific tasks or what a person does. Tool 5-1 shows a job analysis form that is adaptable to any institution. In essence, the job analysis form examines what job is being done, why it is being done, how often it must be done, and how much of the worker's time is required to complete it. In addition, the job analysis form must examine how much authority is required to complete the task, the degree of difficulty or complexity in the task, and the quality and quantity of work required in order to produce the end product. Lastly, the job analysis form examines when the work should be performed, the cost standard to perform the task, the appearance standard of the finished product, and the step-by-step procedure required to actually complete the task (Laliberty and Christopher, 1984).

JOB DESIGN

After job analysis has been completed, the manager utilizes the information in determining what types and numbers of employees are needed. Position requirements must be carefully defined and outlined for each member of that unit. This is called *job design*. Milkovich and Glueck (1985) define job design as integrating the work content (tasks, functions, relationships), the rewards (extrinsic and intrinsic), and the qualifications required (skills, knowledge, abilities) for each job.

Both theory and research indicate that job design has an impact on employee and organization effectiveness (Dunham, 1977). Each employee and manager must have a clear understanding of what each job requires, as well as an understanding of how job requirements differ among positions within the organization.

This distinction between job classifications must be clear and specific. Laliberty and Christopher (1984) identified 12 factors that must be examined in comparing different job classifications within an organization. These factors include the following:

1. *A difference in tasks performed.* Although job classifications may overlap in their tasks to be performed, it is important to identify the extent of these overlaps as well as the specific differences between job classifications. For example, the job description for both the first- and middle-level manager may

include employee performance appraisal; however, their actual roles may be very different. Likewise, the job classification for the registered nurse may include the administration of intravenous medications, which is noticeably absent from the job classification of the licensed practical nurse.

Tool 5-1   Job Analysis Outline

Job _____ Dept. _____ Work unit _____

Specified task being analyzed _____

Prepared by _____ Date _____ Reviewed with employee ____

What is being done? _____

_____

_____

Why? _____

_____

Frequency of performance _____

Percentage of time _____

Degree of delegated authority _____

Degree of difficulty or task complexity _____

_____

Quality required _____

_____

Quantity required _____

_____

Timing _____

_____

Unit cost _____

Appearance required _____

How the Work Is to Be Performed	
Procedures and Steps (in sequence)	*Means or Method* (appropriate to execute step)

Adapted from Laliberty, R., and Christopher, W.I., *Enhancing Productivity in Health Care Facilities*, p. 25. National Health Publishing, Owing Mills, MD, 1984.

2. *Performance frequency and time variations.* Again, although two job positions might include overlapping functions, job analysis may indicate a substantial difference in the amount of time spent on a particular task in one classification as compared to the other, as well as the frequency with which the tasks are performed. Staffing may be a major task in the performance of the nursing supervisor, but only be a minor task in the performance of the charge nurse. Likewise, although the registered nurse and licensed practical nurse may both give medications, there may be a

significant difference in the time required in either classification to do so, depending on the patient care delivery
method that is being utilized.

3. *Different performance procedures or methods.* Although the
two jobs may be described in a similar fashion, the actual
procedure or method used to perform the task may differ.
An example of this might be two middle-level supervisors
who select different teaching modes for their staff's inservice education needs on the same topic. As another example,
the job classifications for registered nurse and licensed
practical nurse might both list the admission of patients as
a procedure to be accomplished, but the registered nurse
might be expected to complete the history and physical
exam whereas the licensed practical nurse might have the
responsibility for orienting patients to their rooms and
hospital policies.

4. *Differences in the intent or purpose of the task.* Job analysis
might indicate that two jobs with the same nature may
require the achievement of somewhat different intents or
purposes. One middle-level nursing manager might request
staff nurse participation on organization committees to
foster subordinate good will and create a motivating climate. Another middle-level nursing manager might seek
staff nurse participation in an effort to reduce the burden of
a substantial work assignment. The nursing assistant
might provide a bath to meet the hygiene needs of the
patient. The registered nurse might utilize the bath as a
physical assessment tool or a stress reduction tool as well as
a means of meeting hygiene needs.

5. *Variant performance standards.* Even the same job may
require different quality of performance, or different economic and time requirements, at different times. For example, the budgetary expertise or refinement expected may
vary considerably among different nursing managers and
nursing units. Likewise, although all registered nurses,
licensed practical nurses, and nursing assistants are expected to do some informal patient teaching, the expectations of the quality and quantity of that teaching varies
with each job classification.

6. *Variant performance requirements for competency factors.*
Because of the prior five factors, different jobs may require
different patterns or degrees of competency, such as responsibility to be assumed, know-how to be achieved, effort to be
applied, or working conditions to be endured.

7. *Relative value differences.* As performance requirements increase, the general availability of qualified applicants decreases. Thus, as performance requirements increase, a concomitant increase in wage value should also be seen. Generally, as the management level increases, so too does the level of expertise required, as well as the economic compensation.

8. *Different costs or economic value.* It is important for the manager to identify conditions that are directly job related and that may increase or decrease the economic cost of the work performance. This may include an assessment of the internal and external environment in the organization. One example may be the economic value of having intra-agency certification for licensed practical nurses to do some types of intravenous therapy.

9. *Cost benefit analysis.* There is always a relationship between the cost and the quality of the performance, so both cost and quality requirements must be examined in assigning each job. The prudent nurse manager must carefully examine the staffing mix to be sure that priority patient needs are being met with the lowest salaried level employee possible to do so. Likewise, the prudent nurse manager must be sure that an acceptable quality of care is not sacrificed in an effort to reduce costs.

10. *Different pathways of advancement and promotion opportunity.* Because of varying combinations of the preceding factors, the lines of advancement and promotion between two jobs may appear to be similar, when in actuality they are very different. The experience gained in continued performance and the learning opportunities inherent in such performance usually result in different patterns of advancement and promotion. The experience and knowledge gained by two first-level supervisors on differing units may vary greatly. Either one may be better qualified for advancement depending on the experiences they have had.

11. *Differences in external job requirements.* Even if two workers have similar competency for a certain task, external factors may impact on their effectiveness and on the question of which worker should be allowed to perform a particular task. Legal, ethical, professional, or moral conditions may influence which worker should perform the task. Equal Opportunity Employment constraints are one such example.

12. *Comparable worth.* It may be very difficult to compare one job classification to another because of prior discrimination in job analysis and job design on the basis of sex. Title VII of the Civil Rights Act of 1964 prohibits discrimination on the basis of sex. The idea of comparable worth was established because many jobs traditionally held by women had been undervalued solely because they were held by women. Comparable worth states that pay for a particular position should reflect the value of that position to the employer.

Table 5-1 is an example of how work responsibilities may be divided into job classifications. This type of listing should be made available to employees in each job classification.

Once the work to be accomplished has been defined and job standards have been established, the nursing manager can design written position statements or job descriptions. Unfortunately, many organizations shortcut the employment planning process in regard to job analysis and job design. Rather than being based on the information gained from the job analysis and job design, and on unit or organizational needs, position descriptions are frequently written based on a prespecified individual's

Table 5-1. Sample Work Responsibilities According to Job Classifications

Procedure	Job Classification		
	RN	LPN	NA
1. Assignment of nursing care	X		
2. Bathing the patient	X	X	X
3. Charting	X	X	X
4. CPR, code teams	X	X	X
5. Gravity chest drainage	X		
6. Decubitus ulcer care	X	X	X
7. Discharge of patients	X	X	X
8. Ear drop instillation	X	X	
9. Gastrostomy feeding	X	X	
10. Levine irrigation	X	X	
11. Oral hygiene	X	X	X
12. Physician orders, noting of	X		
13. Preoperative care	X	X	X
14. Sterile dressing changes	X	X	
15. Report to charge nurse	X	X	X
16. Report to oncoming shift	X		
17. Transfers, interfacility	X		
18. Vital signs	X	X	X

strengths and talents. Although this individual may have tremendous value to the unit, there is great potential for future difficulty in finding another individual to fill this position. If job descriptions are created following a systematic process of job analysis and job design, the work to be accomplished is much clearer, more objective in terms of organizational expectations, and thus much more likely to result in greater employee satisfaction and productivity.

Tool 5-2 shows an outline adapted from Laliberty and Christopher (1984) summarizing the information that should be included in a position or job description. At the top of the form should be the title of the job, the department/unit offering the job as described, the shift/hours required, and the official approval date of the position description. The position description follows. The position description describes what work is to be accomplished and how it is to be done, the purpose of the job, and the level of supervision to be rendered. The third section of the job description form should identify the major responsibilities or tasks essential to completion of the job. Responsibilities should be listed in decreasing order of importance. The fourth section of the form should identify required performance standards, such as quality, quantity, time, cost, and appearance. Lastly, the job description should identify performance requirements relating the compatibility of the work and the worker. Tool 5-3 shows an example of a completed job description that meets these criteria.

Employment process planning is a vital part of the hierarchy of planning required in organizations. The nature of work and how that work is organized plays a critical factor in human resource management. It is necessary to carefully analyze and design work so that employees can be selected who optimally complement the work to be accomplished. Likewise, having clear descriptions about the work to be accomplished and the standards that are required in the end product greatly increases the probability of congruent employee and organizational expectations. Thus personnel planning at the unit level becomes one of the most important facets of optimal human resource management.

Tool 5-2   Position or Job Description
(approval date _____)

I. Identification of the job
   Title:
   Department:
   Shift/Hours:

II. Position description
   A. Brief description of what the worker will do
   B. Brief description of how these activities are performed
   C. Purpose of the job
   D. Degree or level of supervision rendered

III. Responsibilities
   A. Identification of major vs. minor job responsibilities

IV. Performance standards
   A. Quality
   B. Quantity
   C. Time
   D. Cost
   E. Appearance (where it applies)

V. Performance requirements
   A. Responsibility
   B. Knowledge
   C. Skill
   D. Mental application
   E. Dexterity
   F. Accuracy
   G. Experience
   H. Education or formal training
   I. Physical demands, such as physical activity, working conditions,
       or hazards/risks

Adapted from Laliberty, R., and Christopher, W.I., *Enhancing Productivity in
Health Care Facilities*, p. 63. National Health Publishing, Owing Mills, MD, 1984.

Tool 5-3   Sample Job Description — Hospital XX
(approved 4/88)

I. Identification of the job
Title: Registered nurse I — patient care provider
Department: Medical surgical
Shift/Hours: Full time, day shift (0700-1530)

II. Position description
The registered nurse I uses information communicated by the charge nurse in applying the nursing process to direct patient care of a selected group of patients. This nurse is responsible for all aspects of care assigned to these patients. This includes physical care of the patients, verbal and written documentation of care given, and participation in beginning- and end-of-shift reports. The registered nurse I is directly accountable to the charge nurse on the shift.

III. Duties

1. Plans and organizes own daily nursing activities, recognizing priority responsibilities and time limitations.

2. Identifies patient problems based on clinical observations, knowledge, and judgment. Includes learning needs of patient and family in problem identification.

3. Provides effective nursing care in the following skills areas:
   a. Administration of medications
   b. Performance of technical skills required to deal safely and efficiently with dressings, invasive tubes, and supportive equipment

4. Performs ongoing assessments of patient conditions, treatment regimes, and discharge needs.

5. Gives complete and concise verbal and written reports regarding patient condition.

6. Revises patient care plan according to changing needs of the patient.

IV. Performance standards
The registered nurse I must perform the aforementioned duties in a professional and cost-effective manner.

V. Performance requirements

Physical demands — Requires exertion of moderately heavy manual effort such as patient lifting, pushing of heavy medication carts, making of beds, and ambulation of patients. Pregnant nurses or nurses attempting to become pregnant are advised to use appropriate precautions in caring for the high number of patients on this unit undergoing radioactive implants and chemotherapy.

Education — Current registered nursing license in this state.

Experience — No previous experience required for entry into this position.

Skills — This position requires satisfactory completion of at least a 70% accuracy level the Hospital XX medication and IV mastery course, within 2 weeks after beginning employment.

KEY CONCEPTS CHAPTER 5

1. The four primary means of organizing patient care delivery on the unit level are case method or total patient care, functional or task-oriented, team or modular, and primary care nursing.

2. There is no "one best" mode of patient care delivery. The best mode for any particular unit depends on a variety of factors, such as staffing mix available, cost, patient population, level of technology, organizational and unit philosophy, and self-esteem/self-actualization needs of the employees.

3. Changes in the patient care delivery mode should be undertaken only if a change is actually needed; that is, if patient and staff satisfaction are low, quality of work is low, or if work is inefficient.

4. Job analysis is necessary to determine the exact requirements and standards necessary for each job to be completed.

5. Job design integrates work content, rewards, and the qualifications required for each job.

6. Position (job) descriptions should be based on information gathered in the planning phases of job analysis and job design.

7. Written, concise position (job) descriptions increase the probability that employees will be matched to the most appropriate job within the institution. Likewise, clear and

specific position descriptions increase the probability that employee and organizational expectations will be congruent.

8. Careful and well-thought-out personnel planning on the unit level is vital to optimal human resource management in the organization.

REFERENCES

Beyers, M., and Phillips, C., *Nursing Management for Patient Care*, Little, Brown and Company, Boston, 1979.

Dunham, R.B., "Reactions to Job Characteristics: Moderating Effects of the Organization," *Academy of Management Journal*, 20:42–65, 1977.

Hackman, J.R., "The Designing Work for Individuals and Groups," in Hackman, J.R., Lawler, E.E., and Porter, L.W., *Perspectives on Behavior in Organizations*, McGraw-Hill, New York, 1977.

Laliberty, R., and Christopher, W.I., *Enhancing Productivity in Health Care Facilities*, National Health Publishing, Owing Mills, MD, 1984.

Marquis, B., and Huston, C., *Management Decision Making for Nurses*, J.B. Lippincott, Philadelphia, 1987.

Milkovich, G.T., and Glueck, W.F., *Personnel: Human Resource Management—A Diagnostic Approach*, Fourth Edition, Business Publications, Plano, TX, 1985.

ADDITIONAL READINGS

Alexander, J., *Nursing Unit Organization: Its Effects on Staff Professionalism*, UMI Research Press, Ann Arbor, MI, 1982.

Beyers, M., and Phillips, C., *Nursing Management for Patient Care*, Second Edition, Little, Brown and Company, Boston, 1979.

DiVincenti, M., *Administering Nursing Service*, Little, Brown and Company, Boston, 1972.

Ganong, J., and Ganong, W., *Nursing Management: Concepts, Functions, Techniques, and Skills*, Aspen Publications, Germantown, MD, 1976.

Gargal, P., "Modular Nursing: Nurses Rediscover Nursing," *Nursing Management*, 18(11):98–104, 1987.

Hardesty, S.T., "Knowledge Nurses Need to Participate on a Design Team," *Nursing Management*, 19(3):49–57, 1988.

Johnson, M., and McCloskey, J., *Series on Nursing Administration*. Volume 1, Iowa Nursing Administration Series, Addison-Wesley, Menlo Park, CA, 1988.

McFarland, G.K., Leonard, H.S., and Morris, M.M., *Nursing Leadership and Management: Contemporary Strategies*, John Wiley and Sons, New York, 1984.

Mayer, G.G., and Bailey, K., *The Middle Manager in Primary Nursing*, Springer, New York, 1982.

Price, J.L., and Mueller, C.W., *Professional Turnover: The Case of Nurses*, SP Medical and Scientific Books, Spectrum Publications, New York, 1981.

Schuster, F.E., *Human Resource Management: Concepts, Cases and Readings*, Second Edition, Reston Publishing, Reston, VA, 1985.

Strasen, L., *Key Business Skills for Nurse Managers*, Lippincott's Nursing Management Series, J.B. Lippincott, Philadelphia, 1987.

Sullivan, E.J., and Decker, P.J., *Effective Management in Nursing*, Second Edition, Addison-Wesley, Menlo Park, CA, 1988.

6

Human Resource Planning for Staffing and Scheduling

BY NOW the unit manager should have an adequate understanding of the goals and objectives of the organization, how job descriptions are developed, and the criteria for the selection of a patient care delivery mode. In this chapter the focus remains at the unit level, but the planning activity shifts to staffing and scheduling. In some decentralized organizations, a great deal of autonomy is given to first- and middle-level managers, which allows them to set policies regarding scheduling. As was stated in the previous chapter, some organizations have each unit select its own mode of patient care delivery and determine its own nursing care hour needs. Other more centralized organizations provide general guidelines for scheduling and staffing policies but allow managers at the unit level to develop definitive policies. Currently, most organizations utilize some type of patient classification system to determine unit staffing needs, but do allow the unit manager daily or weekly variance for overstaffing or understaffing. At some point, however, the unit manager is held accountable for any significant variance from the documented need.

This chapter will examine appropriate staffing and scheduling policies and types of scheduling patterns. Included will be the advantages and disadvantages of the different types of schedules. Unit fiscal planning will be discussed, with formulas and instructions presented for calculating daily staffing needs. Tools for implementation in this chapter are sample staffing policies, staffing formulas, and sample staffing patterns. Additionally, a check list is included to assist the manager in long-range personnel planning.

LONG-RANGE UNIT LEVEL PERSONNEL PLANNING

If there is one common fault among unit-level managers in personnel planning, it is not developing adequate long-range planning. Many managers operate in a crisis mode. They do not use the available historical patterns to assist them in planning for the future, nor do they examine present clues and projected statistics, commonly called *forecasting*, to determine future needs. Hiring "any warm body" may fill vacant positions, but at best it is only a short-term solution for staffing inadequacies.

In addition to using forecasting and historical perspectives to determine long-range personnel planning, the unit manager can also use certain quantitative methods to assist in determining future needs. For instance, a supervisor could use probability formulas to analyze past termination figures and years of service at termination to estimate when nurses on her unit were likely to terminate. For example, one unit supervisor analyzed her unit terminations over a period of ten years and discovered that nurses had a 65% probability of terminating during their first 18 months of employment. After 2 years of employment the probability dropped dramatically and continued to drop for every year employed, until by the end of 5 years of employment the probability that a nurse would terminate dropped to 5%. The supervisor used this information in two ways. First, she developed a more personalized orientation and induction program for her unit and provided preceptor support for new nurses. Second, she built into her personnel planning a prediction that a percentage of newly hired nurses would need to be replaced.

Lastly, unit managers should be continually aware of the present supply of human resources as they finalize their long-term personnel planning. Managers who were unaware that the current nursing shortage was imminent obviously did not plan appropriately for this event, and therefore, their staffing suffered much more than did that of those managers who had accurately predicted and carefully planned for the future. Two ways to keep current regarding changing availability of human resources are to be an avid reader of professional journals and to be involved with professional organizations. Tool 6-1 provides a check list to assist managers in long-range personnel planning.

SHORT-RANGE UNIT LEVEL PERSONNEL PLANNING

At the unit level, long-range personnel planning is planning that is at least 6 months in the future, while at the department level it is longer, probably 1 to 3 years. Likewise, short-range planning at the department level might be 1 to 6 months, but at the unit level it could be as short as planning staffing needs for an 8-hour shift. Planning to meet monthly staffing needs is considered to be short-range unit personnel planning.

Just as each organization has differing expectations regarding the unit manager's responsibility in long-range planning of human resources, so too do organizations differ in their expectations of the unit supervisor's responsibility for short-range personnel planning. In organizations with decentralized staffing, the unit manager is often responsible for (1) covering all scheduled staff absences, (2) reducing staff during periods of increased patient acuity, (3) adding staff during high patient census or acuity, (4) preparing monthly unit schedules, and (5) preparing holiday and vacation schedules. Other organizations have a centralized, and often computerized, staffing office that takes over many of the staffing and scheduling duties of the unit manager.

There are both advantages and disadvantages to centralized and decentralized unit staffing. One can work as a manager in an organization that has centralized staffing but have decentralized organizational decision-making. The terms *centralized* and *decentralized* staffing are *not* synonymous with centralized and decentralized decision-making, which were discussed in Chapter 5.

Marquis and Huston (1987) have outlined the advantages and disadvantages of these two types of methods for meeting short-term personnel planning. The decentralized staffing carried out by the unit manager allows personnel to make personal

---

Tool 6-1   Personnel Planning Guide

Historical data

1. What is the attrition rate on your unit?
2. Are transfers frequently requested to other areas?
3. What percentage of your staff leave the unit between one and two years after arriving?
4. Are certain months of the year usually understaffed?
5. What months have the highest number of resignations?
6. Which months show high and low numbers of employment applications?
7. Are there historical difficulties with staffing certain shifts?

Current data regarding human resources

1. What is the current enrollment for the schools of nursing in your area? Does this number represent a decline or increase?
2. Are other hospitals in your area experiencing a nursing shortage?
3. What percentage of local graduating RN classes generally apply for positions in your unit?
4. Are there employees in other areas of the hospital that would like to transfer to your unit? How many?
5. How many applications do you receive for positions on your unit during a year? Are they all qualified? Is this number declining or increasing?

---

scheduling requests directly to their immediate supervisors. While this facilitates much flexibility in meeting employees' needs, it also carries the risk that employees will not be treated equally or consistently. Additionally, the unit manager is often viewed as the individual granting rewards or punishments as a result of the staffing schedule, which can be viewed by personnel as either positive or negative. Lastly, it is time consuming for the nurse manager and often promotes more "special pleading" than when staffing is done in a centralized manner.

In centralized staffing an individual or computer does the staffing for the entire department, although the nurse manager continues to have the option to make minor adjustments and provide input. In analyzing centralized staffing Marquis and Huston (1987) state

> This type of staffing is fairer to all employees because policies tend to be employed more consistently and impartially. In addition, the first-level manager is freed to complete other management functions and is more cost effective to the organization.

Marquis and Huston do caution, however, that centralized staffing does not provide as much flexibility for the worker, nor is it able to account for the worker's interests or special needs. Additionally, it is easy for nurse managers to develop a habit of nonresponsiveness to budget control of personnel if they have little to do with staffing.

Even when nurse managers at the unit level have little to do with scheduling, they need to develop an understanding of the scheduling procedures, the various options for scheduling, and their fiscal responsibility for personnel staffing.

STAFFING AND SCHEDULING OPTIONS

Nursing is one of only a few professions that require night, evening, weekend, and holiday work schedules. This frequently results in much frustration for nurses. Scheduling, therefore, becomes a major factor in promoting either job dissatisfaction or job satisfaction for them. Nurses often feel a total lack of control over their work hours. In several recent studies (Hinshaw et al., 1987; Marquis, 1988; Patterson and Goad, 1987) this lack of control contributed to increased attrition rates and feelings of burnout among professional nurses. It becomes obvious that the unit supervisor who strives to develop a perception among the staff that they do have some control over scheduling, shift options, and staffing policies will have done much to improve the nurses' job satisfaction.

There are various options available for scheduling, and each has both positive and negative aspects. It is beyond the scope of this book to provide a complete review of every possible type of creative staffing and scheduling available. It is very important that thorough research be done prior to introducing staffing and scheduling changes and that the staff be very much involved with any proposed change. Additional readings that address various types of staffing and scheduling have been included at the end of this chapter. Since staffing and scheduling is so important to nurses, unit managers should periodically evaluate the satisfaction of the unit nurses with their present system. Following is a partial list of some creative efforts to increase nurse satisfaction, using innovative scheduling and staffing methods, that have been successfully implemented during the past ten years:

1. Use of the 10-hour shift
2. Use of the 12-hour shift
3. Premium pay for weekend work
4. Use of a part-time premium paid pool for weekend shifts
5. Cyclical staffing, which allows very advanced knowledge of nurses' future work schedules
6. Job sharing
7. Allowing nurses to exchange hours of work with each other
8. 7–70 work schedule
9. Use of supplemental nursing agencies for weekend coverage

Included in Tables 6-1 and 6-2 are samples of scheduling patterns; one shows an individual work schedule and the other is a master cyclic staffing pattern.

There are both advantages and disadvantages to the various types of creative scheduling. Some changes involve overtime pay, and any additional cost must be weighed against the high cost of attrition. Long shifts may result in errors in clinical judgment. For this reason many organizations limit the number of consecutive days a nurse can work 12-hour shifts. The excessive use of

Table 6-1.   A Typical Individual 4-Week Cyclic Schedule

Weeks	M	T	W	Th	F	S	S
1	on	on	on	—	—	on	on
2	on	on	on	on	on	—	—
3	on	on	—	on	on	on	on
4	—	on	on	on	on	—	—
Days Worked	3	4	3	3	3	2	2

Total days worked in 4 weeks. . . . . 20 days

Table 6-2. Master Time Schedule: 4-Week Cycle

Position	Name	W I S	W I M	W I T	W I W	W I T	W I F	W I S	W II S	W II M	W II T	W II W	W II T	W II F	W II S	W III S	W III M	W III T	W III W	W III T	W III F	W III S	W IV S	W IV M	W IV T	W IV W	W IV T	W IV F	W IV S
Full time	RN 1				X			X	X					X					X			X	X					X	
Full time	RN 2	X					X					X			X	X					X					X			X
Full time	RN 3			X				X	X				X					X				X	X				X		
Full time	RN 4	X				X					X				X	X				X					X				X
Full time	RN 5				X			X	X			X							X			X	X			X			
Full time	RN 6	X				X							X		X	X				X							X		X
Full time	RN 7		X					X	X	X							X					X	X	X					
Full time	RN 8	X					X							X	X	X					X							X	X
Part time 8 hrs/week	RN 9	ON							ON							ON							ON						
Part time 8 hrs/week	RN 10							ON							ON							ON							ON
Part time 8 hrs/week	RN 11	ON							ON							ON							ON						
Part time 8 hrs/week	RN 12							ON							ON							ON							ON
Total RNs on duty each day		6	7	7	6	6	6	6	6	7	7	6	6	6	6	6	7	7	6	6	6	6	6	7	7	6	6	6	6

Elements: Every other weekend off   Number of split days off each period: 2   X Scheduled day off
Maximum days worked: 4   Operates in multiples of 4, 8, 12,....
Minimum days worked: 2   Schedule repeats itself every 4 weeks

part-time or supplemental nurses can result in poor continuity of nursing care. It is obvious that all scheduling and staffing patterns, from traditional to creative, have shortcomings. Therefore, proposed changes in current policies should be evaluated carefully before they are implemented. It is wise to have a 6-month trial of new staffing and scheduling changes, with an evaluation at the end of that time to determine the impact on financial cost, retention, productivity, risk management, and employee and patient satisfaction.

DEVELOPING STAFFING AND SCHEDULING POLICIES

Nurses will be more satisfied in the work place if staffing and scheduling policies and procedures are spelled out clearly in writing. Written policies also provide a means for greater consistency and fairness for all concerned. It is not enough that policies be written down; it is also vital that such policies be communicated clearly to all employees. Hanson (1983) feels personnel policies represent the standard of action that is communicated in advance so that employees are not caught unaware of personnel decisions. In addition to being standardized, these policies should be written in a manner to allow some flexibility.

Just as other policies are reviewed on a periodic basis, so should personnel policies be updated. When formulating policies, management must examine its own philosophy as well as give consideration to prevailing practices in the community. At the unit level, managers may not be totally involved in formulating organizational personnel policies, but they should have some input as they are reviewed. There are, however, nursing department and unit personnel policies that the unit supervisor will be responsible for developing and implementing. When appropriate and whenever possible, the unit manager should seek input from the staff in developing and revising staffing and scheduling policies.

Not all authorities on staffing and scheduling agree on what should be covered by such policies. Indeed, some authors separate the two and have a set of policies and accompanying procedures related to scheduling and another set of policies related to staffing. Tools 6-2 and 6-3 are sample check lists showing the personnel policies that two different authors (Hanson, 1983;

(Text continued on p. 104)

Tool 6-2   Check List of Employee Staffing Policies

Employee categories

1. Full time
   1.1 Hours worked per week
   1.2 Weekends worked per schedule
   1.3 Benefits calculation

2. Part time
   2.1 Hours worked per week
   2.2 Weekends worked per schedule
   2.3 Benefits calculation

3. Float pool
   3.1 Hours worked status
   3.2 Weekends worked per schedule
   3.3 Scheduling pattern
   3.4 Assignment method
   3.5 Line of authority
   3.6 Salary and benefits paid
   3.7 Differentials paid
   3.8 Orientation provided

4. On-call pool
   4.1 Availability requirements
   4.2 Weekends worked per schedule
   4.3 Assignments method
   4.4 Line of authority
   4.5 Compensation calculation
   4.6 Orientation provided

Scheduling

1. Authority and responsibility

2. Length of cycle rotation

3. Posting time

4. Reporting responsibility

Assignments

1. Placement determination

2. Basic care requirements

Days off

1. Rotation pattern/service

2. Weekend rotation

3. Special requests
   3.1 School schedule
   3.2 Change status

Weekends

1. Definition

2. Family member schedules

Scheduling requests

1. Request/response procedure

2. Weekend requests

3. Educational days

4. Emergency leave

5. Failure to report when scheduled

Trade procedure

1. Acceptable trades

2. Request/response procedure

Vacations

1. Request/response procedure
   1.1 Time to submit
   1.2 Place to submit

2. Approval guidelines
   2.1 Seniority preference
   2.2 Who decides
   2.3 Number limitations

3. Change request

4. Extended vacations

Holidays

1. Paid holidays

2. Request/response procedure

3. Approval guidelines
   3.1 Granting criteria
   3.2 Number limitations

4. Unexcused absence on a holiday

5. Vacation during holiday period

Illness

1. Notification procedure

 2. Extended days

 3. Illness duty

Leave of absence (LOA)

 1. Request/response procedure

 2. Paid leave time interface

Failure to report to work

 1. Consequences

Transfers

 1. Request/response procedure

 2. Approval guidelines

Temporary reassignment

 1. Who will float

 2. Refusal consequences

 3. Equitably

Absenteeism

 1. Percentage acceptable

 2. Disciplinary action

Tardiness

 1. Percentage acceptable

 2. Disciplinary action

Irregular hours worked

 1. Report/return home

 2. Called after shift begins

 3. On-call availability

Low census procedures

 1. Selection process

  1.1 Sequence followed

  1.2 Patient care safety levels

 2. Benefits accrued

 3. Paid hours

Overtime

 1. Payment guidelines

 2. Availability

Family policy

1. **Family member assignment**

2. **Time-off policy**

NOTE: *Although both the check lists in Tools 6-2 and 6-3 appear to be all encompassing, all items are very necessary if employees are to have a clear understanding of staffing and scheduling policies. The result of not having clearly delineated policies in writing are: (1) frequent over- and under-staffing, (2) high staff dissatisfaction, and (3) management frustration.*

Reproduced with permission of West Coast Medical Management Associates, Westlake Village, CA, 1983.

Gillies, 1982) suggest should be written and communicated to all nursing personnel. Middle managers should use these lists to determine if their units have sufficient staffing policies.

As in all planning, managers should be careful that policies they develop at the unit level are not in conflict with personnel policies at a higher level. For example, some states may have labor laws that prohibit 12-hour shifts. Additionally, in organizations with union contracts, many staffing and scheduling policies are incorporated into the contract. In such cases, some staffing changes might need to be negotiated at the time of contract renewal.

THE IMPACT OF STANDARDS OF PRODUCTIVITY ON STAFFING

One of the greatest impacts on staffing is the standard of measurement for productivity that has been adopted by the unit. A unit standard may be expressed in many ways. In the emergency room, the unit for measuring staffing might be in numbers of patients seen per shift. In the operating room, it could be the number of minutes of circulating time, and in a public health agency, it might be the number of home visits per month. Nearly all organizations have a unit of measurement they use to determine staffing and productivity. The unit of measurement for inpatient hospital units is usually in nursing care hours per patient.

Tool 6-3   Gillie's Staffing and Scheduling Policies

1. Person, by title, who prepares time schedules for personnel in each unit
2. Time period to be covered by each on/off-duty schedule
3. Amount of advance notice to be given worker concerning on/off-duty schedule
4. Total required on- and off-duty time for each worker per day, week, or month
5. Day that starts the duty week
6. Beginning and ending time for each duty shift
7. Number of shifts that each worker must rotate
8. Required frequency of shift rotation
9. Necessity of rotating from one unit to another and frequency of such rotation
10. Necessity of scheduling 2 days off each week or an **average** of 2 days off each week
11. Frequency of weekends off for each category of personnel
12. Definition of "weekend off" for night-duty personnel
13. Required incidence of sequential and nonsequential days off
14. Maximum sequential duty days allowable
15. Minimum interval required between sequential duty shifts
16. Number of paid holidays to be granted each employee
17. Required number of holidays per year on which employee must be scheduled off duty
18. Length of advance notice to be given employee regarding holiday on/off-duty schedule
19. Procedure to be followed in requesting to be off duty on a specific holiday
20. Number of paid vacation days to be granted each employee
21. Length of advance notice to be given employee regarding vacation schedules
22. Procedure to be followed in requesting specific vaction time
23. Restrictions of vacation scheduling during Thanksgiving, Christmas, and New Year's holidays

24. Number of personnel of each category to be scheduled for vacation or holiday at one time

25. Procedures for resolving conflicts among personnel in regard to vacation and holiday time requests

26. Procedure for processing "emergency" requests for adjustment of time schedules

Reprinted by permission from Gillies, D.A., *Nursing Management: A Systems Approach*, W.B. Saunders Co., Philadelphia, 1982.

It is important to note that such units of measurement change over time. For instance, a nursing unit might be allotted x hours of nursing care per patient, based on the acuity or level of intensity of care required for each patient. However, the middle-level manager must be alert to other things that affect the needs of her unit and that may not be reflected in the patient care classification system used by the organization. Examples of such extraneous circumstances could be a sudden increase in nursing or medical students using the unit, a lower skill level of new graduates, or cultural and language difficulties of recently hired foreign nurses.

The classification system selected for use by the organization may prove to be inaccurate, or the hours allotted for each category or classification of patient may be inadequate. This does not mean that middle-level managers should not be held accountable for the standard unit of measurement, but they need to be cognizant of justifiable reasons that their unit appears overstaffed or understaffed.

Patient classification is generally defined as the grouping of patients according to some specific characteristics. The reason for using patient classification is that numbers alone have proven to be an inaccurate method on which to base nursing care assignments. Because other variables within the system also have an impact on nursing care hours, it is usually not possible to transfer a patient classification system from one facility to another. Instead, each basic classification system must be modified to fit a specific institution.

Once an organization adopts an appropriate system, hours of nursing care must be assigned for each classification. An appropriate number of hours of care for each classification is suggested by most companies marketing patient classification systems. Each institution, however, makes the final decision regarding the number of care hours it will allot to each classification of patient. It quickly becomes obvious that there are many variables in any chosen system and that no system is without faults. Giovannetti (1979) has stated that it is a mistake for managers to think that patient classification systems will solve staffing problems. She maintains that such systems provide a better definition of problems but that it is up to people in the organization to use the information obtained by the system to solve the problems. A sample classification system can be found in Tool 6-4.

FISCAL ACCOUNTABILITY FOR MIDDLE-LEVEL MANAGERS

Regardless of the associated difficulties, patient classification systems and assignment of nursing care hours remain the best methods that have yet been devised for controlling the staffing function of management. As long as managers realize that all systems have weaknesses, and as long as they periodically evaluate the system in effect, they will be able to initiate change as necessary. It is critical, however, that managers make every effort to use the patient classification system currently in use in their organization as the basis for unit staffing and scheduling. Nursing care remains labor intensive, and appropriate staffing is an effective method for the manager to be fiscally accountable to the organization. Accountability for a prenegotiated budget is a responsibility of the manager.

Fiscal accountability is not the opposite of irresponsibility with respect to patients or staff. It is possible to keep within a staffing budget and meet the needs of patients and staff. However, it is necessary that the supervisor obtain staff when patient acuity increases, as well as decrease staffing when acuity is low; to do otherwise is demoralizing to the staff on the unit. If the unit supervisor keeps a careful accounting of staffing, he or she will be able to make adjustments quickly.

One reason many institutions have adopted centralized staffing offices is because unit managers were not responsive enough to reducing or increasing nursing care hours. Staffing formulas

Tool 6-4   Patient Care Classification System
Using Four Levels of Nursing Care Intensity

Area of Care	Category I	Category II	Category III	Category IV
Eating	Feeds self or needs little food for eating	Needs some help in preparing; may need encouragement	Cannot feed self but is able to chew and swallow	Cannot feed self and may have difficulty swallowing
Grooming	Almost entirely self-sufficient	Needs some help in bathing, oral hygiene, hair combing, etc.	Unable to do much for self	Completely dependent
Excretion	Up and to bathroom alone or almost alone	Needs some help in getting up to bathroom or using urinal	In bed, needing bedpan or urinal placed; may be able to partially turn or lift self	Completely dependent
Comfort	Self-sufficient	Needs some help with adjustment of position or bed (tubes, IVs, etc.)	Cannot turn without help, get drink, adjust position of extremities, etc.	Completely dependent
General health	Good—in for diagnostic procedure, simple treatment, or surgical procedure (D & C, biopsy, minor fracture)	Mild symptoms—more than one mild illness, mild debility, mild emotional reaction, mild incontinence (not more than once/shift)	Acute symptoms—severe emotional reaction to illness or surgery, more than one acute illness; medical or surgical problem, severe or frequent incontinence	Critically ill—may have severe emotional reaction
Treatments	Simple—supervised ambulation, dangle, simple dressing, test procedure preparation not requiring medication, reinforcement of surgical dressing, X-pad, vital signs once/shift	Any Category I treatment more than once/shift, Foley cath care, I & O, bladder irrigations, sitz bath, compresses, test procedures requiring medications or follow-ups, simple enema for evacuation, vital signs every 4 hours	Any treatment more than twice/shift, medicated IVs, complicated dressings, sterile procedures, care of tracheotomy, Harris flush, suctioning, tube feeding, vital signs more than every 4 hours	Any elaborate or delicate procedure requiring 2 nurses, vital signs more often than every 2 hours

Area of Care	Category I	Category II	Category III	Category IV
Medications	Simple, routine, not needing pre- or post-evaluation; PRN; medications no more than once/shift	Diabetic, cardiac, hypotensive, hypertensive, diuretic, anti-coagulant medications, PRN medications, more than once/shift, medications needing pre- or post-evaluation	Unusual amount of Category II medications; control of refractory diabetics (need to be monitored more than every 4 hours)	More intensive Category III medications; IVs with frequent, close observation and regulation
Teaching and emotional support	Routine follow-up teaching; patients with no unusual or adverse emotional reactions	Initial teaching of care of ostomies, new diabetics, tubes that will be in place for periods of time; conditions requiring major change in eating, living, or excretory practices, patients with mild adverse reactions to their illness (depression, overly demanding, etc.)	More intensive Category II items; teaching of apprehensive or mildly resistive patients; care of moderately upset or apprehensive patients; confused or disoriented patients	Teaching of resistive patients, care and support of patients with severe emotional reaction

and staffing terminology for calculating nursing care hours and patient days are found in Tool 6-5.

It is recommended that unit managers keep shift totals, 24-hour totals, weekly totals, and monthly totals of their staffing. The accounting department will send each supervisor timely print-outs of the monthly and year-to-date patient care hours. This ledger sheet will indicate whether the manager is over or under the total budgeted care hours. The accounting office uses an average figure of budgeted nursing care hours, so its figures might be slightly different than those kept by the unit. The unit's more accurate records of shift acuity are useful for negotiating an increase in the total budgeted nursing care hours. Table 6-3 is an example of the records of a supervisor on a 30-bed unit. The budgeted nursing care hours were 5 nursing care hours per patient. Using the patient classification system

---

Tool 6-5   Staffing Formulas and Terminology

TERMINOLOGY

Acuity index – a weighted statistical measurement that refers to severity of illness of patients for a given time. Patients are classified according to acuity of illness, usually in one of four categories. The acuity index is determined by taking a total of acuities and then dividing by the total number of patients.

Full-time equivalent (FTE) – the number of hours of work for which a full-time employee is scheduled for weekly period. For example, 1.0 FTE-five 8-hour days of staffing, which equals 40 hours of staffing per week. One FTE can be divided in different ways. For example, two part-time employees, each working 20 hours per week, would equal 1 FTE. If a position requires coverage for more than 5 days or 40 hours per week, the FTE will be greater than 1.0 for that position. Assume a position requires 7-day coverage, or 56 hours, then the position requires 1.4 FTE coverage (56 divided by 40 = 1.4). This means that more than one person is needed to fill the FTE positions for a 7-day period.

Hours per patient day (HPPD) – the hours of nursing care provided per patient per day by various levels of nursing personnel. HPPD are determined by dividing total production hours by the number of patients.

$$NCH/PPD = \frac{\text{nursing hours worked in 24 hrs}}{\text{patient census}}$$

Patient classification system – a method of classifying patients. Different criteria are used for different systems. In nursing, patients are usually classified according to severity of illness.

Production hours – the total amount of regular time, overtime, and temporary time. This may also be referred to as actual hours.

Staffing Distribution – a determination of the number of personnel allocated per shift. Example – 45% days, 35% evenings, and 20% nights. Hospitals vary on how staff is distributed.

Staffing mix – the ratio of RNs to other personnel. For example, a shift on one unit might have 40% RNs, 40% LVNs, and 20% other. Hospitals vary in their staffing mix policies.

Variable costs — costs that vary with the volume.

STAFFING FORMULAS

- To determine average patient census:

$$\frac{\text{Census figures per day}}{\text{Numbers of days}}$$

- To determine average daily acuity levels (acuity index):

$$\frac{\text{Total acuities}}{\text{Number of patients}}$$

- To determine average monthly patient days:

$$\frac{\text{Average daily census} \times \text{days in calendar year (365)}}{\text{Number of months in a year (12)}}$$

- To determine the actual hours of care being provided:

$$\frac{\text{Total hours of care}}{\text{Number of staff}}$$

- To determine the number of FTEs required:

FIRST: Projected hours of care × average daily census = hours of care/day
SECOND: Hours of care/day × number of days in year (365) = hours of care/year
THIRD:
$$\frac{\text{Hours of care needed per year}}{\text{Hours of 1 FTE per year (2080)}}$$

- To determine the average percentage of nonproductive time:

$$\frac{\text{Hours of 1 FTE (2080)}}{\text{Hours off}}$$

- To estimate rate of turnover:

$$\frac{\text{Number of employees leaving}}{\text{Total number of employees}} \times 100$$

---

adopted by the institution, the supervisor was able to show that she was justified in exceeding the budgeted nursing care hours.

Certain staffing functions remain the responsibility of unit management, regardless of whether the organization has centralized or decentralized staffing. The following are always responsibilities of management:

Table 6-3.   Use of Patient Classification System to Justify New NCH/PPD

Budgeted hours (5.0) × 10,000 patient care days = 50,000 hours of care

Actual acuity stated that Class I required 4 hours of care per patient day, Class II required 5 hours per day, Class III required 6 hours, and Class IV required 7 hours.

A new assessment of patients presently in each category revealed the following:

$$\begin{array}{ll} \text{CLASS I} & = 1000 \text{ PT. DAYS} \\ \text{CLASS II} & = 4000 \text{ PT. DAYS} \\ \text{CLASS III} & = 4000 \text{ PT. DAYS} \\ \underline{\text{CLASS IV}} & = \underline{1000 \text{ PT. DAYS}} \\ & 10000 \text{ PT. DAYS} \end{array}$$

$$\begin{array}{llll} \text{CLASS I} & 4 \times 1000 & = & 4,000 \\ \text{CLASS II} & 5 \times 4000 & = & 20,000 \\ \text{CLASS III} & 6 \times 4000 & = & 24,000 \\ \text{CLASS IV} & 7 \times 1000 & = & \underline{7,000} \end{array}$$

Total NCH 55,000 ÷ 10,000 patient days = 5.5

Interpretation: The unit had a budgeted figure of 5 nursing care hours per patient day. This is the overall average figure for the unit. By using the hospital's patient classification system, the nursing supervisor was able to show that the patient acuity had become more acute and was able to support the need for increasing the budgeted nursing care hours. *The supervisor should request a new projected budget of 5.5 NCH/PPD.*

When the needed nursing care hours per year (55,000) are compared to the budgeted care hours (50,000), it shows that the supervisor needs 5000 more nursing care hours per shift. Using the standard annual working hours per nurse of 2085 per FTE, it is apparent that the *unit needs two more full-time nursing personnel.*

1. Establish and control the personnel budget.

2. Develop a master staffing plan based on the needs of the patients.

3. Develop a method of staffing that allows the unit mode of delivery of patient care to be effectively implemented.

4. Establish the requirements for each position.

5. Assist in the development of each employee to meet job requirements.

6. Use effective management skills to hire, fire, promote, discipline, and counsel employees to ensure that staffing is of high quality.

Supervisors who work in organizations with decentralized staffing have additional responsibilities. Following are the responsibilities of the centralized staffing office in organizations with centralized staffing or of the unit manager in organizations with decentralized staffing:

1. Gather facts and figures to assist with the budgeting process.
2. Schedule employees according to established staffing and scheduling policies.
3. Implement the unit's and the organization's established written procedures for the reallocation of staff as the acuity and patient classification system warrant.
4. Maintain records as necessary on vacation accrual, absenteeism, etc. (Many personnel departments keep such records, but the person responsible for scheduling should be aware of the information.)
5. Implement established procedures for position control.
6. Maintain open and effective communication with the central nursing service administration, the personnel department, and the payroll department.

The effective nursing manager must be able to stay within the staffing budget and still meet the needs of the staff and patients. A manager needs to look at all components of productivity, rather than focusing solely on the number of personnel.

TEAM BUILDING FOR STAFFING EFFECTIVENESS

A major focus of this book is the impact of effective supervision on the resulting productivity of staff. This is never more apparent than in the staffing and scheduling functions of management. Over the years, we have witnessed many superhuman efforts of nursing staff during periods of short staffing with little complaining, simply because the staff believed in their supervisors and in the organization. Yet, just as often, the opposite has occurred: Staff who were only moderately short staffed spent an inordinate amount of time and energy complaining about their plight. The difference between the two examples has much to do with trust — trust that such conditions are the exception, not the norm; trust that real solutions and not Bandaid approaches to problem solving will be used to plan for the future; trust that the management team will work just as hard as the staff in meeting patient needs; and lastly, trust that the organization's overriding philosophy is based on patient interest and not on financial gain.

KEY CONCEPTS CHAPTER 6

1. The unit manager should provide adequate staffing to meet patient care needs.

2. Historical data and current events should both be used to assist in planning for adequate numbers of staff at the unit level.

3. Efforts must be made to avoid under- and over-staffing as patient census and acuity fluctuate.

4. Fair and uniform staffing and scheduling policies and procedures must be written and communicated to all staff.

5. Staffing and scheduling policies should not violate labor laws or union contracts.

6. Existing staffing policies must be examined periodically to determine if they are satisfactory to both the staff and the organization.

7. The patient classification system should be reviewed periodically to determine if it is a valid and reliable tool to measure staffing needs.

8. Managers should continue to examine creative and flexible methods of staffing and scheduling.

9. The middle-level manager should not forget that efforts used for team building will become very useful when there are staffing shortages.

REFERENCES

Gillies, D.A., *Nursing Management—A Systems Approach*, W.B. Saunders, Philadelphia, 1982.

Giovannetti, P., "Understanding Patient Classification Systems," *JONA*, 8(2):4–8, 1979.

Hanson, R.L., *Management Systems For Nursing Staffing*, Aspen Systems, Rockville, MD, 1983.

Hinshaw, A.S., Smeltzer, C.H., Atwood, J.R., "Innovative Retention Strategies for Nursing Staff," *JONA*, 17(6):8–16, 1987.

Marquis, B.L., "Attrition: The Effectiveness of Retention Activities," *JONA*, 18(3):25–29, 1988.

Marquis, B.L., Huston, C.J., *Management Decision Making for Nurses: 101 Case Studies*, J.B. Lippincott, Philadelphia, 1987.

Patterson, S.W., Goad, S., "Incentives for Retention," *Nursing Management*, 18(2):69–70, 1987.

ADDITIONAL READINGS

Barnes, R.M., *Motion and Time Study Design and Measurement of Work*, Sixth Edition, John Wiley and Sons, New York, 1986.

Colt, A.M., "What Nurses Think of the 10 Hour Shift," *Hospitals*, 48:134, 1974.

Eusanio, P.L., "Effective Scheduling—The Foundation for Quality Care," *JONA*, 8(1):12–17, 1978.

Gahan, R., Talley, R., "A Block Scheduling System," *JONA*, 5:39, 1975.

Hanson, R., "Staffing Statistics: Their Use and Usefulness." *JONA*, 12:28, 1982.

Jelinek, R.C., Linn, T.K., Brya, J.R., "Tell the Computer How Sick the Patients Are and It Will Tell How Many Nurses They Need," *Modern Hospitals*, 121:6, 1973.

Williams, M.A., "Quantification of Direct Nursing Care Activities," *JONA*, 7(8):15–18, 1977.

▪ UNIT THREE
External Constraints Affecting Human Resource Management

IN UNIT 2, mention was made of the need to examine the external environment to determine the constraints and assets that are present. This unit examines the two potential constraints that affect personnel planning at the department and unit level of nursing management. These two potential constraints are collective bargaining and legislation concerning employment practices. It is possible to maximize these constraints, making them positive rather than negative influences. In order for management to accomplish this task, however, it must first have an understanding of the issues underlying the growth of unionization in the health care industry and in the proliferation of legislation regarding employment practices.

It is necessary that managers be able to see collective bargaining from four perspectives: (1) the viewpoint of the organization, (2) the viewpoint of the worker, (3) a general historical and societal viewpoint, and (4) a personal viewpoint. Managers able to gain this broad perspective of unionization and collective bargaining will have made great progress in understanding how management and unions can work together for the good of the organization. This is an accomplishment of many other industrialized countries, but an achievement not often realized in the United States.

This is not to say that being a manager in an organization with unions makes the task of management simple. Indeed, it takes much maturity and talent to be a successful manager in an organization with a strong union. Additionally, the type of union leadership displayed will strongly affect how effectively the organization and the union are able to work together.

In assessing the external environment, as well as in all personnel planning, the manager must consider the presence or absence of unions and collective bargaining. The manager must be able to forecast how his or her management position will be influenced by such events.

Likewise, the prudent manager of human resources develops an understanding of the legal issues involved in personnel functions. Legal constraints on employment practices have greatly proliferated in the last 20 years. One of the greatest advantages of being a nurse manager in an organization with a good personnel department is the understanding gained regarding employment legislation. A word of advice with respect to dealing with employee vs. organization rights: *Always* confer with an authority prior to making a decision regarding a sensitive employment issue that might have long-term consequences.

The effective manager of human resources needs to acquire both knowledge and a historical understanding of legislation that affects human resource management functions. Such legislation is often viewed as cumbersome by management, and it does make some aspects of management more difficult; but when it is viewed from a historical perspective, it becomes evident that such legislation was necessary at certain points in the development of this country to right past wrongs. Once such legislation has become ancient history, such as the child labor laws of the 1900s, modern management looks back with awe that such laws were necessary to produce such obviously needed reforms. It is hoped that in 50 years managers of the 2000s will look back in wonder that it was necessary in the 1970s and 1980s to enact legislation that gave certain employment rights to women and minorities.

7
Unions and Collective Bargaining

COLLECTIVE BARGAINING may be defined as those activities occurring between organized labor and management that concern employee relations. Such activities include the negotiation of formal labor agreements and the day-to-day interactions between the union and management. Middle-level managers may have little to do with the negotiation of the labor contract, but they have a great deal to do with the day-to-day implementation of the contract. It has often been said that it is the middle manager who has the greatest impact on the quality of the relationship that develops between labor and management.

Because unions play a prominent role in our society as a whole, it is important that managers develop an understanding of the sociology of unionization. This chapter gives a short history of the labor movement, with emphasis on the events and growth of unions within the health care industry.

Although it is not part of the formalized job description of managers, most nonunionized organizations feel that it is the responsibility of all of management to prevent unionization. Therefore, a section of this chapter will include information to assist managers in recognizing early union activity. Included will be a discussion of why individuals reject or embrace unionization and suggestions on how the effective middle manager can tip the balance toward the rejection of unions by employees.

Because so many health care organizations are currently unionized, the majority of this chapter will be used to depict how management can coexist effectively in an organization with unions. This chapter includes an assessment tool for managers to determine if their organization is adequately prepared to resist union activity and a tool to assess the presence of union activity in the environment. A list of collective bargaining terminology and bargaining agreement content is also included.

HISTORICAL PERSPECTIVE ON UNIONIZATION IN AMERICA

Unions have been present in America since the 1790s. Early unionizers were skilled craftsmen, who formed unions to protect themselves from wage cuts during the highly competitive era of the industrialization of the United States. An examination of the history of the union movement reveals that union membership and activity increase sharply during high employment and prosperity and decrease sharply during economic recessions and layoffs (Allen and Keavenly, 1983).

Presently, in the health care industry, nurses are in demand and the country is experiencing economic stability. Therefore, using historical events as a means to forecast the future, we are able to predict that the next few years will show increased union activity in all areas where nurses are employed. At present, only two events can prevent the rapid unionization of nursing in America. The first event would be the occurrence of a moderate to severe recession, and the second event would be a dramatic improvement in nurses' perceptions of the quality of their supervision. Recent polls taken of nurses' perceptions of management reveal that, in overwhelming numbers, nurses feel that management does not listen to them or care about their needs ("Job Satisfaction," 1987). This provides a fertile ground for union organizers. Unions thrive in a climate where the employees perceive the organizational philosophy to be insensitive to the worker.

For many reasons, collective bargaining was slow in coming to the health care industry. Until amendments to labor laws were made, it was not legally possible for unionization to occur.

The long history of nursing as a service commodity also contributed to the delay in labor organization.

Collective bargaining in the nursing profession initially took place in health care organizations that were in some manner deemed government or public organizations. This was made possible by President Kennedy's Executive Order 10988, which he authored in 1962. This order lifted the restrictions preventing public employees from organizing. Therefore, in the 1960s collective bargaining by nurses began at city, county, and district hospitals and health care agencies.

In 1974, following Kennedy's executive order, Congress made amendments to the Wagner Act, which extended national labor laws to private, nonprofit hospitals, nursing homes, health clinics, health maintenance organizations, and other health care institutions. The Wagner Act amendment of 1974 opened the doors to much union activity for both the professional and the public employee sector. Indeed, if the figures of union membership are reviewed, it becomes readily apparent that since 1960 most collective bargaining activity in the United States has taken place in the public and/or professional sector of industry. There has been little growth of unionization in the private and/or blue collar sector since membership peaked in the 1950s.

From 1962 through 1983, there has been a slow, but steady, increase in the number of nurses represented by collective bargaining agents. In 1983 the American Nurses' Association (ANA) estimated that 130,000 of the nurses in the United States were represented by a collective bargaining agent. This type of consistent steady increase in union membership is also seen in other professions, most notably among faculty at institutions of higher education, teachers at primary and secondary levels, and physicians.

Various unions represent nurses and other health care workers. The following are the major organizations that act as collective bargaining agents in the health care industry. They are listed in order from those representing the largest number to those representing the least number of nursing members: (1) American Nurses' Association, (2) National Union of Hospital and Health Care Employees of Retail, Wholesale, and Department Store Union, AFL-CIO, (3) Service Employees International Union, AFL-CIO, (4) American Federation of Government Employees, AFL-CIO, (5) American Federation of State, County, and Municipal Employees, AFL-CIO, and (6) American Federation of Teachers, AFL-CIO (ANA, 1983).

THE AMERICAN NURSES' ASSOCIATION AND COLLECTIVE BARGAINING

One of the difficult issues facing nurse managers that is not typically encountered in other disciplines is due to the dual role of their professional organization, the American Nurses' Association.

This organization is recognized by the National Labor Relations Board (NLRB) as a collective bargaining agent. In 1980, Barbara Nichols, then ANA president, stated that the ANA represented more registered nurses at the bargaining table than all of the other collective bargaining agents combined (Nichols, 1980).

The use of state nurses associations as bargaining agents has long been a divisive issue among American nurses. Some nurses in management feel they have been disenfranchised by their professional organization. For many other members of the nursing profession this issue presents no conflict. Regardless of individual values, there does appear to be some conflict in loyalty. Sullivan and Decker (1985) pose the question, How can managers, who are charged with the administration of the union contract, belong to the same organization that serves as the bargaining agent for their subordinates? There are no easy solutions to the dilemma created by the dual role held by the American Nurses' Association. Clarifying some of these issues begins by having nurse managers examine the motivation of nurses to participate in collective bargaining activity. Managers must make an effort to at least hear and understand the employee's point of view.

MOTIVATION TO JOIN OR REJECT UNIONS

Knowing that human behavior is goal directed, it is important to examine what drives are fulfilled by union membership. Nurse managers often tell each other that health care organizations are different from other types of industrial organizations. This is a myth, however; in reality, most nurses work in large, impersonal organizations. The nurse frequently feels powerless and vulnerable as an individual alone in a complex institution.

Therefore, one of the primary motivations for joining a union is to *increase the power of the individual*. Employees know that they are essentially dispensable. Since a large group of employees is much less dispensable, the individual nurse greatly increases his or her bargaining power, and reduces vulnerability, by joining a union.

Because of the current nursing shortage, nurses of 1989 feel less vulnerable than nurses of 1982. Therefore, the motivator driving 1989 nurses toward unionization might be *the need most individuals have to communicate their aims, feelings, complaints, and ideas to others*. Beach (1980) maintains that the need to make the organization listen is often a reason individuals join unions.

Since unions emphasize equality and fairness, individual nurses often join a union because they are *driven by a need to eliminate discrimination and favoritism*. This might be an especially strong motivator in groups that have had past experience with discrimination, such as women and minorities.

A variety of social factors also act as motivators to nurses regarding union activity. Peer pressure often culminates in a *social need to be accepted*. Sometimes this social need occurs as a result of family pressures. Many working-class families have a long history of strong union ties, and individuals are frequently raised in a cultural milieu that promotes unionization.

Lastly, nurses sometimes are motivated to join unions because *it is a part of the union contract that all nurses belong to the union*. Although this driving force has been a big motivator among blue-collar workers, the closed shop has never become prevalent in the health care industry. Most health care unions have open shops, allowing nurses to choose whether they want to join.

There are also many reasons why nurses have a need to reject unions. Perhaps one of the strongest is cultural factors. Many people in the United States distrust unions, feeling that unions promote the welfare state and stand in opposition to the American system of free enterprise. Therefore, nurses rejecting unions for these reasons, might have *a need to demonstrate that they can get ahead on their own merits*.

Professional employees have been slow in forming unions for several reasons to do with class and education. They have argued that unions are appropriate for the blue-collar worker, but not for the university professor, physician, or engineer. Nurses rejecting unions on this basis usually are driven by *a need to demonstrate their individualism and social status.*

Beach (1980) states that many employees tend to identify themselves with management and that they frequently adopt the management viewpoint toward unions. Such nurses would reject unions because they have *a need to favorably impress their immediate supervisors.*

A great number of employees reject unions because they fear reprisal from their employers. Although employees are protected under the National Labor Relations Act, they often harbor fear about the possible consequences of their actions. Nurses who reject unions on this basis could be said to be motivated most of all by *a need to keep their jobs.*

Once managers understand the drives and needs behind a union movement, they can begin to address those needs. It is certainly within their power to meet the first three needs for joining unions. They can ascertain that subordinates have a feeling of power by allowing them input into decisions that are made about their work. Managers can listen to ideas, complaints, and feelings, and they can take positive steps to ensure that favoritism and discrimination are not part of their management style. Additionally, managers can strengthen the drives and needs that make nurses reject unions. By building a team effort, by sharing ideas and future plans from upper management with the staff, and by encouraging employees' individualism, managers facilitate identification of workers with management.

It is more likely that organizations with unfair management policies will become unionized. However, organizations offering liberal benefits packages and fair labor practices may still experience union activity if certain societal and cultural factors are present. If managers have tried to meet their employees' needs as described and union activity still occurs, there are specific employee and management rights that managers must be aware of so that the National Labor Relations Act is not violated by either managers or their employees.

MANAGER'S ROLE DURING UNION ORGANIZING

Because of the great increase in unionization within the health care industry, it is probable that most managers will be involved with unions in some manner. Managers who are not presently employed in a unionized health care organization should anticipate that there will be an attempt by one or more unions to organize the nurses in their organization within the next few years. The climate is ripe for union activity, and it will occur. Tool 7-1 is a list of management functions that should occur *prior* to union activity. If the organization waits until the union arrives, it will be too late to perform these functions.

There are also certain behaviors that employees frequently engage in that can alert managers that a union is organizing. Employees have a right to participate in union organizing, and managers must not interfere with this right. However, if the astute manager picks up early clues of union activity, the organization can sometimes take action that will prevent the union from being successful in its attempts to have employees sign membership cards. The union must be able to show an adequate desire for unionization by the employees before an election can be held. Tool 7-2 is a list of employee behaviors that indicate possible union activity and that the manager should be alert for.

Managers should never attempt to deal with union-organizing activity independently. They should always seek assistance and guidance from higher level management and the personnel department. The entire list of rights for both management and labor during the organizing phase of unionization is beyond the scope of this book, but managers need to know that over many years of legislation, Congress has amended various labor acts and laws so that there is a balance of power between management and labor. At times the balance of power has shifted to management or labor, but Congress, in its wisdom, eventually enacts laws that return the balance. Managers must ensure that the rights of both management and employees are protected.

MANAGER'S ROLE IN COLLECTIVE BARGAINING

Once an organization is unionized, managers have specific responsibilities regarding the union contract. Usually first- and middle-level managers have very little to do with the negotiation of the labor-management agreement. The middle-level manager, however, has a great deal to do with implementation of the

(Text continued on p.128)

Tool 7-1 Before the Union Comes

I. Board-approved policy on unionization

- Address the issue with the Board of Directors
- Provide administration with guidance and direction
- Let employees know the Board's attitude (handbooks, orientation)
- Review policy periodically and keep preventive actions current

II. Establish personnel policies

- Write the policy
- Administer fairly and consistently
- Communicate the policy
- Keep policy up-to-date
- Separate policy from procedure
- Monitor the "effect" of the policy
- Include rules and regulations

III. Communication

- Utilize all media
- Hold *regular* employee meetings
- Develop feedback—and react
- Remember to include *all* employees—evening and night shifts too
- Letter to homes at least anually

IV. Supervisory effectiveness

- The first line supervisor is *THE* most important person in maintaining nonunion status
- Conduct relevant supervisory training
- Effective supervisors *not* super techs
- Objective oriented supervision
- Keep supervision informed and involved

V. Employee problem-solving procedure

- Develop and publish a formal procedure
- Educate management and supervision (eliminate threatening nature)
- Basic compensation for grievances
  - Have procedure in writing
  - Include several (three or four) levels of review

        — Establish time limits
        — Reduce grievance to writing after Step 1
        — Consider independent final step
- Make procedure work

VI. Competitive compensation programs
- Keep in line with the community
- Publish rate ranges and all benefit provisions
- Merit pay must be based on effective performance appraisal system
- Explain the "benefit of the benefit"
- Maintain an adequate program (minimum of annual reviews) — don't wait for employees to complain

VII. Effective performance appraisal
- Based on work performance
- Avoid "halo" or "horns" effect
- Make this the responsibility of the supervisor
- Eliminate marginal employees

VIII. Selection, promotion/transfer procedures
- Watch for union organizers
- Maintain stable work records
- Check references
- Promote from within when possible
- Base promotions on merit and performance and *not on seniority*
- Explain reason for not transferring/promoting

IX. Job security
- "Guarantee" job security on basis of adequate
        — job performance
        — adherence to rules/regulations
        — availability of work
- Be sure managers are firm but fair regarding discipline
- Guarantee use of the grievance procedure
- Give seniority proper consideration
        — Layoffs/reductions
        — Vacation preferences

X. Know your employees
- Care about your employees. "If management doesn't care, then the union will."
- Develop your "sources of information"
- Recognize early signs of union organization activity
- Audit your organization periodically

Tool 7-2   Signs of Union Activity

---

1. Small gatherings of employees, perhaps in an unusual part of the facility.

2. Employees getting together in atypical ways

3. The usual grapevine suddenly dies.

4. A former employee periodically shows up after work and talks with a variety of employees.

5. A great deal of "busyness" occurs during breaks and after work.

6. New groups form and new informal leaders emerge.

7. People who are deep in conversation suddenly stop talking when a member of management approaches.

8. There is a sudden increase in questions regarding the organization policies and benefits.

9. Groups of employees appear to become more assertive.

10. People who are usually amiable become uncommunicative.

11. A formerly poor employee with a poor work performance suddenly becomes a model employee.

12. A previously popular employee suddenly becomes unpopular.

13. Graffiti appears that is critical of the organization.

14. Restrooms suddenly become very popular.

15. There is an unexplained reduction in work performance.

---

contract. Tool 7-3 lists the content most commonly found in union contracts. Nurse managers must become familiar with the contract and seek guidance in those areas where interpretation is ambiguous. Tool 7-4 provides managers with a list of collective bargaining definitions and terminology with which they should become familiar when dealing with a union contract.

The two most sensitive areas of any union contract, once wages have been agreed upon, are the areas of discipline and the grievance process. Because of the importance of these two subjects to human resource management, two separate chapters have been devoted to these issues. Chapter 21 discusses employee discipline, and Chapter 22 reviews the grievance process.

Tool 7-3   Content of Collective Bargaining Agreements

 I. Union recognition and scope of bargaining unit
 II. Management rights
 III. Union security
 IV. Strikes and lockouts
 V. Union activities and responsibilities
   A. Dues collection
   B. Union officers and shop stewards
   C. Union bulletin boards
   D. Wildcat strikes or slowdowns
 VI. Wages
   A. General wage adjustments
   B. Wage structure
   C. Merit increases
   D. Call pay and reporting in pay
   E. Shift differentials
 VII. Working-time and time-off policies
   A. Regular hours of work
   B. Holidays and vacations
   C. Overtime and premium pay
   D. Leaves of absence
   E. Rest and break periods
   F. Meal and periods
 VIII. Job rights and seniority
   A. Seniority regulations
   B. Transfers and promotions
   C. Lay-offs and recalls
   D. Job posting and bidding
 IX. Discipline, suspension, and discharge
 X. Grievance handling and arbitration
 XI. Health and safety
 XII. Insurance and benefit programs
   A. Group life insurance
   B. Health insurance
   C. Pension program
   D. Supplemental unemployment benefits

Tool 7-4   Collective Bargaining Terminology

Collective bargaining – The relations between employers, acting through their management representatives, and organized labor.

National Labor Relations Board – A labor board formed to implement the Wagner Act. Its two major functions are to (1) determine who should be the official bargaining unit when a new unit is formed and who should be in the unit, and (2) adjudicate charges of employer unfair labor practices.

Supervisors – A supervisor is defined as someone who has the authority to hire, fire, transfer, and promote another employee. Supervisors are excluded from protection under the Taft-Hartley Act and cannot be represented by a union.

Professionals – Professionals have the right to be represented by a union, but cannot belong to a union that represents nonprofessionals unless a majority of them vote for inclusion in the nonprofessional unit.

Free speech – The law states that "the expressing of any views, argument, or dissemination thereof, whether in writing, printed, graphic, or visual form, shall not constitute or be evidence of an unfair labor practice under any provisions of this Act, if such expression contains no threat of reprisal or force or promise of benefit." (Public Law 101, Sec. 8.)

Union shop – Also called a "closed shop." All employees are required to join the union and pay dues.

Agency shop – Also called an "open shop." Employees are not required to join the union.

Strike – Strikes are concerted withholdings of labor supply in order to bring about economic pressure upon employers and to cause them to grant employee demands.

Lockout – A lockout consists of the closing of a place of business by management in the course of a labor dispute for the purpose of forcing employees to accept management terms.

Grievance – A perception on the part of a union member that management has failed in some way to meet the terms of the labor agreement.

Arbitration – The terminal step in the grievance procedure. Always indicates the involvement of a third party. Arbitration may be voluntary on the part of management and labor, or imposed by the government in a compulsory arbitration.

Conciliation and mediation – Synonymous terms. They refer to the activity of a third party to help disputants reach an agreement.

However, unlike an arbitrator, this individual has no final power of decision-making.

Fact finding — Rarely used in the private sector but used frequently in labor management disputes that involve government-owned companies. In the private sector fact finding is usually performed by a Board of Inquiry.

MANAGER'S ROLE IN PRODUCING EFFECTIVE LABOR-MANAGEMENT RELATIONS

Prior to the 1950s labor-management relations had a turbulent history. History books are filled with various battles, strikes, mass picketing scenes, and brutal treatment on both sides. In the last 30 years employers and unions have substantially improved their relationships. Although there is growing evidence that modern management has come to accept the reality that unions are here to stay, U.S. businesses are still less comfortable with unions than their counterparts in many other countries. Likewise, unions have come to accept the fact that there are times when organizations are not healthy enough to survive aggressive union demands.

Once management is faced with dealing with a bargaining agent, they have a choice of either accepting or opposing the unions. They may actively oppose the union by using various "union-busting" techniques, or they may take a more subtle form of opposition by using any attempt to discredit the union and win employee trust. Acceptance may also run along a continuum. The company may accept the union with reluctance and suspicion. The managers know that the union has legitimate rights, but feel they must continually be on their guard against further encroachment by the union into traditional management territory.

Lastly, there is the type of union acceptance that Beach labels *accommodation*. Accommodation, according to Beach, is becoming increasingly common and is characterized by a complete acceptance of the union by management, with both union and management showing mutual respect for each other (Beach, 1980).

When these latter conditions exist, there can be a climate where labor and management can establish mutual goals, especially in the areas of safety, cost reduction, efficiency, elimination of waste, and improvement of working conditions. Admittedly, such labor-management cooperation represents the most mature and advanced type of labor-management relations.

Beach maintains that the attitudes and the philosophies of the leaders in management and the union determine what type of relationship develops between the two parties in any given organization (Beach, 1980). Middle-level managers have a great deal of influence on the type of relationship that operates between union and management.

Some advice to the manager dealing with unions: Be flexible. Do not try to overwhelm others with power. Do not ignore issues. Do use a rational approach to problem solving.

Unionization of the health care industry will undoubtedly expand. It is important for managers to learn how to overcome this constraint to effective human resource management. Managers must learn to work with unions and must learn the art of using unions to assist the organization in building a team effort to meet organizational goals.

KEY CONCEPTS CHAPTER 7

1. Historically, union activity is greatest during labor shortages and economic upswings.
2. The American Nurses Association acts as the collective bargaining agent for the largest number of nurses.
3. Individuals are motivated to join or reject unions as a result of many needs and values.
4. The middle-level manager has the greatest influence on preventing unionization in a nonunion organization.
5. The middle-level manager has a very important role in establishing and maintaining effective management-labor relationships.
6. It is possible to create a climate in which labor and management can work together to accomplish mutual goals.

REFERENCES

Allen, R.E., and Keavenly, T.J., *Contemporary Labor Relations*, Addison-Wesley, Reading, MA, 1983.

American Nurses Association, *Collective Bargaining and the Nursing Profession*, 1983.

Beach, D., *Personnel: The Management of People at Work, Fourth Edition*, Macmillan, New York, 1980.

"Job Satisfaction: What Nurses Have to Say," *California Nursing Review*, 9(4):14–18, 1987.

Marquis, B.L., Huston, C.J., *Management Decision Making for Nurses: 101 Case Studies*, J.B. Lippincott, Philadelphia, 1987.

Nichols, B., "Belonging to Your Professional Organization: A Commitment to Your Personal Growth and Professional Development." *Imprint*, 27(4):18, 1980.

Public Law 101, 80th Congress, June 23, 1947.

Sullivan, E., and Decker, P., *Effective Management in Nursing*, Addison-Wesley, Menlo Park, CA, 1985, p. 443–457.

ADDITIONAL READINGS

Cleland, V.S., "The Supervisor in Collective Bargaining," *JONA*, 4:33, 1974.

Huston, C.L., "Preparing for Student Grievances," *Imprint*, 34(6):304, 1986.

Lorenz, F.J., "Nursing Administration and Undivided Loyalty." *Nurs Adm Quart*, 6(2):67, 1982.

National Commission on Nursing, *Summary Report and Recommendations*, American Hospital Association, Chicago, 1983.

Sain, T.R., "Effects of Unionization," *Nursing Management*, 15(1):43, 1984.

Sargis, N., Collective Bargaining: Serving the Common Good in a Crisis," *Nursing Management*, 16:23, 1965.

Taylor, B.J., and Whitney, F., *Labor Relations Law*, Second Edition, Prentice-Hall, Englewood Cliffs, NJ, 1983.

Taylor, V.E., "The Dynamics of a Strike," *Supervisor Nurse*, 12:51, 1981.

Telesco, M., "Let's Say Yes to Unions." *RN* 41:29, 1978.

Legal Constraints of Human Resource Management

THE SECOND constraint on the management of human resources is due to the many legal issues involving hiring and employment. These constraints are a factor regardless of the presence of unions.

The U.S. industrial relations system is regarded as one of the most legalistic in the Western world (Howard and Towney, 1975). No major aspect of the employment relationship is free from detailed regulation by either state or federal law. In order to provide managers with a basic legal reference, the regulations will be categorized in this chapter. Many of these regulations relate to specific aspects of personnel management, such as the laws that deal with collective bargaining or the equal employment laws that regulate hiring. When more appropriate, some personnel regulations have been discussed in previous chapters and others will be discussed in subsequent chapters.

Some observers believe that employment and labor-management laws have become so prescriptive that they preclude experimentation and creativity on the part of management. Others believe that, like collective bargaining, the proliferation of employment laws must be viewed from a historical standpoint in order for one to gain a true understanding of the need for such laws (Beach, 1980). Regardless of whether one feels such laws and regulations are necessary, they are a fact of life that each manager must deal with.

Being able to handle the legal requirements of management effectively requires an understanding of labor laws and their interpretation. The manager who embraces the intent of laws that bar discrimination and provide equal opportunity becomes a role model for fairness. The feeling that the employer is fair to all will set the stage for the type of team building that is so important in increasing productivity and retention.

Employment laws fall into one of the following five categories:

1. *Labor standards*. These laws establish minimum standards that employers must maintain with respect to working conditions. These standards apply regardless of the presence or absence of a union contract. Included in this set of laws are the minimum wage, health and safety, equal pay, and other labor standards.

2. *Labor relations*. Some of these laws were discussed in the preceding chapter on collective bargaining. These laws relate to the rights and duties of unions and employers in their relationship with each other.

3. *Equal employment*. These are laws dealing with employment discrimination and will be discussed again in Chapter 10, Interviewing.

4. *Civil and criminal law*. These are statutory and judicial laws that prescribe certain kinds of conduct and establish penalties.

5. *Other legislation*. There are various legal responsibilities of a nursing supervisor that may or may not apply to other industrial managers. For instance, there is a requirement that licensed personnel have a current, valid license from the state in which they practice. Additionally, most states require that employers report certain types of substance abuse to the state licensing boards.

This chapter will give a brief overview of the personnel legislation that has the greatest impact on managers in the health care industry. Tools included in this chapter are a check list to evaluate the organizational environment for employment discrimination and a model of an affirmative action program.

LABOR STANDARDS

Labor standards are regulations dealing with the conditions of the employee's work, including physical conditions, financial aspects, and number of hours worked. There is some overlap in state and federal legislation, and as a general rule the employer must abide by the stricter of the two regulations. The following are the major labor standards:

Minimum Wages and Maximum Hours. More than 85% of all nonsupervisory employees are now covered by the Fair Labor Standards Act (FLSA). This law was first enacted by Congress in 1938 and established a minimum wage of 25 cents an hour. Since that time it has been amended numerous times, most recently in California in 1987, when the current wage was raised to $4.35, to be effective July, 1988.

It is often said that, in addition to putting a "floor under wages," the FLSA also puts a "ceiling over hours." The latter statement, however, is not quite accurate. The FLSA sets a maximum number of hours in any week beyond which a person may be employed *only if he or she is paid an overtime rate*. Some states have enacted a law that makes an exception to this weekly rule on overtime. The exception is an 80-hour pay-period ceiling, after which the employee must receive overtime. The difference in overtime pay can be significant, so it is imperative that middle managers know which standard their organizations is operating under.

The "hours worked" include all the time the employee is required to be on duty. Therefore, mandatory classes, orientation, conferences, and so on must be recorded as duty time and are subject to the overtime rules. The FLSA does not require time clocks but does require that some record be maintained of hours worked.

The FLSA also regulates the minimum amount of overtime pay, which is at least 1½ times the basic rate. State and federal laws may differ on when overtime pay begins. Remember that the stricter rule will usually apply. Some union contracts also have stricter agreements in regard to overtime pay than the FLSA.

The federal labor laws exempt certain employees from the minimum wage and overtime pay requirements. Executive employees, administrative employees, and professional employees are the three more notable "white-collar" exemptions. It is the functions of the position rather than the title, or the fact that the employees are paid a monthly wage, that makes them "exempt" employees. Certain students, apprentice learners, and other special employees may also qualify for an exemption to FLSA regulations. The personnel department in any large organization is especially helpful to the manager in assisting with implementation of these labor laws. The middle-level manager, however, should be cognizant of such laws and have a general understanding of the restrictions they place on staffing and scheduling policies.

Other parts of the labor standards that impact less on nursing are those that deal with the basic minimum age for employment. The minimum age of 16 is waived only for certain occupations.

Equal Pay. The Equal Pay Act of 1963 requires that men and women performing equal work receive equal compensation. This law had a great impact on nursing management when it was enacted. For many years prior to 1963, male "orderlies" were routinely paid at a higher wage than female "aides" performing the identical duties. This fact seems incredible in the 1980s, yet women managers condoned this widespread practice of blatant wage discrimination. Most health care agencies now call these employees "nursing assistants," whether they are male or female, and all are paid the same wage. There are four equal pay tests: equal skill, equal effort, equal responsibility, and similar working conditions.

LABOR-MANAGEMENT RELATIONS LAWS

In addition to the laws regarding collective bargaining discussed in Chapter 7, the manager needs to be aware of one section of the Wagner Act of 1935 and the Taft-Hartley Act of 1947 that deal with unfair labor practices by employers and unfair labor practices by unions.

The initial Wagner Act listed five unfair labor practices, which were henceforth prohibited. These five practices are as follows:

1. To interfere with, restrain, or coerce employees in a manner that interferes with their rights as outlined under the act. Examples of the type of activity that was prohibited was

spying on union gatherings, threatening employees with job loss, or threatening to close down a company if the union organized.

2. To interfere with formation of any labor organization or to give financial assistance to a labor organization. This provision was included to prohibit "employee representation plans" that were primarily controlled by management.

3. To discriminate in regard to hiring, tenure, and so on in order to discourage membership in the union.

4. To discharge or discriminate against an employee who filed charges or testified before the NLRB.

5. To refuse to bargain in good faith.

The original Wagner Act gave much power to the unions, and it was necessary in 1947 to pass additional federal legislation to restore a balance of power to labor-management relations. The Taft-Hartley Act retained the provisions under the Wagner Act that guaranteed employees the right to collective bargaining, but the Taft-Hartley Act added the provision that employees had the right to *refrain* from taking part in unions. In addition to that provision, the Taft-Hartley Act added the following six unfair labor practices of unions that would be henceforth prohibited:

1. Requiring an individual to join a union.

2. Forcing an employer to cease doing business with another person. This placed a ban on secondary boycotts, which were then prevalent in unions.

3. Forcing an employer to bargain with one union when another union has already been certified as the bargaining agent.

4. Forcing the employer to assign certain work to members of one union rather than members of another.

5. Charging excessive or discriminatory initiation fees.

6. Causing or attempting to cause an employer to pay for unnecessary services. This prohibited *featherbedding*, which is a term used to describe union practices that prevented the displacement of workers due to advances in technology.

EQUAL EMPLOYMENT OPPORTUNITY LAWS

Under the American free enterprise system, employers have historically been able to hire whomever they desire. Today the transplanted employer of the 1920s might be shocked to see that racial and ethnic minorities, women, the aged, and the handicapped have acquired substantial rights in the work place. The first legislation in the area of employment hiring practices occurred as a result of years of discrimination against minorities. More recent legislation has been aimed at eliminating discrimination that occurs because of sex, age, and handicaps.

Many profound changes have taken place in the American work place as a result of equal employment opportunity. Women, minorities, and the handicapped have been very successful in jobs that had previously been denied them. Beach (1980) states that if the government had not applied pressure through legislation to increase employment opportunities for these groups, it is highly unlikely that such a change would have occurred. He suggests, however, that such legislative protection may result in a type of reverse discrimination and that this problem may never be solved to the satisfaction of all the involved parties.

The manager should be knowledgeable regarding the following equal employment opportunity (EEO) laws:

1. *Civil Rights Act of 1964.* This act laid the foundation for equal employment opportunity in the United States. The section of this act known as "Title VII" has had an impact on a wide range of employment practices. Many aspects of this act will be discussed in specific detail in Unit 4. The thrust of Title VII is twofold. It prohibits discrimination based on factors not related to job qualifications, and it promotes employment based on ability and merit. The areas of discrimination specifically mentioned are race, color, religion, sex, and national origin. This act was strengthened by President Lyndon Johnson's Executive Order 11246 in 1965 and his Executive Order 11375 in 1967.

   The executive orders seek to correct past injustices. Because the government felt that some groups had a long history of being discriminated against, they wanted to build in a mechanism that would assist those groups in "catching up" with the rest of the American work force. Therefore, they created an affirmative action component that applies to all government contracts. Affirmative action plans are not specifically required by law but may be required by court order. In most states affirmative action plans are voluntary unless government contracts are involved. Many organizations, however, have voluntarily put affirmative action plans in place. Affirmative action differs from equal opportunity. Equal opportunity legislation is aimed at preventing discrimination.

Affirmative action plans are aimed at *actively seeking* to fill job vacancies with those groups that are underemployed, i.e., women, minorities, and the handicapped. Affirmative action forms and guidelines are presented in Tools 8-1 and 8-2.

The Equal Employment Opportunity Commission (EEOC) is responsible for enforcing Title VII. The investigatory responsibility of the EEOC is broad. When it finds reasonable cause that a charge of discrimination is justified, the agency attempts to reach an agreement through persuasion and conciliation. When the EEOC is unable to reach an agreement, it has the power to bring a civil action against the employer. When discrimination is found, the courts will order the restoration of rightful economic status. This means that the employer may be ordered to restore back pay for a period of 2 years. In health care organizations in which discrimination has been found (e.g., unequal pay for men and women in nursing assistant jobs), financial awards in class action suits have been extraordinarily expensive. Middle-level managers should be on the alert for any such discriminatory practices in their organizations.

2. *State Fair Employment Acts.* Some states have fair employment legislation that is more strict than the federal act. A reminder is given again that the stricter regulations always apply. Managers need to be aware of the fair employment regulations in their states.

3. *Age Discrimination and Employment Act (ADEA).* The ADEA was enacted by Congress in 1967. Its purpose is to promote the employment of older persons based on ability rather than age. In early 1978 the ADEA was amended to increase the protected age to 70 years. In 1987 Congress voted to remove even this age restriction, except in certain job categories. Many individuals have viewed the removal of mandatory age retirements with alarm (Ross, 1978). Statistics show that there has been a trend toward early retirement, rather than a trend toward later retirement (Ross, 1978). However, if this trend is reversed, it may have serious consequences for some organizations. In particular, it could have a significant impact on organizations that are labor intensive. This is especially true if those labor-intensive organizations also have demanding physical requirements such as nursing.

4. *The Rehabilitation Act of 1973.* This act requires all employers with contracts over $25,000 to take affirmative action to recruit, hire, and advance handicapped persons who are qualified. Similar, but less aggressive, affirmative action steps are required for other companies doing business with the federal government, with specific requirements

---

Tool 8-1   Affirmative Action Reporting Form

TOTAL NUMBER OF FULL- AND PART-TIME EMPLOYEES _____

Number of males _____ % _____

Number of females _____ % _____

Number of blacks _____ % _____

Number of Hispanics _____ % _____

Number other nonCaucasians _____ % _____

Number of handicapped _____ % _____

Number of employees over age 65 _____ % _____

Number of Caucasians _____ % _____

REPORT OF AFFIRMATIVE ACTION HIRES

Number of interviews conducted in last calendar year _____

Number of individuals hired in last calendar year _____

Number of minorities interviewed _____ % hired _____

Number of handicapped interviewed _____ % hired_____

Number of men interviewed _____ % hired _____

Number of women interviewed _____ % hired _____

To be completed by unit or department supervisor.

---

depending on the size of the company and the dollar amount of the contract. The Department of Labor has been charged with the enforcement of this act. Although there was initially very slow movement in getting companies to hire the handicapped, there has been steady progress. Many companies now find that they successfully utilize the handicapped in positions that previously would not have been open to them (Beach, 1980).

Tool 8-2   Guidelines for an Affirmative Action Program

---

1. **Policy statement**
   The CEO must issue a statement that the organization will not discriminate because of race, color, religion, national origin, sex, or physical handicap in recruitment, hiring, training, compensation, and promotion.

2. **Communication of policy**
   The commitment to Equal Employment Opportunity policy must be disseminated to recruitment sources, such as colleges and universities, and to appropriate unions and employees.

3. **Assignment of responsibility**
   A top-level administrator should be given the responsibility to plan, coordinate, and evaluate the program. This is usually the personnel officer.

4. **Analysis of work force**
   The present work force should be examined to determine the number of each minority type, women, and handicapped that are in each job classification, pay step, and department or unit. There should also be an analysis to determine if some groups are being underutilized.

5. **Goals and timetables**
   Numerical goals should be set for each underutilized group in a reasonable relationship to their availability in the labor market. Target dates should be set for reaching these goals. This is a controversial part of affirmative action.

6. **Implementation**
   There must be detailed policies for implementation, with retrievable proof that the action was taken. Examples would be copies of letters sent to nursing schools that communicated the health organization's desire to hire minorities. Other examples of implementation would be specific policies for maternity leave and nondiscriminatory polices on promotions.

7. **Internal audit and system for reporting**
   Data needs to be gathered and evaluated on a quarterly basis, with a determination of how goals are being met and with suggestions for corrective action when goals are not met.

8. **Supporting company and community programs**
   Middle-level management should have training in the requirements for affirmative action and the implementation of the company's program.

Job and career guidance should be made available to employees. The organization should cooperate with other community agencies in regard to child care, transportation, and housing.

Adapted from Federal Regulations: Title VII of the Civil Rights Act of 1964.

---

5. *The Vietnam Era Veterans Readjustment Assistance Act.* This act provides re-employment rights and privileges for veterans to positions that they held prior to their entry in the armed forces. This act was used by nurses during the nursing surplus of 1983 to 1984. Some nurses worked a short time following graduation from nursing school prior to being commissioned in the armed services. On their discharge from the armed forces, they sought positions from their prior employer and, even if there were no positions available, the hospitals were required by this act to reinstate them to their former positions.

OTHER LEGISLATION AFFECTING HUMAN RESOURCE MANAGEMENT

Several other federal and state regulations have an impact on the management of human resources. Only those that the manager needs to be especially cognizant of are listed.

1. *The Occupational Safety and Health Act (OSHA).* This broadly written piece of legislation speaks to the requirements of the employer to provide a place of employment that is free from recognized hazards that may cause physical harm. The Department of Labor enforces this act. It is impossible for the Department of Labor to physically inspect all facilities; therefore, most of their inspections are brought about because of an employee complaint or at the request of an employer to conduct an inspection. The act does allow for fines to be levied if employers continue with unsafe conditions.

Since its inception, many companies have been vehement in their criticism of the act, specifically its administration. They have also charged that the economic cost of meeting OSHA standards has been an excessive burden for American business.

In contrast, unions have charged that the federal government has never staffed or funded the Occupational and Health Administration adequately. They have charged that OSHA has been negligent in setting standards for toxic substances, carcinogens, and other disease-producing agents. This view is supported in the 1977 report of the Comptroller General of the United States, who reported that 390,000 new cases of occupational disease occur each year and that 100,000 people die from them.

Since the risk of discovery, and the fine if discovered, are both low, employers often choose to ignore unsafe working conditions. Nurse managers are in a unique position to call attention to hazardous conditions in the work place and should communicate such concerns upward to higher authority. Public health scientists have estimated that 80% of all cancers are caused by exposure to environmental factors (Ashford, 1976).

Most states also have occupational and safety regulations. Here again, the more stringent regulations are those with which the employer must comply. Many of the state licensing boards have additional health regulations, which may differ in some manner from the federal regulations.

2. *State Health Facilities Licensing Boards.* In addition to health and safety requirements, many state boards have regulations regarding staffing requirements. It is the ultimate responsibility of top-level management to maintain the state license that permits them to operate. However, nurse managers are responsible for knowing and meeting the regulations that apply to their units or departments. For example, if the manager of an intensive care unit has a state staffing level that mandates 12 hours of nursing care per patient and also requires that the ratio of registered nurses to other staff be 2:1, the supervisor is obligated to staff at that level or above. If, during times of short staffing, supervisors are unable to meet this level of staffing, they must apprise upper level management so that there can be joint decision-making to resolve the situation.

Variations in state licensing requirements make a discussion of them outside the scope of this book. It is important, however, for nurse managers at every level to be knowledgeable about state licensing regulations that pertain to their levels of supervision.

THE LIABILITY OF SUPERVISION

There are three specific areas of liability where the manager is particularly vulnerable. The first is in the broad area of supervision itself. Fiesta (1988) maintains that "failure to supervise in accordance with the standard expected of a professional nurse may be viewed with negligence." This would not remove personal liability from the individuals directly involved with exercising the standard; rather, it extends that liability to include the supervising individual.

One way to avoid liability in this area is for supervisors to fulfill the duties of the supervisory positions that are listed in their job descriptions. Seeking consultation in "gray areas" of supervision is another good method to prevent liability. Before taking action in sensitive legal issues, the manager should discuss the problems with the personnel department and with higher authority.

The second duty for which the supervisor may be held liable is in the area of inadequate staffing. If nurses make errors due to unsafe staffing, the nurses may not be held liable, if it can be proven that the supervisors were aware of the problem (Fiesta, 1988).

The last area of supervisory liability is in delegation or assignment of work. The supervisor is responsible for assigning work at the competence level of the employee. Again, this does not remove the personal liability of individuals who have accepted a work assignment beyond their level of competence. Assignments beyond the training, education, or competence of the employee that result in injury could lead to a charge of negligence on the part of both the employee and the supervisor.

THE LEGAL PRACTICE OF NURSING

The final area of legal constraints that concern the nurse manager lies in the professional practice of nursing. Nurse managers are legally responsible for both their own and their staffs' professional practices. This is another area where there is joint liability (i.e., personal and supervisory), since supervisors are responsible for seeing that all nurses under their supervision maintain a current license and are competent in their field.

Managers should be aware of the nurse practice act in their states, as well as the legal rights of patients. If they are supervising other types of licensed workers, they should have knowledge of the limitations of their practices.

Marquis and Huston (1987) also maintain that nurse managers have some legal responsibility for quality control of nursing practice on their units. Included among these legal responsibilities are checking credentials and qualifications of their staff, carrying out appropriate discipline, and reporting substandard medical care.

Additional legal responsibilities of nurse managers are to ensure client confidentiality, report required public health information, and report suspected elder, child, and patient abuse.

The legal constraints will seem less burdensome to managers if they remember that most laws were enacted to protect the rights of patients and employees. If managers perform their jobs well and work for organizations that desire to "do the right thing" by accepting their social responsibility, then they need not fear the legal aspects of human resource management.

KEY CONCEPTS CHAPTER 8

1. There are many state and federal laws and regulations that influence how human resources are managed.

2. Much of the human rights legislation concerning employment practices resulted because of documented discrimination in the work place.

3. Although legislation makes the job of managing people more difficult for managers, it has resulted in increased job fairness and job opportunities for women, minorities, the aged, and the handicapped.

4. Affirmative action differs from equal opportunity in that the former seeks to correct past injustices, while the latter only prevents present discrimination.

5. The middle-level manager is in a good position to detect health hazards in the work place.

6. Managers are more vulnerable to liability than their workers, due to the added responsibilities inherent in any supervisory role.

7. Nursing managers have additional liability not found in all management roles, due to the responsibilities that arise out of their accountability to their clients and their professional practice.

REFERENCES

Ashford, N.A., *Crisis In The Workplace: Occupational Disease and Injury*, MIT Press, Cambridge, MA, 1976.

Beach, D.S., *Personnel: The Management of People at Work*, Fourth Edition, Macmillan, New York, 1980.

Comptroller General of the United States, *Delays in Setting Workplace Standards for Cancer Causing and Other Dangerous Substances*, General Accounting Office, Washington, D.C., May 10, 1977.

Fiesta, J., *The Law and Liability: A Guide For Nurses*, Second Edition, John Wiley and Sons, New York, 1988.

Howard, A.H., Towney, D.P., *Labor Law and Legislation*, Fifth Edition, Southwestern Publishing, Cincinnati, 1975.

Marquis, B.L. and Huston, C.J., *Management Decision Making for Nurses: 101 Case Studies*, J.B. Lippincott, Philadelphia, 1987.

Public Law 101, 80th Congress, June 23, 1947.

Ross, I., Retirement at Seventy: "A New Trauma for Management," *Fortune* 97(9):102–106, 1978.

Wagner Act, 298 U.S. 238, 1935.

ADDITIONAL READINGS

Bruce, J.A.C., *Privacy and Confidentiality of Health Care Information*, American Hospital Publishers, Chicago, 1984.

Decker, L.R., and Peed, D.A., "Affirmative Action for the Handicapped," *Personnel*, 53(3):64–69, 1976.

Fine, E.R., "What to Do When the Doctor is Wrong," *Nursing Life*, 2(6):22–24, 1982.

Hollander, J., "A Step by Step Guide to Affirmative Action," *Business and Society Review*, 1(14):67–73, 1975.

Page, J.A., and O'Brien, M.W., *Bitter Wages*, Grossman, New York, 1973.

Robertson, D.E., "New Directions in EEO Guidelines," *Personnel* 57:360, 1978.

· UNIT FOUR
The Employment Process

THIS UNIT will examine the employment process. All too often in the past, organizations placed little value on the process of selecting employees. This occurred because the organization could replace nurses who left the organization fairly easily, often with novice nurses at a lower salary. The supply was adequate and turnover was considered to be a noncontrollable cost. Organizations today, in an age of cost containment and widespread nursing shortages, recognize the need to proactively recruit highly skilled individuals for positions, to select the most qualified applicant for a particular position, and to create a work environment that promotes retention. An organization can not prosper and grow, and may not survive, without adequate human resources (Lopresto, 1986). Likewise, the successes and failures of an organization are usually determined by the quality of its work force. Therefore, the methods and procedures the organization utilizes to obtain that work force is one of the most vital components of human resource management.

This unit will focus primarily on three components of the employment process: recruitment, interviewing, and selection. Recruitment involves influencing the size and quality of the applicant pool by making more people aware of job openings and enticing them to apply. Having established the applicant pool, the recruiter begins the process of narrowing the pool by sifting out unqualified applicants and applicants who do not fit with the culture of the organization (Milkovich and Glueck, 1985).

After the applicant list has been narrowed to appropriate candidates for a particular position, organizations most frequently utilize interviews as their primary selection tool. Interviewing refers to the verbal interaction between a prospective employee and a representative of an organization. Both the applicant and the organization attempt to gain as much information about the other as possible. If applicants have a clear idea of the job requirements, the rewards offered, and the organizational goals, they can better assess whether a specific job offers a "good match" with their own needs and abilities (Milkovich and Glueck, 1985). Likewise, if the organization gains a better understanding of an applicant's strengths and weaknesses, it can better plan a training and orientation program for that applicant as an employee. Interviews, when conducted appropriately, should yield information about which applicant would be best suited for which position.

Selection is the process of choosing from among applicants the best qualified individual(s) for a particular position. Proper selection of employees requires the matching of applicant qualifications and job requirements as well as organizational and employee expectations. Selection criteria may include standardized testing of job applicants. Lastly, the selection phase of the employment process includes the completion of pre-employment paperwork and physical screening of employees.

The employment process puts the human resource plan into action. Effective managers do not look on personnel functions in their jobs as merely a potpourri of isolated tasks. Planning and implementation of recruitment, interviewing, and selection must be integrated in thought and design by all managers in the organization. This holistic approach to personnel management enhances both the organization's objectives and the satisfaction that individual employees receive.

REFERENCES

Lopresto, R.L., "Recruitment Sources and Techniques" in Famularo, J.J., *Handbook of Human Resources Administration*, Second Edition, McGraw Hill, New York, 1986.

Milkovich, G.T., and Glueck, W.F., *Personnel/Human Resource Management: A Diagnostic Approach*, Business Publications, Plano, TX, 1985.

9
Recruitment

THE ABILITY of the organization to meet its goals and objectives is directly related to the quality of the individuals it recruits and employs. Wise managers will surround themselves with people who have ability, motivation, and promise. Managers who recruit, identify, and hire gifted individuals prevent stagnation in the organization, increase productivity, and increase their own value to the organization (Marquis and Huston, 1987).

Recruitment is the process of actively seeking out and bringing in qualified applicants for existing job positions in organizations in a cost-effective manner. Recruitment requires long-term planning and continuous effort if the organization is truly going to be proactive in recruiting and retaining a highly qualified staff. Unfortunately, many institutions fail to proactively assess their staffing needs and thus are required to take swift and expensive action. Many hospitals respond to acute staffing shortages with gimmicks, including new cars, shift and recruitment bonuses, paid vacations, and other costly incentives. Although these gimmicks generally bring about a quick resolution to the acute shortage, they are almost always very expensive and provide only a short-term solution to the staffing shortage. It is imperative, then, that organizations have a clear concept of the components of a proactive and productive recruitment process.

This chapter will examine recruitment in terms of the steps in the recruitment process, variables affecting recruitment, the recruitment resources available to most health care organizations, the role of the nurse recruiter, organizational competition for qualified applicants in a nursing shortage, and recruitment methods and strategies. Tools for implementation include excerpts from recruitment position announcements for use in developing recruitment literature. A check list is also included to assist in developing recruitment advertisements for professional journals.

STEPS IN THE RECRUITMENT PROCESS

Lyles and Joiner (1986) identified the following five steps in the recruitment process:

1. Organizational policies regarding recruitment should be reviewed prior to the advertisement of a job position. These policies should examine both internal and external recruitment. Internal recruitment policies might examine issues such as intraunit or interunit promotions, length of time required for posting, and how notices should be posted for vacant positions. External policies might include timelines, required numbers of applicants for a position to be closed, and affirmative action and hiring requirements. It is important that the organization continually reassess these policies for fairness and consistency. Wolf (1981) stated that administrative philosophy and policies contribute more than any other factor to a high turnover rate, and this is a direct result of inadequate attention to retention and staff satisfaction.

2. All relevant sources of potential applicants must be identified. This requires that the nurse supervisor or recruiter assess the specific job requirements and the qualifications needed to be successful in that position. The more specific the requirements, the fewer sources will be available to the recruiter for the applicant pool. For example, hiring staff for specialty units or upper management positions would normally draw less qualified applicants.

3. The optimum mode of communicating job vacancies must be determined. Communication modes may include personal contact, letters, telephone calls, and so on.

4. The recruitment needs and qualifications required must be communicated. It is imperative that the hiring needs be understood by potential applicants and that communication and cooperation be continuous and ongoing. Organizations will often provide overt or covert misrepresentations about the job description or behavioral expectations in an effort to increase their applicant pool. This usually results in employee mistrust, dissatisfaction, and even rapid turnover. Ilgen and Seely (1974) found significantly lower turnover rates among recruits who had been given realistic written information about their jobs than among those who had not. Accurate job descriptions and behavioral expectations may dull some interest initially but will assure greater job satisfaction later, as well as serve the needs of both the applicant and the organization (Vogt et al., 1983). Qualified applicants will thus be identified and can be encouraged to go forward with the processes of interviewing and selection.

5. Evaluate the response to the recruitment effort and adjust as needed. Too few applicants limit management from hiring the most qualified individuals. In contrast, applicants from too large a pool are discouraged from reapplying in the future. In addition, having enormous numbers of inappropriate, underqualified or overqualified applicants reflects poor recruitment. Recruitment must be both efficient and effective if it is to be successful.

VARIABLES AFFECTING RECRUITMENT

Because recruitment needs are not static, human needs forecasting requires a constant determination of both present and future supply. In forecasting supply, the manager needs to estimate the number of personnel currently working on individual units that will need to be replaced by a given period of time. The manager must then determine how much of this estimated need will require recruitment from outside the agency and how much can be successfully recruited from within. Much of this human resource planning is affected by variables beyond the control of the manager.

Conditions in the labor market are one such major variable. Strauss and Sayles (1972) define a labor market as a geographical area in which the forces of supply (people looking for work) and demand (employers looking for people to hire) interact and thus affect the price of labor (wages and salaries). The actual boundaries of the market depend on the type and number of applicants being sought. For example, in nursing, when the national economy worsens, nurses have returned to the work setting. When this occurred in 1979, it resulted in a nursing surplus that virtually eliminated positions for new graduate nurses (White, 1984).

In contrast, when the economy improves, the nursing shortage has increased. During such periods of worker shortages, the manager must plan more elaborate and prolonged recruitment strategies to meet the demand. When an abundant supply of nurses is available, informal recruiting methods may be more than adequate to attract an adequate work force.

Another variable affecting recruitment is the size of the applicant pool. If recruiters consider all individuals having passed the registered nurse licensing examination as potential candidates, then their pool is truly limitless. More frequently, organizations limit the applicant pool by establishing criteria for each position that exceed the minimum necessary for the legal practice of nursing. For example, the organization might have a philosophy or policy that limits the hiring of novice or inexperienced nurses or part-time nurses, or it might have a philosophy that discourages inactive nurses from returning to the work setting.

Marquis and Huston (1987) identified additional variables that influence successful recruitment of an adequate work force:

1. Available resources for advertisement, recruitment literature, and visits to career-day programs
2. Available numbers of new and experienced nurses
3. Competitiveness of the organization's salaries and benefits
4. Attractiveness to the potential work force of the setting where the organization is located
5. The reputation of the organization regarding past employment practices and the quality of patient care
6. The status of the national and local economy

Given unlimited recruitment monies, a local school of nursing, a progressive community with a moderate climate, and an organization that has a reputation for fair employment practices, quality patient care, and generous compensation, few organizations would have any difficulty recruiting an adequate staff. Unfortunately, it is more common for many or all of these variables to be lacking, making recruitment very difficult and very expensive.

RESOURCES FOR RECRUITMENT

The sources utilized to find an adequate number of job applicants varies with elements such as management policy, the type of positions open, the supply of labor in relation to demand, and the nature of the existing labor market (DiVincenti, 1972). One recruitment source that both is inexpensive and has a more rapid turn-around time is the organization itself. Intraorganization recruitment methods include the organization's informal and formal communication network. Position announcements may be posted on appropriate bulletin boards or may be listed in organizational newsletters. Open positions may also be announced at management and unit meetings or may be passed informally between employees.

Recruitment methods using external sources generally require greater time, effort, and cost. Examples of external recruitment sources cited by Lyles and Joiner (1986) include:

1. Nonemployed nurses
2. Public employment services
3. Private employment agencies
4. Direct hiring
5. Friends and relatives
6. Advertising in newspapers
7. Professional associations or journals
8. Colleges and universities
9. High schools
10. Vocational colleges
11. Referrals of past and present employees
12. Transfers from other organizations
13. Walk-ins
14. Rehires/re-employed
15. Doctor's offices
16. Unions
17. National professional meetings or conferences

The organization must capitalize on as many sources as possible to ensure an adequate applicant pool. Recent research, however, has indicated that the source of the referral may be at least as important in successful recruitment as an adequate number of applicants. Research done by Breaugh (1981) demonstrated that the recruitment source plays an important role in subsequent employee performance. Employees recruited through college placement offices were found to be lower in performance quality, job involvement, dependability, and supervisory satisfaction than recruits from other sources. Employees solicited from newspaper advertising had almost twice the absenteeism of recruits from other sources.

Decker and Cornelius (1979) also found that the recruitment source has a direct impact on employee turnover. Applicants hired by informal means (rehires, walk-ins, and employee/friend referrals) remained with the organization longer than those who were recruited through external and more formal sources (newspaper ads, employment agencies, etc.). In addition, they were generally more satisfied with their jobs, as their pre-employment expectations more closely matched the real work situation. Given that where one looks for applicants may have significant consequences in turnover, the organization should, whenever possible, assess which sources have provided them with the most qualified applicants. Additionally, there should be complete follow-up evaluations regarding the relationship between the recruitment source and subsequent employee performance. In addition to identifying and evaluating sources for recruitment, the wise organization will use specific recruitment methods to attract candidates for job openings, such as the following (Marquis and Huston, 1987):

1. *Advertising*. Advertising may be done locally through newspapers or nationally through nursing journals. National searches can be expensive and time consuming due to the lag time for publication but may be required when the pool of applicants with the desired qualifications is small. National searches are also indicated when a specific target group is identified (Lewis and Spicer, 1987). Thus the recruiter is able to reach the most appropriate market of readers. Tool 9-1 provides a check list for developing recruitment advertisements for professional journals.

   Generally, most health care institutions attempt, at least initially, to advertise locally. There is often a pool of "in-active

Tool 9-1   Check List for Developing Professional Journal Recruitment Advertisements

Selecting the best advertising source

1. Any advanced skills, education, certification, or training necessary to meet the position requirements should be identified. This determines your target audience. Is a more specialized audience necessary?

2. Professional journals that reach the target audience should be identified.

3. Circulation, cost, frequency of journal publication, and delay time in submission and publication should be compared among appropriate journals. Do certain journals have higher regional circulation?

4. The style and format, if any, of advertisements in each journal must be identified.

5. Determine how much money is available to use for journal recruitment advertisements. Is it more beneficial to buy fewer large advertisements or to buy smaller advertisements in several different journals? How many positions must be filled? How successful has journal advertising been in the past in increasing the applicant pool?

Design of the advertisement

1. Determine whether professional advertising or design specialists are needed to assist you with the advertisement layout. Determine the cost of professional design. Does a current employee have special skill in this area? Has the nurse recruiter or any other individual involved in the personnel process already developed specific ideas for recruitment advertisements?

2. Determine the greatest drawing factors your organization has (i.e., geographic focus, reputation or quality of nursing care, salary and benefits).

3. The drawing factor(s) should be highlighted as a major feature of the advertisement.

4. The advertisement must be eye-catching. Combine pictorial and verbal messages whenever possible to draw the interest of a greater number of readers. Alter typeface and print size to increase visual appeal. Photographs must be clear and legible.

5. Follow journal specifications exactly regarding display space to be utilized, typeset, spacing, etc. Ascertain journal deadlines for publication.

6. The advertisement should identify a contact person in the organization, to whom all inquiries should be directed, by name. This will reduce the possibility of inquiries being lost or misdirected.

nurses" locally who might be recruited under the right conditions (i.e., under difficult economic conditions) (Decker, Moore, and Sullivan, 1982). The local newspaper advertisement should be employee centered. It should deal with the specifics of company projects and achievements and relate them to the advantages they create for the person who joins the company (Deutsch, 1979).

In addition, recruitment flyers are another local advertising source that are frequently sent to schools of nursing for placement on recruitment bulletin boards or to potential applicants. The flyer or brochure must convey a positive message and should briefly describe specifics regarding the organization and what it offers to those who join the team. The brochure should be designed for easy mailing and for posting at nursing conferences, job fairs, and professional meetings (Lewis and Spicer, 1987).

2. *Career days.* Career days provide another local and fairly inexpensive recruiting strategy. Many schools of nursing offer career-day programs, to which a recruiter is often sent. Organizations that do not have a recruiter often attract potential nurses by having volunteer staff attend the career-day programs. A good endorsement for a particular agency is to have an employee who is a recent graduate of a school of nursing return to that school on career day.

3. *Recruitment literature.* One successful method of recruitment is to have printed materials available to give to potential applicants or to mail out on request. These brochures should list the salaries, benefits, philosophy of the organization, and something about the community where the health care facility is located.

4. *Use of resources in the organization.* Some health care organizations attempt to reduce recruitment costs by using less expensive means of recruitment. One of the best ways to maintain an adequate employee pool with minimal recruitment costs is to attract potential employees by word of mouth through their own satisfied and happy employees. Employees who are recruited informally following a referral by friends or employees usually remain longer with an organization than those who are hired following formal recruitment methods such as advertising and employment agencies (Decker and Cornelius, 1979). Other less expensive ways of using resources within the organization are to have open houses for nurses in the community or to use educational resources to recruit, especially at the local level.

ROLE OF THE NURSE RECRUITER IN THE ORGANIZATION

Although there have been temporary, and isolated, shortages in some parts of the country, the nurse applicant pool has traditionally been adequate to meet the needs of most organizations. Thus, until 15 years ago, limited effort had gone into the recruitment of registered nurses. With increasingly widespread nursing shortages, organizations have placed a greater priority on the need to proactively assure an adequate number of well-qualified staff. Often this has resulted in the creation of one or more nurse recruiter positions.

The determination of whether an organization will utilize nurse recruiters or will delegate recruitment to lower level nursing managers, depends on several factors. These factors are (1) the size of the institution, (2) the existence of a separate personnel department within the organization, and (3) use of centralized or decentralized management (Marquis and Huston, 1987). Larger organizations typically can more easily justify the use of nurse recruiters because of their large RN staff. Smaller health care organizations tend to centralize the recruitment and hiring in their facility within a personnel department, as the recruitment and selection of RNs does not financially justify a full-time nurse recruiter position.

As nursing management becomes more decentralized, personnel management becomes more complex and the involvement of lower level managers becomes greater in the selection of nursing personnel for their own units. Regardless of the extent of involvement of nurse managers in the recruitment and selection of personnel, it is important for all nurse managers to be aware of the constraints of management (Marquis and Huston, 1987). Likewise, nurse recruiters and nurse managers who coordinate recruitment must understand and adhere to the policies that have been established by the organization's personnel department (Lewis and Spicer, 1987). Furthermore, recruiters must understand the organization's philosophy and goals and be aware of what the organization is attempting to accomplish through recruitment. Recruiters should also have an understanding of current legal and labor restraints affecting the recruitment process.

Administratively, the cost of a nurse recruiter's salary may be reflected solely in the personnel department or the nursing service budget, or it may be borne by all nursing departments. Expenses for brochures, travel, and recruitment aids must also be considered in the recruitment budget.

Recruiting is a difficult management position, and the individual selected for this position requires special characteristics. Bowin (1987) states that the successful recruiter requires intelligence, enthusiasm, communication skills, self-confidence, persistence, a mind for detail, and an ability to represent the organization. The importance of these personal characteristics cannot be underemphasized. Studies by Alderfer and McCord (1970) demonstrated that supportive, interested recruiter behavior may result in positive applicant reaction. Certain recruiter traits and behaviors are also related to the stated likelihood of an applicant's accepting a job offer.

THE APPLICANT POOL—COMPETITION FOR EMPLOYEES

Two basic sources of applicants exist: internal (current employees) and external (those not currently affiliated with the organization) (Milkovich and Glueck, 1985). Whether the employer decides to go inside or outside for applicants depends on such factors as availability of qualified people in both sources, the economic conditions and plans of the organization, how quickly the vacancy needs to be filled, and relative costs. Inhouse recruiting can be done in three ways: transferring an employee from other units within the organization, promoting an employee, or upgrading the educational or skill level of an employee now holding a certain position (Schuster, 1985).

Inhouse recruiting may result in wider organization disruption, because each position filled creates another opening (Vogt et al., 1983). It may also result in an inbreeding of values and ideas, which contributes to stagnation within the organization. It does, however, provide an important outlet for employee recognition and motivation. It is also much less expensive and usually results in a more productive employee in a shorter period of time, due to the reduction in orientation and socialization time that would be required for an employee who is new to the organization. DiVincenti (1972) suggests that in promotions the majority of vacancies should be filled from within, but external recruitment should be utilized in situations where qualified individuals are not available within the organization. She also suggests, however, that in order to suggest new ideas, consideration should be given to filling a moderate percentage of management positions from the outside.

With the current nursing shortage, most hospitals must recruit externally to have an adequate work-force pool. External recruiting is generally more expensive and requires personal socialization and professional orientation of new employees. At least part of the reason hospitals must do so much external recruiting is the lack of emphasis currently placed on retention. Although retention is not the primary focus in this chapter, it is important to remember that retention and recruitment are very closely linked. Longo and Uranker (1987) stated that hospitals should adopt the premise, "a nurse retained is a nurse recruited" and that the retention of a nurse exemplifies the hospital's protection of its investment. Figure 9-1 depicts the interdependence of recruitment and retention (Wall, 1988). In this figure, recruited nurses provide feedback regarding their

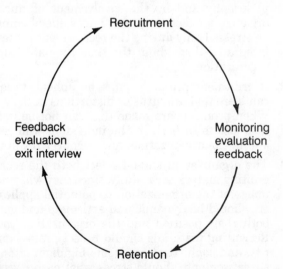

FIGURE 9-1. *Sequential interdependent nurse recruitment-retention loop (From Wall, L., "Plan Development for a Nurse Recruitment-Retention Program," JONA 18(2):21, 1988.)*

career wants and needs so that the organization can make an effort to meet the needs of the nurses. Further evaluation then occurs regarding whether these efforts have been successful in increasing retention. If retention has been positive, nurses with compatible interests or career goals can be recruited for the same units or positions. This relationship is sequential in that recruitment must be successful before retention can be initiated. Many organizations could greatly decrease the need for external recruitment if retention-recruitment programs were more closely aligned and given equal priority.

STRATEGIES FOR RECRUITMENT

In a nursing shortage, the wise employer will use the following strategies to ensure a successful external recruitment program:

1. Evaluate and make organizational changes that meet employee needs and expectations whenever possible. These may include establishment of variable work schedules, a specific mode of patient care management, and on-site child care or educational benefits.

2. The value of employees to the organization should be stressed, and this should be reflected in the organizational philosophy and by the involvement of nurses on major organizational committees. This value of employees cannot be stressed only during the recruitment process; it must be integrated throughout the time they are employed by the organization.

3. Recruitment promises must be upheld. Frequently applicants are told untruths or distortions in the zeal to recruit. When promises are made that can not be upheld, individuals lose faith both in the individual who recruited them and in the organization, and turnover results.

4. The organization should select both the recruiter and recruiting materials carefully, since they will present the first image of the organization to potential applicants. Recruiters should be dynamic and articulate and genuinely enjoy both their position and the organization they represent. Recruiting materials should reflect professionalism, integrity, and sophistication. Items highlighted on recruitment advertisements should stress what each organization feels are its greatest drawing factors. Tools 9-2, 9-3, and 9-4

Tool 9-2 Recruitment Advertisements: Geographic Focus

"We have a hospital by your place in the sun" — Hospital Corporation of America — Florida Connection

"Registered Nurses, Take Advantage of Florida Sun" — Highlands Regional Medical Center

"I'm proud to be part of the Iowa Team" — University of Iowa Hospitals and Clinics

"Palm Springs: Some nurses really know how to live. Ahhh, Palm Springs!" — Palm Springs Desert Hospital

"Let Maryland Touch You" — Maryland Hospital Association

"When you move to Atlanta, plan on spending a lot of time under an umbrella" — Georgia Baptist Medical Center

"Big city hospital experience set in a resort community" — Sarasota Memorial Hospital, Sarasota, Florida

"They say you can spend a lifetime in Washington and never see it all. Like to give it a try?" — Providence Hospital, Washington D.C.

"Travel to the beautiful Northwest — Seattle/Tacoma area." — MRA Staffing Systems, Chicago, Illinois

---

represent highlights from sample recruitment ads in a March issue of *Nursing 88*. These highlights have been grouped into three categories frequently used in marketing: geographical motivators, the reputation or quality of nursing care at the organization, and salaries and fringe benefits, respectively.

5. Recruitment must at all times be ethical. In periods of acute nursing shortages, some organizations attempt to undercut or "steal" employees away from other organizations. This is at best unprofessional and usually results in only short-

Tool 9-3   Recruitment Advertisements: Reputation/Quality of Nursing Care

"High tech hasn't made us lose our touch" — Army Nurse Corps

"The ideal habitat for an endangered species" — North Carolina Baptist hospital

"Nurses are the heart of Pitt County Memorial Hospital and we never forget it" — Pitt County Memorial Hospital, Greenville, North Carolina

"Caring: High touch from special people" — New Hanover Memorial Hospital, New Hanover, North Carolina

"Special People Satisfying Special Needs" — Health Force Inc.

"Children with special needs need special nurses" — Texas Children's Hospital

"We're not just looking for nurses. We're looking for decision makers — Saint Joseph's Hospital of Atlanta

"You can make a difference at Memorial Sloan-Kettering Cancer Center" — Memorial Sloan-Kettering Cancer Center, New York

"What's happening in nursing tomorrow is happening at Cedars-Sinai" — Cedars Sinai Medical Center, Los Angeles, CA

"Kimberly has some very tough shoes to fill" — Kimberly Nurses, Kansas

"Advance to excellence" — Fairfax Hospital, Virginia

"Name one place that cares about its nurses" — Medlantic Healthcare Group, Washington D.C.

"It took us 100 years to get here. You could be here tomorrow" — University of Virginia Medical Center

Tool 9-4   Recruitment Advertisements: Salary/Benefits/Flexible Staffing/Career Options

"Best Travel Opps"—MRA Staffing Systems

"RNs—Looking for More than Room and Bored?"—MRA West and East

"Nurse America's Working Vacation"—Nurse America

"Feel warm and wealthy"—Memorial General Hospital, New Mexico

"What have we got to offer? Simply everything"—North Broward Hospital District, Florida

"And who's monitoring *your* most important needs?"—Western Medical Services, California

"Career Challenges and Exciting Lifestyle are available to nurses at Eisenhower Memorial Hospital"—Eisenhower Memorial Hospital California

"Broaden your horizons—Travel with America's finest team"— American Mobile Nurses

"What do birthdays, boomerangs, and Florida hospital nurses have in common? They all keep coming back"—Florida Hospital, Orlando, Florida

"Nurses get the experience of a lifetime, serving part-time in the Air Guard"—Air National Guard

"Call me in the morning, or in the evening. And, only one weekend a month"—HCA Southern Hills Medical Center, Tennessee

term recruitment success, since the individuals recruited are apt to again be drawn away when a better offer comes along.

Well-planned recruitment lays the foundation for successful implementation of the employment process in organizations. If organizations desire high productivity and retention in their staffs they must be willing to make a philosophical and financial commitment to recruiting quality staff and to creating an environment that meets their needs.

KEY CONCEPTS CHAPTER 9

1. The ability of the organization to meet its goals and objectives is directly related to the quality of the individuals it recruits and employs.

2. During periods of worker shortages, more elaborate and prolonged recruitment strategies are required to meet the demand. This requires both internal and external recruiting.

3. Nurse recruiters and nurse managers who coordinate recruitment must understand the philosophy and goals of the organization as well as the policies of the personnel department. As in all planning, these policies must be congruent with all other planning in the hierarchy.

4. There is often a pool of "inactive nurses" locally who may be recruited under the right conditions.

5. National advertising searches are expensive and time consuming but may be required when a specific target group is indicated and the applicant pool having the desired qualifications is small.

6. Research has shown that there is a relationship between the recruitment source and subsequent employee performance. Each organization must individually evaluate which recruitment sources are most productive for the organization in terms of the number of employees brought into the organization and their subsequent productivity and retention rates.

7. Retention and recruitment, although not synonymous, are very closely linked. Organizations must begin to refocus on meeting employee needs in an effort to promote retention. Satisfied, productive employees, in turn, reduce the need for future recruitment as well as create an environment that is conducive to attracting new nurses.

REFERENCES

Alderfer, C.P., and McCord, C.G., "Personal and Situational Factors in the Recruitment Interview," *Journal of Applied Psychology*, 54:377–385, 1970.

Bowin, R.B., *Human Resource Problem Solving*, Prentice-Hall, Englewood Cliffs, NJ, 1987.

Breaugh, J.A., "Relationship Between Recruiting Sources and Employee Performance, Absenteeism and Work Attitudes," *Acad. Management Journal*, 24(1):145, 1981.

Decker, P.J., and Cornelius, E.T., III, "A Note on Recruiting Sources and Job Survival Rates," *Journal of Applied Psychology*, 64:463, 1979.

Decker, P.J., Moore, R.C., Sullivan, E., "How Hospitals Can Solve the Nursing Shortage," *Hospital Health Services Administration*, 27(6):12, 1982.

Deutsch, A.R., *The Human Resources Revolution*, McGraw Hill, New York, 1979.

DiVincenti, M., *Administering Nursing Service*, Little, Brown and Company, Boston, 1972.

Ilgen, D.R., and Seely, W., "Realistic Expectations as an Aid in Reducing Voluntary Resignation," *Journal of Applied Psychology*, 59:452–455, 1974.

Lewis, E.M., and Spicer, J.G., *Human Resource Management Handbook*, Aspen Publishers, Rockville, MD, 1987.

Longo, R.A., and Uranker, M.M., "Why Nurses Stay: A Positive Approach to the Nursing Shortage," *Nursing Management*, 18(7):78–79, 1987.

Lyles, R.I., and Joiner, C., *Supervision in Health Care Organizations*, John Wiley and Sons, New York, 1986.

Marquis, B., and Huston, C., *Management Decision Making for Nurses: 101 Case Studies*, J.B. Lippincott, Philadelphia, 1987.

Milkovich, G.T., and Glueck, W.F., *Personnel/Human Resource Management: A Diagnostic Approach*, Business Publications, Plano, TX, 1985.

Nursing 88, 18(3), 1988.

Schuster, F.E., *Human Resource Management: Concepts, Cases and Readings*, Second Edition, Reston Publishing, Reston, VA, 1985.

Strauss, G., and Sayles, L.R., *Personnel: The Human Problems of Management*, Third Edition, Prentice-Hall, Englewood Cliffs, NJ, 1972.

Vogt, J.F., Cox, J.L., Velthouse, B.A., and Thames, B.H., *Retaining Professional Nurses: A Planned Process*, C.V. Mosby, St. Louis, 1983.

Wall, L.L., "Plan Development for a Nurse Recruitment-Retention Program," *JONA*, 18(2):20–26, 1988.

White, C.H., "The Shrinking Hospital Workplace," *CHA Insight*, 8(26):1, 1984.

Wolf, G.A., "Nursing Turnover: Some Causes and Solutions," *Nursing Outlook*, 29(4):233–236, 1981.

10
Interviewing

THE INTERVIEW is the most widely used method of selecting applicants for hire. Although other selection tools such as testing and reference checks are also used, the interview remains the foundation for selection.

In the last 20 years much research has been done on the validity of interviews, and the findings have led to improvement in how interviews are conducted. Although interviews will always have many pitfalls, it is possible to reduce the errors inherent in the interview process. This chapter will discuss many of the hazards of interviewing and will provide various tools that assist in eliminating or reducing these hazards.

Because there are specific questions that may not be asked during the interview, this chapter will also discuss the legal constraints of the interview. Additionally, information will be provided on interpretation, closure, and follow-up of the interview.

GOALS OF THE INTERVIEW

An interview may be defined as a verbal interaction between individuals for a particular purpose. Beach (1980) maintains that the purpose, or goals, of the selection interview are three-fold: (1) the interviewer seeks to obtain enough information about applicants to determine their suitability for the available position, (2) applicants obtain information to assist them in making an intelligent decision regarding the selection or acceptance of the job, should it be offered, and (3) the interviewer seeks to conduct the interview in such a manner that, regardless of the end result of the interview, applicants will continue to have respect and good will toward the company.

LIMITATIONS OF INTERVIEWS

The major defect of the interview is its subjectivity. The individuals making the decisions following an interview are using their own judgments, biases, and values, and they are making decisions based on a short interaction with an applicant in an unnatural situation. The applicant is trying to create a favorable impression and may be unduly influenced by the interviewer's personality. Many authorities on the interview process suggest that most candidates for employment should be interviewed more than once. One of the justifications for multiple interviews is that the interview itself, although widely used, is full of hazards.

The research findings on the validity and reliability of interviews have not been consistent. However, the following results have been found repeatedly (Bouchard, 1976; Ghiselli, 1966; Jablin, 1975; Mayfield, 1964):

1. The same interviewer will consistently rate the same interviewee the same. Therefore, the *intra-rater reliability* is said to be high.

2. If two different interviewers conduct an unstructured interview of the same applicant, they will not have consistent ratings. Therefore, the *inter-rater reliability* is extremely low in unstructured interviews.

3. *Inter-rater reliability* is satisfactory if the interview is structured and the same interview format is used by both interviewers.

4. Even if the interview has *reliability* (i.e., it measures the same thing consistently), it still may not be valid. *Validity* occurs when the interview measures what it is supposed to measure, which in this case is a potential productive employee.

5. High *interview assessments* are not related to subsequent high-level performance on the job.

6. *Validity* increases when there is a team approach to the interview.

7. The attitudes and *biases* of interviewers have a great influence on how candidates are rated, and although methods can be taken to reduce *subjectivity*, it cannot be entirely eliminated.

8. The interviewer is more influenced by unfavorable than by favorable information. In other words, *negative information is weighed more heavily* than positive information about the applicant.

9. Interviewers tend to make up their minds regarding hiring applicants very early in the job interview. *Decisions are often formed in the first few minutes of the interview.*

10. In *unstructured interviews the interviewer tends to do most of the talking*, while in structured interviews the interviewer does only about 50% to 60% of the talking.

Regardless of its pitfalls, interviewing remains a widely used and accepted method of selecting from among many applicants for a limited number of positions. By knowing the limitations of interviews and by using the knowledge obtained from current research, the manager should be able to conduct interviews in such a manner that they will have a positive and predictive value.

OVERCOMING INTERVIEW LIMITATIONS

Interview research has been very helpful to managers because the findings have allowed them to develop strategies to overcome many of the limitations inherent in the interview. The following guidelines will assist the manager in developing an interview process that results in increased reliability and validity:

1. *Develop a structured interview format for each job classification.* Because each job has different position requirements, structured interviews must be tailored to fit the position. The same structured interview should be used for all employees applying for the same job classification. A good structured interview uses open-ended questions and provides ample opportunity for the interviewee to talk. The advantage of the structured interview is that it allows the interviewer to be consistent and prevents the interview from becoming sidetracked. Tool 10-1 is an example of a structured interview.

2. *Conduct multiple interviews.* Having more than one person interview the job applicant reduces the bias that is the

(Text continued on p. 176)

Tool 10-1   The Structured Interview

Motivation
Why did you apply for employment with this company?

Physical
Do you have any limitations that might prohibit you from accomplishing the job? If so, what are they?

How many days have you been absent from work during the last year of employment?

Education
What was your grade-point average in the last school setting you attended?

What were your favorite and least-liked subjects?

What were your extracurricular activities? Offices held?

For verification purposes, are your school records listed under the name on your application form?

Professional
In what states are you licensed to practice?

Do you have a copy of your license with you to show us?

What certifications do you hold?

In what professional organizations do you currently participate that would be of value in the job you are applying for?

Military experience
What military assignments do you think would be of value for you in applying for this job (if in the military service)?

What are your current military obligations?

Present employer
How did you secure you present position?

What is your current job title, and what was your job title when you began your present job?

What supervisory responsibilities do you currently have?

How would you describe your immediate supervisor?

What are some examples of the success that you have achieved at your present job?

How do you get along with your present employer?

How would you describe how you get along with your present peer group?

What do you like least about your present job?

What do you like most about your present job?

May we contact your present employer?

Why do you want to change jobs?

For verification purposes only, is your name the same as it was while employed with your current employer?

Previous positions
Similar questions should be asked about the employment that occurred just prior to the present employment, depending on the time span and type of other positions held in the past. The interviewer does not usually go back to review employment history that took place beyond the position just prior to the current one.

Specific questions for registered nurses
What do you like most about nursing?

What do you like least about nursing?

What is your philosophy of nursing?

Personal characteristics
What personal characteristics are your greatest assets?

What personal characteristics cause you the most difficulty?

Professional goals
What are your career goals for the future?

Where do you see yourself ten years from now?

Contributions to organization
What do you feel you have to offer this organization?

Questions for interviewer
What questions do you have about the organization?

What questions do you have about the position?

What other questions do you have?

Evaluation
Note: Comments evaluating the applicant should be objective and relate to the applicant's qualification for the position for which he or she is being interviewed.

normal part of individual personalities. For this technique to be most effective, the applicant should be interviewed on two separate days. This prevents the interviewee from being accepted or rejected merely because he or she was having a good or bad day.

3. *Use a team approach.* Many organizations use a hiring committee or a hiring panel to interview job applicants. This can become expensive for the personnel department, since it involves much employee time. Organizations need to weigh the amount of time involved in the personnel interview process with the outcomes. If attrition rates are particularly high, an organization should look very carefully at the process used for selection.

4. *All individuals performing interviews should be given some training in the technique of effective interviewing.* The training should include skills in communication, as well as advice on planning, conducting, and controlling the interview. It is unfair to expect head nurses to make appropriate hiring decisions based on interviews if they have never had adequate training in interview techniques. Vogt and associates (1983) maintain that practice in interview techniques should be part of any management training program.

PLANNING, CONDUCTING, AND CONTROLLING THE INTERVIEW

Planning the interview will help make it successful. Decide what type of interview format is to be used and make sure that if others are to be present they will be available at the appointed time. Allow adequate time for the interview. The application should be thoroughly reviewed and notes made of any questions concerning information on the application. Although it takes considerable practice, the consistent use of a planned sequence in the interview format will eventually yield a relaxed and spontaneous process. The following is a suggested format for the interview:

1. Introductions and greetings

2. A brief statement about the company and about the positions that are available

3. Have the applicant state what position(s) he or she desires

4. Discussion of the application and clarification or amplification of information on the application

5. Discussion of employee's qualifications and other factors and considerations of employment

6. If the applicant appears qualified, more specific discussion about the company and the position

7. Discussion and arrangement of subsequent procedures for hiring (e.g., employment physical, hiring date). If the applicant is not hired at this time, discuss how he or she will be notified of the result of the interview and when.

8. Termination of the interview

If you have achieved a good opening and managed to put the applicant at ease, the interview will usually proceed smoothly. As you are conducting the interview, be sure that you pause frequently to allow the applicant to ask questions. Your interview format should always include ample time for questions from the applicant, and such questions should be encouraged. The interviewer can often gain much insight about the applicant by the types of questions that he or she puts forth.

Keeping the conversation going, covering the questions on the structured interview guide, and keeping the interview pertinent, but friendly, becomes easier with experience. Methods that appear to be effective in reaching the goals of the interview are as follows:

1. Use open-ended questions that require more than a yes-or-no answer.

2. Pause a few seconds after the applicant has seemingly finished before asking the next question. This gives the applicant a chance to talk further.

3. Return later in the interview to topics the applicant offered little information on initially.

4. Ask only one question at a time.

5. Restate part of the applicant's statement in a question if you seek elaboration. For instance, if the applicant stated, "I did not like my former employer because the agency had a low RN staffing ratio," you could repeat in a questioning tone, "The hospital had a low RN staffing ratio?"

6. Ask questions clearly, but do not indicate what the correct answer is, either verbally or nonverbally. The astute job applicant learns to watch for nonverbal clues. By watching the interviewer's eyes and observing other body language, the interviewee learns which answers are desired.

7. The interviewer's manner should always reflect interest. The interview should never be interrupted, and the interviewer's words should never imply criticism of, or impatience with, the applicant.

8. The more personal questions in an interview should come later in the interview, after a rapport has been established.

9. Language should be used that is appropriate for the applicant. Do not use terminology or language that makes applicants feel you are either "talking down" to them or talking "over their heads."

Tool 10-2 lists sample questions that may be used in an interview, with an explanation of the importance of the question.

A written record should be kept of all interviews. Note-taking is necessary to ensure accuracy, as well as to serve as a written record to use to recall the applicant. It is advisable to keep the note-taking or use of a check list to a minimum so that an uncomfortable climate is not created.

As the interview draws to a close, the interviewer should check that all questions have been answered and that all pertinent information has been obtained. Usually an applicant is not offered a job at the end of an evaluation interview unless he or she is clearly qualified and the labor market is such that another applicant would be difficult to find. In most cases the interviewer needs to analyze his or her impressions of the applicant, compare these perceptions with those of other members of the selection team, and incorporate those impressions with other available data about the applicant. Frequently, the interviewer needs to consult with others in the organization before a job offer can be made. It is important, however, to let applicants know if they are being seriously considered for the position and how soon they can expect to hear the final outcome of the job interviews.

When it is obvious that the applicant is not qualified, the interviewer needs to be extremely tactful in advising the individual that he or she does not have the proper qualifications for the position. It is important that such applicants not feel they have been treated unfairly, and the interviewer should maintain records of the exact reasons for rejection in case of later charges of discrimination.

EVALUATION OF THE INTERVIEW

The interviewer should build into the plan additional time post-interview to evaluate the applicant's interview performance. Often notes are taken in a shorthand style, which becomes

Tool 10-2   How to Develop an Interview Guide

Note: All questions on the application form and questions asked at the interview should have a specific purpose. Application forms and structured interviews should be reviewed periodically and revised as necessary. Some examples of questions and explanations for their inclusion are given below. Managers should be able to provide similar explanations for all questions on their application forms and all questions asked at the interview.

Question: *How did you hear about us?*
> This question might be asked to gather statistics that would identify the effectiveness of various recruiting methods used by the organization. If the organization is having difficulty with recruitment or wants to know what recruitment method is producing the best results, then this would be an important question to include on the application form or at the interview.

Question: *Is there any reason why you might not be able to work on a regular schedule?*
> By asking this question the interviewer is able to elicit information that would indicate any possible impediments to dependable attendance. The information could have relevance to shift assignments.

Question: *In what community and/or professional activities are you involved?*
> The interviewer may find this information helpful in identifying leadership capabilities in applicants. Additionally, this question may serve to create a common ground of communication and induce a more relaxed atmosphere in which to conduct the interview.

Question: *What kind of references do you expect to get from your previous employers?*
> This question should be asked to give the applicant the opportunity to discuss any possible problems that might be expected in obtaining references.

Question: *What was your attendance record at your previous job?*
> Due to the necessity for dependability required in most health care organizations, the interviewer should be interested in

soliciting information about past attendance. Asking this question also provides the applicant an opportunity to discuss any previous attendance problems and state if these have been resolved.

---

difficult to read at a later date. To avoid this problem, the notes taken during the interview should be reviewed, and, where necessary, clarified or amplified. It is advisable to use some type of form to record the interview evaluation. An example of such a form is shown in Tool 10-3. The final question on the interview report form is a recommendation for or against hiring. In answering this question, two things carry the most weight:

1. *The requirements for the job.* Regardless of how interesting or friendly an applicant is, without the basic skills for the job he or she will not be successful at meeting the expectations of the position. Likewise, someone who is overqualified for a position will usually be unhappy in the job.

2. *Personal bias.* Since it is impossible to eliminate completely the personal biases of the interviewer, it is important that the interviewer examine any negative feelings that came up during the interview. Often, when they are analyzed, the interviewer will discover that such negative feelings have no relation to the criteria necessary for success in the position.

LEGAL ASPECTS OF INTERVIEWING

The organization must ascertain that its application form does not contain questions that violate various employment acts. Likewise, managers must avoid any unlawful inquiries during the interview. In addition to federal legislation, many states have specific laws pertaining to information that can lawfully be obtained during interviews. New York state prohibits asking-about a woman's ability to reproduce or her attitudes toward family planning. Table 10-1 lists those subjects that are most frequently a part of the interview process or application form, with examples of both acceptable and unacceptable inquiries.

Occasionally, reference checks will reveal unsolicited, potentially negative information regarding an applicant. It is important to note that information you receive should be used only if

---

Tool 10-3   Sample Interview Evaluation Form

Interviewer's recommendation about applicant

Interviewer #1 _____

_____

_____

_____   Accept _____ Reject _____

Pending_____

Date_____   Interviewer's signature _____

Interviewer #2 _____

_____

_____   Accept _____ Reject _____

Pending_____

Date_____   Interviewer's signature _____

---

it is applicable and relevant to the job requirements. For example, if the applicant volunteers information that he or she has credit problems, or if this information is discovered by other means, it cannot be used to reject that potential employee. In this example, the applicant could justifiably be disqualified on the basis of this information only if the position required someone with a good credit rating.

Managers who maintain records of their interviews and who receive each applicant with an open and unbiased attitude will

Table 10-1. Legal Interview Inquiries

Subject	Acceptable Inquiries	Unacceptable Inquiries
Name	Have you ever worked for this company under a different name? Are your school records under another name? Have you ever been convicted of a crime under another name?	Inquiries about name that would indicate lineage, national origin, or marital status
Marital and family status	Whether applicant can meet specified work schedules or has commitments that may hinder attendance requirements; inquiries as to anticipated stay on the job	Any inquiry asking applicant's marital status, number or age of children; information of child care arrangements; any questions concerning pregnancy
Address or residence	Place of residence and length resided in city or state	Former addresses; names or relationship of persons with whom applicant resides or if owns or rents home
Age	If over age 18 or statement that hire is subject to age requirement; can ask if they are between 18 and 70	Inquiry of specific age or date of birth
Birthplace	Can ask for proof of U.S. citizenship	Birthplace of applicant or spouse or any relative
Religion	No inquiries allowed	
Race or color	Can be requested for affirmative action but not as employment criteria	All questions about race are prohibited.
Character	Inquiry into actual convictions that relate to fitness to perform job	Inquiries relating to arrests
Relatives	Relatives employed in company; names and addresses of parents if applicant is a minor	With whom do you reside? Do you live with your parents? Number of dependents
Notice in case of emergency	Name and address of a *person* to be notified	Name and address of a *relative* to be notified
Organizations	What professional organizations do you belong to?	Requesting a list of all memberships
References	Professional and/or character references	Religious reference
Physical condition	All applicants can be asked if they are able to carry out the physical demands of the job.	Employers must be prepared to justify any mental or physical requirements. Specific questions regarding handicaps are forbidden.
Photographs	Statement that a photograph may be required *after* employment	Requirement that a photograph be taken prior to interview or hiring

National origin	Languages applicant speaks, reads, or writes (if necessary to perform job)	Inquiries about birthplace, native language, ancestry, etc.; date of arrival in U.S. or, "What is your mother tongue?"
Education	Academic, vocational, or professional education; schools attended; ability to read, speak and write foreign languages	Inquiries into racial or religious affiliation of a school; inquiry into dates of schooling
Sex	Inquiry or restriction of employment is only for bona fide occupational qualification, which is interpreted very narrowly by the courts	

have little to fear regarding charges of discrimination. Remember, the third goal of the interview process is for each applicant to feel good about the company when the interview is over; regardless of the final outcome of the interview, each applicant and interviewer should remember the experience as a positive one.

KEY CONCEPTS CHAPTER 10

1. Interviews are widely used as a method of selecting which applicants to hire.
2. The interview should meet the goals of the applicant as well as those of the manager.
3. Interviews have many limitations and are not always reliable or valid.
4. There are many proven ways to overcome the limitations of interviews.
5. The structured interview reduces some of the bias in the interview process.
6. It is important that the manager have skill in planning, conducting, and controlling the interview.
7. Applicants should be evaluated in some written form as soon as possible following the interview.
8. Due to numerous federal acts that protect the rights of individuals seeking jobs, managers must be cognizant of the legal constraints of interviews.

REFERENCES

Beach, D.S., *Personnel: The Management of People at Work*, Fourth Edition, Macmillan, New York, 1980.

Bouchard, T.J., "Field Research Methods: Interviewing Questionnaires, Participant Observation, Systematic Observation, Unobtrusive Methods," Dunnette, M.D. (ed.), *Handbook of Industrial and Organizational Psychology,* Rand McNally, Chicago, 1976.

Ghiselli E.E., "The Validity of the Personnel Interview," *Personnel Psychology*, 19(4):389–394, 1966.

Jablin, F., "The Selection Interview: Contingency Theory and Beyond," *Human Resource Management* 4(1):243–249, 1975.

Marquis, B.L., and Huston, C.J., *Management Decision Making for Nurses: 101 Case Studies*, J.B. Lippincott, Philadelphia, 1987.

Mayfield, E.C., "The Selection Interview: A Re-evaluation of Published Research," *Personnel Psychology* 17(2):239–260, 1964.

Vogt, J.F., Cox, J.L., Velthouse, B.A., and Tyhames, B.H., *Retaining Professional Nurses*, C.V. Mosby, St. Louis, 1983.

ADDITIONAL READINGS

Goodale, J.G., *The Fine Art of Interviewing*, Prentice-Hall, Englewood Cliffs, NJ, 1982.

Lopez, F.M., *Personnel Interviewing: Theory and Practice*, Second Edition, McGraw-Hill, New York, 1975.

Minner, M.G., and Miner, J.B., *Employee Selection Within the Law*, Bureau of National Affairs, Washington D.C., 1978.

Robertson, D.E., "New Directions in EEO Guidelines." *Personnel* 57:360, 1978.

Rogers, J.L., and Fortson, W.L., *Fair Employment Interviewing*, Addison-Wesley, Reading, MA, 1976.

Sullivan, E.J., and Decker, P.J., *Effective Management in Nursing*, Addison-Wesley, Menlo Park, CA, 1985.

11

Selection and Placement

SELECTION IS the process of choosing the best qualified individual(s) for a particular position or job from a group of applicants. Selection assumes knowledge of the organization, its jobs, its philosophy and mission, and its atmosphere (Vogt et al., 1983).

Selection, as the last step in the employment process, can be successful only if recruitment and interviewing have been done appropriately. Successful recruitment yields an adequate pool of qualified applicants. A carefully implemented interview process provides invaluable feedback to both the employer and the applicant regarding the expectations of the position and the unique strengths, weaknesses, needs, and desires of each applicant. Some employers choose to elicit feedback for selection decisions other than that obtained in the interview process. One such method of feedback is pre-employment testing. The information gathered in interviewing and testing is then used to select the employee whose talents best match the job requirements.

Legal issues greatly affecting employee selection, such as affirmative action hiring and equal opportunity employment, have already been covered in Chapter 8. Thus, Chapter 11 will examine selection procedures aimed at matching applicant qualifications and job requirements. The use of preemployment testing will be discussed in detail, including the current legal implications of such testing. The paperwork and documentation involved in employee selection will also be discussed, and suggestions for streamlining the application process will be given. Lastly, the obligations of the organization and the employee in the selection process will be compared. Tools for implementation include assessment questions to be used by the organization and individuals involved in making selection decisions to evaluate the selection process and a listing of some commonly used preemployment testing materials.

SELECTION AS A TOOL FOR INCREASING PRODUCTIVITY

The first step in achieving excellence in human resource management is to hire the right person for the right job; that is, to match the person's abilities, motivations, interests, and skills with the demands of the job and the "personality" or climate of the work group and company (Kern et al., 1987). This is not an easy process and, in fact, much of the waste and mismanagement of human resources can be attributed to mistakes made in the selection process. The organization must pay the price for selection of inappropriate personnel in terms of financial costs (recruitment, orientation, salaries and benefits, turnover, etc.) as well as the cost of time and motivation of other employees. Attempting to "make the mismatched employee fit the job" requires endless hours of unrewarded supervisory time and reduces personal and department morale as well as productivity.

Research has shown that the selection procedure utilized in the hiring of employees may be related to or predictive of subsequent work behavior in the employee. Schmidt and associates (1979) demonstrated that using work-related selection procedures can result in significant improvements (up to 40%) in productivity and financial rewards.

THE SELECTION PROCESS

Figure 11-1 illustrates a typical selection process. The applicant pool is generated in response to recruitment and should yield an

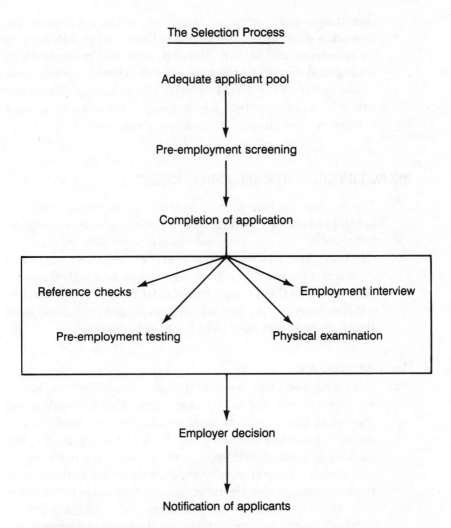

FIGURE 11-1. *The selection process*

adequate number of qualified and motivated applicants. The applicant pool then undergoes pre-employment screening. This screening typically is done on a one-on-one basis (although it may be done in small groups) and involves the employer sharing information about minimum qualifications needed of potential applicants, as well as a brief outline of employer expectations for a given position. If both the employee and employer feel that there is a match between expectations, the potential employee should continue through to completion of the application. Information given in the application is then used in following up on references and in the interview process. Pre-employment testing and physical examinations are other screening tools utilized prior to the actual selection of the best-qualified individual for a given position. The last step of the selection process is employer decision and notification of applicants.

THE PAPER TRAIL OF THE SELECTION PROCESS

The selector has four primary sources of information available to utilize in the selection process. These include the application form and/or résumé, interview impressions, test results, and references from past employers (Vogt et al., 1983). No one source of information should be given sole weight or weighed disproportionately in the selection decision. Of these four sources, two compose most of the paper trail. These are the application form and/or résumé, and references from past employers.

The Application Form

The application blank is one of the oldest procedures in personnel selection and is used by most employers. A well-designed application blank requires applicants to organize data in a format that helps to eliminate generalities and fuzzy details. The application form should request information about the applicant's work history such as titles, duties, salaries, dates, names, and addresses. It also should request demographic information such as social security, driver's license, and nursing license numbers. Lastly, the application should request the educational history, degrees, and addresses (Lotito and Kostenbauer, 1981).

The application form must also meet federal and state laws and guidelines and *cannot* include items that are discriminatory in nature or application, that could be interpreted as disproportionately screening out members of a minority group or specific gender, or that are not valid predictors of successful job performance (Miller, 1980).

The wise manager should remember that in the pressure to obtain a job, some individuals will provide false or misleading information on the application blank. Goldstein (1971) found

that almost two thirds of applications held inaccurate information primarily in the areas of duration of previous employment
and previous salary earned. All information given on the application blank should be reverified in the interview and through
references.

The application form can also provide subtle information to
the employer regarding the applicant's accuracy, attention to
detail, clarity, organization, honesty, conciseness of expression,
and neatness. In fact, the application form often provides the
employer with the first impression of the potential employee.

The Résumé

In hospitals, résumés are ranked second only to interviews as
the most important screening mechanism to help employers
make hiring decisions (Lotito and Kostenbauer, 1981). The
résumé is used primarily to summarize employee education and
experience. It is important for the selector to assess past work
experience in terms of the depth and range of responsibility the
applicant had in former jobs, the length of time employed at
those jobs, evidence of career progression, and the relevance of
skills obtained or demonstrated in employment prior to the
current position. For novice nurses, the selector should consider
the educational preparation of the nurse in terms of the quality
of the nursing curriculum, grade-point average achieved in nursing courses and cumulatively, and the reputation of the school
for producing quality graduates.

It is more difficult for the manager to draw clues about the
organizational skills, creativity, and writing skills of the prospective employee from the résumé than from the application blank.
This is because résumés are increasingly written by professional
employment consultants whose writing skills may exceed those
of their clients (Bowin, 1987). All résumés should be preceded by
a cover letter introducing the applicant and specifying the job
that is being sought, the applicant's qualifications for that job,
and available times for the follow-up interview. Determining
which applicant has the best fit with a particular job (i.e., skill,
aptitude, experience) is generally done using the application,
references, and results of pre-employment occupational skill
testing. The match between the applicant and the social and
climatic aspects of the position (i.e., personal characteristics,

leadership skills, motivation, and interpersonal relationships) should generally be judged by the interview and/or psychological testing (Lorsch and Morse, 1976).

References

Traditionally, as part of the selection process, applicants have submitted names of references who could supply information about their past performances at certain jobs or their potential abilities to function in specific positions. These references should be considered an important source of information for the organization, and all references should be followed up and verified.

Lewis and Spicer (1987) identified six points that should be examined in both verbal and written references:

1. Data from the application blank should be compared with reference information for congruence.

2. The applicant's performance in previous positions should be compared to the actual job expectations of those positions.

3. The reference should be reviewed in terms of the interview format questions used. Is the reference congruent with the applicant's interview response?

4. What is the relationship between the applicant and the person giving the reference? How long has that person known the applicant?

5. The reference should be used to check absenteeism, attendance, and tardiness.

6. The candidate's reasons for leaving the last position should be assessed.

Although references can provide valuable information in the selection process, the wise employer will keep in mind that the use of references as a valid selection tool is unproven. Research has demonstrated their rather low correlation with job success. However, correlation does increase somewhat in the case of unstructured letters of recommendation requested from employers, as opposed to the use of a standardized questionnaire (Bowin, 1987).

Many reference letters received about applicants offer little helpful information in the selection decision. Often, reference letters are not tailored to the specific job the applicant is seeking. Other problems with validity occur because most applicants volunteer only references who perceived their prior performance in a positive manner. Likewise, many individuals writing references are reluctant to discuss negative aspects of the applicant because they fear that the applicant will read the references (Milkovich and Glueck, 1985). This fear is not unfounded; the Privacy Act of 1974 gave applicants the right to examine reference letters concerning themselves unless they give up the right to do so (Milkovich and Glueck, 1985). Because of legal fears of slander or defamation, many employers will give only limited objective reference information about previous employees, such as dates of employment and verification of salary. The hiring organization should obtain written permission from applicants to check prior work references.

Prudent managers will quickly learn to "read between the lines" on letters of reference, although managers must always be cautious in their interpretations. Individuals making selection decisions should be suspect of purposefully vague or superficial references. Ambiguous language often covers weaknesses. For example, a 1962 study by Peres and Garcia (1962) found that "congenial" and "cooperative" were the most frequently used adjectives in reference letters to describe inept behavior and lack of ability. Reference letters with any overt criticism should be taken very seriously. Managers may gain more information about a prospective employee by what is not written in reference letters than by what is.

The manager who is unsure of the accuracy of what he or she has perceived in a letter of reference is encouraged to clarify these perceptions either through telephone follow-up or, when possible, in person. Although there is little motivation to tell the truth to strangers, many organizations with applicants from the same industry develop reciprocal confidential relationships with other organizations (Mandell, 1964). The prudent supervisor will work to establish such relationships with other health care agencies in the area as well as regional schools of nursing.

The paper trail is complicated because of the amount of information that must be gathered and processed for each applicant. Unfortunately, the paper trail often becomes even more complex and time consuming because organizations are not selective about which potential employees should complete the entire application process. Employee selection programs should be based on the "successive hurdles technique" (Beach, 1975).

This means that, to be hired, applicants must successfully pass each and every screening device (e.g., application blank, interview, pre-employment testing, physical examinations). Candidates who do not meet or who exceed the requirements of a hurdle should be rejected at that hurdle.

For example, all applications should be screened for completeness and for confirmation that the applicant is qualified for the position *prior* to the scheduling of interviews. References should be requested and former employment verified. Completion of these steps prior to interviewing and selection are important so that valuable supervisory and applicant time are not wasted when applicants are inadequately qualified or are inappropriate for a position. The practice of interviewing candidates who do not meet all the selection criteria is not cost effective for the organization or fair to the applicant.

PRE-EMPLOYMENT TESTING AS A SELECTION TOOL

In an effort to reduce subjectivity in the selection process, many employers have begun utilizing pre-employment tests as a more objective means of predicting future work performance and success. Pre-employment testing is utilized as part of the selection process only when testing has a direct relationship to the ability to perform a specific job. When it is included, the testing generally consists of standardized tests that have been developed by personnel departments in large-scale organizations (Lyles and Joiner, 1986). The items on the test must specifically relate to actual job qualifications. General knowledge tests are inappropriate unless the general knowledge covered in the test directly relates to the requirements of a specific job (Lyles and Joiner, 1986).

Two types of pre-employment testing are actually incorporated with the application form. These include the biographical information blank (BIB) and the weighted application blank (WAB) (Milkovich and Glueck, 1985). The BIB asks multiple-choice questions, asking opinions about values, interests, attitudes, hobbies, social relations, and health, followed by multiple-choice answers. The employer correlates each item on the form with measures of job success. Those items that predict the best outcome for a position are used to help select applicants for that position.

The WAB is a scored application form that relates the characteristics of applicants to success on the job. Each organization looks at its current employees and divides them into arbitrary groups such as high-, middle-, or low-level achievers. Characteristics of high-, middle-, and low-level performers in the organization are then identified, and applicants are weighted according to these characteristics. For example, an applicant might be weighted 0 (showing no difference) in mathematical accuracy compared to a specific level of performer. The weights then are totaled for all applicants, and the one with the highest positive score is hired (Milkovich and Glueck, 1985). The WAB is also used in determining salary increases, absenteeism, and job turnover (Bowin, 1987).

Other pre-employment tests include ability tests, which assess the individual's aptitudes and achievements (Hunter and Schmidt, 1982). Aptitudes are personal characteristics that give an indication of an individual's potential to acquire a skill with training or education (Milkovich and Glueck, 1985). Examples of aptitudes that can be measured include perceptual accuracy, cognitive abilities, spatial and mechanical ability, and psychomotor skills. Achievement tests measure the effects of training and experience, such as the learning acquired in apprenticeship training or in specific courses (Milkovich and Glueck, 1985). In contrast to aptitude testing, achievement testing examines what the individual already knows and focuses on measuring the knowledge presumed necessary for specific work behaviors.

Personality tests were not originally designed for use in employment selection, and their validity as predictors of job performance has not been well established (Cronbach and Schaeffer, 1981). Interest tests assess applicant preferences and interests. Although interests tests are not usually utilized as a selection tool, employers may use their results to match employee wants and likes with the most appropriate department within the organization.

The types and numbers of pre-employment tests used as selection tools are immense. Tool 11-1 presents a very limited list of some ability, achievement, personality, and interest tests utilized in the selection process.

Pre-employment testing, when implemented properly and for appropriate reasons, can be a valid and useful predictor of

(Text continued on p. 199)

Tool 11-1 Sample Pre-employment Tests

Ability tests

Aptitude Tests

1. Job Tests Program; 1947–81
   Joseph E. King and H.B. Osborn, Jr.
   Industrial Psychology, Inc.
   515 Madison Ave.
   New York, NY

   This aptitude-intelligence test is composed of a series of 15 tests measuring aptitudes such as judgment, fluency, memory, precision, dexterity, motor skills, perception, and numbers.

2. ETSA (formerly called Apitest); 1959–1984
   S. Trevor Hadley and George A.W. Stouffer, Jr.
   Psychological Services Bureau
   Educators-Employer's Tests and Services Associates
   P.O. Box 4
   St. Thomas, PA 17252

3. The Adherence to Chain-of Command Scale
   Larry Wigdor/Bernard M. Baruch College
   R.J. House, Faculty of Management Studies
   Univ. of Toronto, 246 Bloor St. West
   Toronto 181
   Ontario, Canada

   This test measures the effectiveness of various management and organizational characteristics on employee satisfaction and performance as a function of the employee's need for independence.

4. Nursing Orientation Survey (N.O.S); 1972
   Thomas C. Greening
   Psychological Services Association
   1314 Westwood Blvd.
   Los Angeles, CA 90024

   This test measures attitudes regarding the role of feelings in nursing situations and was designed primarily for assessing and creating sensitivity among nurses to the feeling dimension of their interactions with patients.

5. Mental Health Professional's Responses
   to the Mentally Ill Questionnaire; 1971

Mel Karmen
Mental Health Rehabilitation and Research, Inc.
Hill House
Cleveland, OH, 44130

This instrument was designed to measure the reactions of mental health professionals to potential clients. The questionnaire was designed primarily to understand the nature of the initial response by professionals to potential clients and the relationship of this response to other variables.

6. George Washington University Series Nursing Tests; 1931–1950
Thelma Hunt
Center for Psychological Service
1835 Eye Street N.W.
Washington, DC 20006

This series is composed of the following five tests for prospective nurses:

1. Aptitude test for nurses, F.A. Moss, 1931–1950
2. Arithmetic test for prospective nurses, 1940–1950
3. Reading comprehension test for prospective nurses, 1940–1950
4. General science test for prospective nurses, 1944–1950
5. Interest preference test for prospective nurses, 1944–1950

7. Nurse Attitudes Inventory (NAI); 1965–1970
John R.Thurston, Helen L. Brunclik, and John F. Feldhusen
Nursing Research Associates
3752 Cummings St.
Eau Claire, WI 54701

This multiple-choice test is based on Luther Hospital sentence completions. The nine scores measure attitudes: nursing, self, home-family, responsibility, others-love, marriage, and academics. (May no longer be in print.)

Achievement Tests

1. Scale for Evaluating Health Service Professionals
Gary B. Brumback and M.A. Howell
Office of Personnel Training, Policy and Evaluation Division
330 Independence Ave, S.W.
Rm 4273, N. Building
Washington, D.C., 20201

This achievement test consists of performance rating scales that were developed as part of a Public Health Service project to evaluate performance in health-related work functions.

2. Quick Word Test; 1957–1978
   Edgar F. Borgatta and Raymond J. Corsini
   F.E. Peacock Publishers Test Division
   Itasca, IL 60143

   This 100-item test measures verbal ability. It is highly reliable and correlates reasonably well with other group and individual intelligence tests.

3. Iowa Tests of Educational Development (ITED)
   Science Research Associates
   115 N. Wacker Drive, PO Box 5380
   Chicago, IL 60680-5380

   The ITED attempts to measure broad intellectual skills and interests, and understanding of and ability to use what has been learned, rather than mastery of standard subject material or knowledge of specific facts.

Personality tests

1. Guilford-Zimmerman Temperament Survey; 1949–1978
   J.P. Guilford and W.S. Zimmerman
   Sheridan Psychological Services, Inc.
   P.O. Box 6101
   Orange, CA 92667

   This test measures personality traits including general activity, restraint, aggressiveness, sociability, emotional stability, objectiveness, friendliness, etc.

2. Work Values Inventory (WVI); 1968–1970
   Donald E. Super/Teachers College
   Riverside Publishing Company
   8420 Bryn Mawr Ave.
   Chicago, IL 60631

   The WVI assesses goals and values that affect the motivation to work. It also measures the satisfactions that men and women seek in work and the satisfaction that may be the concomitant or outcome of work.

3. The Response to Power Measure (RPM); 1972
   Arthur B. Sweney
   Center for Human Appraisal and Communication Research
   Wichita State University
   Wichita, KS 67208

   The RPM measures superior and subordinate role performance. It enables the prediction of superordinate and subordinate role behaviors resulting from various combinations of the superordinate-subordinate role types.

4. Edwards Personal Preference Schedule; 1954, 1959
A.L. Edwards
The Psychological Corporation
7500 Old Oak Blvd.
Cleveland, OH 44130

The EPPS was developed primarily as an instrument for research and counseling purposes that provides quick and convenient measures of a number of relatively independent, normal personality variables. This test features a forced-choice item format designed to control the social desirability of items.

5. Minnesota Multiphasic Personality Inventory; 1940
S.R. Hathaway and J.C. McKinley
University of Minnesota Press – 1943
Psychological Corporation – 1945
7500 Old Oak Blvd.
Cleveland, OH 44130

This test measures both personality integration and traits as they relate to vocational choice and adjustment.

6. Myer Briggs Type Indicator (MBTI); 1943–1976
Katharine Briggs and Isabel Briggs Myer
Consulting Psychologists Press, Inc.
577 College Ave.
Palo Alto, CA 94306

This test provides scores in four areas:
1. Extraversion vs. introversion
2. Sensation vs. intuition
3. Thinking vs. feeling
4. Judgment vs. perception

Interest tests

1. Brook Reaction Test of Interests; 1968–1969
A.W. Heim, K.P. Watts, and V. Simmonds
NFER–Nelson Publishing Co. Ltd.
Darville House, 2 Oxford Rd. East
Windsor, Berkshire SL4 1DF
England

This test measures vocational interests as well as temperamental predisposition. It is used for vocational and educational guidance.

2. J II – CAL Occupational Interests Guide; 1980
   P.R. MacClean and M.V. Walker
   Hodder and Stoughton Educational
   P.O. Box 702, Dunton Green
   Sevenoaks, Kent TN
   England
   This test measures the examinee's preference among work activities.

3. Job Activity Preference Questionnaire; 1972–1981
   Robert C. Mecham, Alma F. Harris, Ernest J. McCormick, and P.R. Jeanneret
   PAQ Services Inc.
   1625 North 1000 East
   Logan, UT 84321
   This test measures vocational preferences and experience.

4. Strong-Campbell Interest Inventory; 1927–1981
   E.K. Strong. Revised by D.P. Campbell.
   Stanford University Press
   Distributor: Consulting Psychological Press, Inc.
   577 College Ave.
   Palo Alto, CA 94306

   This test is one of the oldest and most well-established interest inventories and predicts adjustment to dozens of occupations. Scores are expressed in terms of the similarity of the applicant's interests to the interests of people in each occupation and groups of occupations, and measures the individual's likes, dislikes, or indifference to certain activities, school subjects, behaviors of people, and jobs.

5. Kuder Preference Record – Vocational; 1934–1976
   Science Research Associates
   115 N. Wacker Drive, P.O. Box 5380
   Chicago, IL 60680-5380

   The Kuder Preference Record is a commonly used test that scores for ten broad interest areas of clusters. Profiles for a considerable number of occupations have been developed empirically in terms of these ten interest areas.

References

Comrey, A.L., Backer, T.E., and Glaser, E.M., *A Sourcebook for Mental Health Measures*, Report to the National Institute of Mental Health, Human Interaction Research Institute, Los Angeles, CA, 1973.

Mandell, M.M., *The Selection Process: Choosing the Right Man for the Job*, American Management Association, New York, 1964.

Mitchell, J. (ed.), *Tests in Print III*, Buros Institute of Mental Measurements, Univ. of Nebraska Press, Lincoln, NB, 1983.

Mitchell, J. (ed.), *The Ninth Mental Measurements Yearbook*, Univ. of Nebraska Press, Lincoln, NB, 1985.

Super, D.E., and Crites, J.O., *Appraising Vocational Fitness by Means of Psychological Tests*, Revised Edition, Harper and Row, New York, 1962.

Zachai, J., Test Officer, California State University, Chico, CA.

---

future job performance (Sackett and Wilson, 1982). When several of the tests are administered together in a battery, their usefulness and validity are greater than when individual tests are utilized.

Legally, however, improper implementation and interpretation of pre-employment testing has been alleged. Suits have been brought against employers who utilized pre-employment testing, charging that the testing discriminated against certain employees in some specific way. Some have charged that certain tests are standardized for only a specific gender or nationality. Other suits have claimed that the very essence of pre-employment testing violates the constitutional right to privacy or that the interpretation of testing results requires high-level testing expertise and education, which is not available in most health care organizations.

Many of these concerns were legitimized by the 1964 Duke Power vs. Griggs landmark legal decision, which required "test validation" prior to test use (Kern et al., 1987). Test validation is a procedure that measures the relationship between the test being used and some criteria for success. Profiles of success must be based on the performance of current employees; test results of new applicants can then be compared against this profile and the probability of "likeness" calculated.

The use of testing as a selection tool is currently gaining popularity in major corporations, since it increases the odds of hiring an individual who possesses the same individual characteristics that have resulted in success for previous and current employees. It should never, however, be used as the sole basis for the selection decision; it should be considered only one additional piece of information that might increase the likelihood of selecting the best individual for a given position. It cannot be stressed enough that there are *many* dangers inherent in the use of testing as a selection tool. Employers must carefully consider the ethical and legal ramifications of testing as a selection tool. Can the information garnered in testing be gathered in any other way? Does the tool have established validity and reliability? Is there adequate expertise to accurately interpret and evaluate the results of pre-employment testing? Employers may wish to consider using testing not as a selection tool, but as a tool to use after employment has been granted, to provide information about how best to place the employee in the organization.

PHYSICAL EXAMINATIONS/TESTING

Pre-employment physical examinations are an almost universal requirement for hiring. The principal components of the pre-employment physical examination include medical history; height and weight measurements; general examination of skin, musculature, and joints; vision and hearing tests; clinical examination of eyes, ears, nose, throat, and teeth; auscultation of heart and lungs; blood pressure screening; urinalysis; tuberculin skin testing; and chest x-rays (Beach, 1975).

These tests provide a baseline measure of employee health and identify major physical and/or mental limitations that might impede job performance. They may also be used to identify applicants who have unfavorable attendance records or who may have excessive future claims against health insurance (Sullivan and Decker, 1988). Beach (1975) identified four additional purposes of pre-employment physical examination:

1. To reject those whose physical qualifications are insufficient to meet the requirements of the work they are being considered for

2. To obtain a record of the physical condition at the time of hiring in the event of a worker's compensation claim for an injury that occurs later

3. To prevent the employment of those with contagious diseases

4. To properly place those who are otherwise employable but whose physically handicapped condition requires assignment to specified jobs only

MATCHING APPLICANT QUALIFICATIONS AND JOB REQUIREMENTS

A primary factor in positive employee retention is careful and conscientious consideration during the selection process to match the qualifications of the applicant with the expectations of the organization. This is not an easy task when one considers that the very basis underlying selection is that the nature of individuals (abilities, experience, motivation, and interests) and the jobs (requirements) differ (Milkovich and Glueck, 1985). In selection, individual differences are often used as the basis for job determination. Because of the uniqueness of individuals, the selection process requires considerable creativity and flexibility to accommodate two sets of needs and even to see that accommodation is possible (Vogt et al., 1983).

Placement of the employee in an appropriate place in the organization is an end result of a carefully implemented selection process. It is an active process and is vital to the functioning of the organization. Faulty placement can result in sacrifices to organizational efficiency, threats to organizational integrity, frustration of personal and professional ambitions, and feelings of failure. Conversely, proper placement occasions growth, effectiveness, satisfaction, stability, and prosperity for both organization and individuals (Vogt et al., 1983). Ideal placement represents an integration of organizational and individual goals and is obvious by the subsequent productivity and success of the employee and the meeting of organizational goals.

APPLICANT AND ORGANIZATIONAL OBLIGATIONS DURING THE SELECTION PROCESS

Because selection involves a process of reduction—that is, diminishing the number of candidates for a particular position—the individual making the final selection for the organization has two vital concerns: control and responsibility (Vogt et al., 1983)

The "control" element refers to the control the organization has in selecting the employees that it wants. The individuals making the selection decision have control over decisions that have a tremendous impact on individual lives. It is imperative that selectors recognize how much power they have and guard against any unethical use of their power. This control by the organization is given up when a commitment is made to the applicant.

The "responsibility" element refers the responsibility the organization has to treat all applicants fairly. This means that all applicants should be judged by the same standards in the selection process and that these standards should reflect the needs of a specific job. Having clear-cut, pre-established standards reduces the impact of the preferences and value judgments of the person making the selection (Marquis and Huston, 1987). Any flexibility in the criteria should be outlined ahead of time, and all individuals should be judged with the same flexibility.

However, it is important to remember that the final selection decision involves human beings and thus is never a totally objective process. There are always circumstances that modify selection as a scientific process, such as urgency of need, ratio of applicants to number of openings, rigidity of the selection criteria, and the appeal, promises, and needs of the applicants (Vogt et al., 1983). It is imperative, however, that the organization and the individuals involved in the selection process be aware of the values and beliefs that affect selection. Tool 11-2 provides a list of pertinent questions for the organization, the individual making the selection decision, and staff or unit members involved in the selection process.

The organization also has a responsibility to bring complete and timely closure to the selection process. All applicants should be notified of the selection decision in writing in as timely a manner as possible. Individuals being offered positions should receive formal notification at the same time as those who are not.

Applicants also have responsibilities in the selection process. Applicants have the responsibility to be honest and forthright regarding their qualifications, needs, and wants.

Selection, the final step in the employment process, epitomizes the goals of human resource planning. When an employee is selected and placed appropriately in the organization, goals become shared and worker satisfaction is high. Employee and organizational productivity is high and retention increases.

Tool 11-2   Assessing the Selection Process

For the organization

1. What is your selection/accuracy ratio?
2. How many appropriate candidates respond to your appeals?
3. At what stage are applicants most frequently lost?
4. How many applicants refuse your offers?
5. How open to creative selection is the organization?
6. Is the organization's community reputation consistent with the types of applicants you would select?
7. Have enough time and effort been devoted to establishing the correct criteria?
8. Are you demonstrating challenge, opportunity, and support?
9. Are your expectations realistic?
10. What is your reputation?
11. How much time elapses between application and decision? Is an adequate time allowed for each candidate?

For the individual making the selection decision

1. What are your biases? How obvious are they?
2. What is your success ratio?
3. How are your interviewing skills?
4. Where do you make common mistakes?
5. What feedback have you gathered?
6. How have your selection failures affected the units? How have they affected you?
7. Do you always bring formal closure to all applications?
8. Which would you prefer in hiring—a false positive (candidates who are selected fail) or a false negative (persons who are not selected who would have succeeded)?

For the staff member (unit)

1. Have you clearly defined your personnel needs?
2. Are you helpful in interviewing?
3. Have you been actively involved in the selection process?

4. Do you prefer anyone or do you wait for a good fit in the selection of employees? Have you communicated this desire to the individual making selection decisions?

Reproduced by permission from Vogt, J.F., et al., *Retaining Professional Nurses: A Planned Process*, p. 57. St. Louis, 1983, The C.V. Mosby Co.

KEY CONCEPTS CHAPTER 11

1. Selection is the process of choosing the best qualified individual(s) for a particular position or job from a group of applicants.

2. Research has shown that the selection procedure utilized in the hiring of employees may be related to or predictive of subsequent work behavior in the employee.

3. No one source of information should be given sole weight or weighed disproportionately in the selection decision.

4. The paper trail in the selection process is complex and time consuming because of the information that must be gathered for each applicant. In order to avoid wasting valuable supervisory time, as well as the time of inadequately qualified applicants, all applications should be screened for completeness and confirmation that the applicant is qualified for the position *prior* to the scheduling of interviews.

5. Pre-employment testing is utilized as part of the selection process only when testing has a direct relationship to the ability to perform a specific job.

6. A primary factor in positive employee retention is careful and conscientious consideration during the selection process to match the qualifications of the applicant with the expectations of the organization.

7. It is imperative that individuals making selection decisions recognize how much power they have and guard against any unethical use of their power.

8. Because the final selection decision involves human beings, it is never a totally objective process. Selectors can, however, reduce the impact of their values and biases on the selection decision by judging all applicants by the same job-related standards in the selection process.

REFERENCES

Beach, D.S., *Personnel: The Management of People at Work*. Third Edition, Macmillan, New York, 1975.

Bowin, R.B., *Human Resource Problem Solving*, Prentice-Hall, Englewood Cliffs, NJ, 1987.

Cronbach, L.J., and Schaeffer, G.A., *Extensions of Personnel Selection Theory to Aspects of Minority Hiring*, Stanford University: Institute for Research or Educational Finance and Governance, Palo Alto, CA, 1981.

Goldstein, I.L., "The Application Blank: How Honest Are Responses?" *Journal of Applied Psychology*, 55:491–492, 1971.

Hunter, J.E., and Schmidt, F., "Ability Tests: Economic Benefits Versus the Issue of Fairness," *Industrial Relations*, 21:293–308, 1982.

Kern, J.P., Riley, J.J., and Jones, L.N., *Human Resources Management*, Marcel Dekker, New York, and ASQC Quality Press, Milwaukee, WI, 1987.

Lewis, E.M., and Spicer, J.G., *Human Resource Management Handbook – Contemporary Strategies for Nursing Managers*, Aspen Publications, Rockville, MD, 1987.

Lorsch, J.W., and Morse, J.J., *Organizations and their Members: A Contingency Approach*, Harper and Row, New York, 1976.

Lotito, M.S., and Kostenbauer, J., *Advance: The Nurse's Guide to Success in Today's Job Market*, Little, Brown and Company, Boston, 1981.

Lyles, R.I., and Joiner, C., *Supervision in Health Care Organizations*. John Wiley & Sons, New York, 1986.

Mandell, M.M., *The Selection Process*, American Management Association, New York, 1964.

Marquis, B., and Huston, C.J., *Management Decision Making for Nurses: 101 Case Studies*, J.B. Lippincott, Philadelphia, 1987,

Milkovich, G.T., and Glueck, W.F., *Personnel, Human Resource Management: A Diagnostic Approach*, Fourth Edition, Business Publications, Plano, TX, 1985.

Miller, E., "An EEO Examination of Employment Applications," *The Personnel Administrator*, March:64, 1980.

Peres, H., and Garcia, J.R., "Validity and Dimensions of Descriptive Adjectives Used in Reference Letters for Engineering Applicants," *Personnel Psychology*, 15:279–286, 1962.

Sackett, P.R., and Wilson, M.A., "Factors Affecting the Consensus Judgment Process in Managerial Assessment Centers," *Journal of Applied Psychology*, 67(1):10–17, 1982.

Schmidt, F.L., Hunter, J.E., McKenzie, R., and Muldrow, T.W., "The Impact of Valid Selection Procedures on Workforce Productivity," *Journal of Applied Psychology*, 64(3):609–626, 1979.

Sullivan, E.J., and Decker, P.J., *Effective Management in Nursing*, Second Edition, Addison-Wesley, Menlo Park, CA, 1988.

Vogt, J.F., Cox, J.L., Velthouse, B.A., and Thames, B.H., *Retaining Professional Nurses: A Planned Approach*, C.V. Mosby, St. Louis, 1983.

ADDITIONAL READINGS

Comrey, A.L., Backer, T.E., and Glaser, E.M., *A Sourcebook for Mental Health Measures*, Report to the National Institute of Mental Health, Human Interaction Research Institute, Los Angeles, CA, 1973.

Mitchell, J. (ed.), *The Ninth Mental Measurements Yearbook*, Univ. of Nebraska Press, Lincoln, NB, 1985.

Mitchell, J. (ed.), *Tests in Print III*, Buros Institute of Mental Measurements, Univ. of Nebraska Press, Lincoln, NB, 1983.

Super, D.E., and Crites, J.O., *Appraising Vocational Fitness by Means of Psychological Tests*, Revised Edition, Harper and Row, New York and Evanston, 1962.

▪ UNIT FIVE
The Employee Indoctrination Process

INDOCTRINATION, AS an employment subfunction, refers to the planned, guided adjustment of a new employee to both the organization and the work environment. Many management and personnel texts use a variety of terms to describe the functions of indoctrination. The words *induction* and *orientation* are frequently used to describe these functions, and some feel that these terms are synonymous. However, for the purposes of this discussion the indoctrination process will be divided into three separate phases: induction, orientation, and socialization.

In defining indoctrination, it becomes apparent that the word denotes a much broader approach to the process of new employment adjustment than either induction or orientation. *Induction* is usually defined as "leading or bringing into" and *orientation* as "familiarizing with," while *indoctrination* is defined as "to instruct in doctrines, theories, beliefs or principles" (Webster, 1979).

Organizations that merely induct and/or orient employees neglect the critical function of socialization. *Socialization* is defined as being able "to adjust to the common needs of a group" or "to make fit" (Webster, 1979).

All parts of indoctrination, however, serve important functions and are effective in reducing subsequent attrition. The impressions new employees form during their adjustment period will remain with them for a long time. If the impressions are positive, they will be remembered even during the difficult times that will ultimately occur during any long tenure of employment.

Indoctrination has many purposes. It seeks to establish favorable employee attitudes toward the organization, the unit, and the department. Indoctrination procedures help instill a feeling of belonging and acceptance, which in turn helps generate enthusiasm and high morale. Beach (1980) maintains that the by-products of effective indoctrination programs are higher productivity, fewer rule violations, less attrition, and greater employee satisfaction.

The amount of time, effort, and money spent on employee indoctrination should be at least equal to that spent on recruitment, selection, and placement functions. Good indoctrination programs are a wise financial decision.

Employee indoctrination should be a joint effort of the personnel department, the staff development or inservice training department, and the manager of the unit or department where the employee has been assigned. The division of responsibility should be clearly delineated and not assumed or left to chance. Organizations should decide what is to be included in the indoctrination process and who is to perform the various functions. Managers often neglect their role in this process and expect the personnel and education departments to play the major role in new employee indoctrination.

There is perhaps no other part of human resource management that has as great an influence on retention and productivity as does the indoctrination process. This time provides the manager with the opportunity to mold a team and to build loyalty in the new employee.

REFERENCES

Beach, D., *Personnel: The Management of People at Work*, Fourth Edition, Macmillan Company, New York, 1980.
Webster New Twentieth Century Dictionary, Second Edition, Simon and Schuster, New York, 1979.

12

The Induction/Orientation Process

MANY FACTORS affect the success of employees besides their ability to do the job. The induction and orientation functions of the indoctrination process should be used by the organization to provide additional information to new employees that will assist them in having a successful employment tenure. The induction and orientation process is an ideal time to educate new employees about the desired behaviors and expected goals of the organization.

Chapter 12 will address the specific information that should be included in the induction and orientation process. It is often difficult to know where placement and pre-employment functions end and where induction begins. As long as certain elements are included, it really does not matter what the function is called. Induction is the first phase of the indoctrination process and includes all the activities that take place after the employee has been selected, but before the employee has started to perform the job. Many of the induction activities are often included as part of the orientation functions.

Both positive and negative aspects of many different types of orientation structure will be given. This chapter also discusses which individuals should be included in the orientation and the desired content of the orientation process. The importance of legal considerations in such things as employee handbooks, fire safety, and documentation of the employee's knowledge of the grievance process will be included. The need for goal planning for meeting the needs of different groups and types of employees will be stressed.

Some content is provided on flexibility and variability of the length of the orientation. Tools included in this chapter provide an example of the content that should be covered during induction and orientation and a sample orientation appropriate for an experienced nurse.

COMPONENTS OF INDUCTION

Although many management authors include induction as part of the orientation process, Holle and Blatchley (1987) see them as separate entities and feel that the employee suffers if either kind of program is omitted. Labeling is less important, however, than identifying the content to be included. The induction process includes all those activities that educate new employees about the company and provides them with adequate information about employment and personnel policies and procedures.

Following is a list of the information and activities that should be included for new employees during the induction process:

1. The history of the organization should be discussed.

2. A copy of the mission, purpose, and philosophy of the organization should be given to all new employees.

3. A copy of the employee handbook should be given to each employee, and it should be reviewed.

4. All personnel functions, such as employee physicals, income tax withholding forms, life insurance forms, and health insurance forms, should be completed as part of the induction process. This may be done prior to the first day of work or on the first day of work.

5. Where there is unionization, a copy of the contract is provided by the union, but labor-management relations should be a part of the induction process.

6. The various department heads should be introduced, with a small presentation on what their roles are in the organization. This may be carried out via a media presentation.

The employee handbook is an important part of the induction. This handbook is usually developed by the personnel department, but all department heads should have input into their development. Most employee handbooks contain a form that must be signed by employees, stating that they have been given an employee handbook and are responsible for knowing the information in it. This signed form is then placed in their personnel files. Suggested content for an employee personnel handbook is included in Tool 12-1.

Beach (1980) has stressed that just providing an employee with a personnel handbook is not sufficient to provide real understanding. Policies need to be followed up with discussion by various individuals during the employment process, such as the personnel manager and the staff development personnel during orientation. Probably the most important link in promoting real understanding of personnel policies lies with the first-line supervisor.

TYPES OF ORIENTATION STRUCTURE

Organizations have a wide variety of orientation programs to choose from, and many large organizations offer more than one type of orientation program. For example, a hospital might have a first-day orientation conducted by the personnel department, which would include a tour of the hospital, in addition to all of the induction items listed above. The next phase of the orientation program might take place in the staff development department where aspects of concern to all employees, such as fire safety, accident prevention, and health promotion, would be presented to all new employees. The third phase would be the individual orientation for each department. At this point the dietary, pharmacy, and nursing departments would each be responsible for developing their own specific programs of orientation.

Tool 12-1   Employee Indoctrination Content

---

1. Company history, mission, and philosophy
2. Company service and service area
3. Organizational structure, including department heads, with an explanation of functions of various departments
4. Employee responsibilities to the company
5. Company responsibilities to the employee
6. Payroll information, including how increases in pay are earned and when they are given. (Progressive and/or unionized companies publish pay scales for all employees.)
7. Rules of conduct
8. Tour of the company and of the assigned department
9. Work schedules, staffing, and scheduling policies
10. When applicable, a discussion of the collective bargaining agreement
11. Benefit plans, including life insurance, health insurance, pension, and unemployment
12. Safety and fire programs
13. Staff-development programs, including inservice, and continuing education for relicensure
14. Promotion and transfer policies
15. Employee appraisal system
16. Workload assignments
17. Introduction to charting
18. Review of important policies and procedures
19. Specific legal requirements, such as maintaining current license, reporting of accidents, etc.
20. Introduction to fellow employees
21. Establishment of a feeling of belonging and acceptance, showing genuine interest in the new employee

Note: Much of this content could be provided in an employee handbook, and the fire and safety regulations could be handled via a media presentation. *Appropriate* use of videotapes or film strips can be very useful in the design of a good orientation program. All orientation programs should be monitored to see if they are achieving their goals. Most programs need to be revised at least annually. Lastly, it is of vital importance that all departments work together to provide a good orientation program. There must be cooperation between the personnel department, the staff development department, and the unit where the new employee is to be assigned. *All* must take responsibility for the success or failure of the orientation.

Because induction and orientation involve many different individuals from a variety of departments, it must be carefully coordinated and planned so that it achieves its preset goals. The overall goals of induction and orientation include helping employees by providing them with information that will smooth their transition into the new work setting. According to Cherniss (1980), research has shown the orientation process to be a successful method of preventing burnout among human service professionals. In citing justifications for orientation programs, Cherniss states that new employees taking part in a formal orientation program reach independent and adequate functioning sooner and remain in the organization longer than do employees who receive no orientation. Therefore, other goals for orientation programs would be reducing turnover and increasing productivity.

It then is important to look at productivity and retention as the orientation program is planned and structured. The entire organization needs to periodically review its induction and orientation program to determine whether it is meeting organizational goals and how the program might be improved.

Too often the various individuals having partial responsibility for induction and orientation "pass the buck" regarding failure of, or weaknesses in, the program. It is the joint responsibility of the personnel department, the staff development department, and the nursing service unit to work together in providing an orientation and induction that meet employee and organizational needs.

Following is a list of various induction and orientation points, with suggestions on which department should best fill each role:

1. *Personnel department:* Pay and payroll functions, insurance forms, physical exams, income withholding forms, tour of the organization, employee responsibilities to the organiza-

tion and organizational responsibilities to the employee, additional labor-management relationships, and benefit plan.

2. *Staff development department:* Hand out and review employee handbook, discuss organizational philosophy and mission, review history of the organization, show media presentation of various departments and how they function (if media presentation is not available, introduce various department heads and discuss how departments function), discuss organizational structure, discuss fire and safety programs, do CPR certification and verifications, discuss educational and training programs available, review selected policies and procedures, and discuss general charting, medication, and treatment policies.

3. *The individual unit:* Tour of the department, introductions, review of specific unit policies that differ in any way from general policies, review of unit scheduling and staffing policies and procedures, work assignments, promotion and transfer policies, review of appraisal system, and establishment of a feeling of belonging and acceptance. Establishing a feeling of belonging and acceptance is part of the socialization phase of indoctrination and will be discussed in detail in Chapter 13.

For some time in health care organizations, especially in hospitals, many managers did not fulfill their proper role in the orientation of new employees. Nursing managers assumed that, between the personnel and staff development, or inservice department, new employees would become completely oriented. This often resulted in much frustration on the part of new employees because, although they received an overview of the organization, they received little indoctrination to the specific unit. Since each unit has many idiosyncrasies, new employees often feel inadequate and incompetent. The latest trend in orientation has been for the nursing unit to take a greater responsibility for individualizing the orientation to that unit (Bastien, 1987; Sovie, 1982; Tucker, 1987).

Beach (1980) elaborates by stating that the supervisor plays a key role in the orientation of new employees. Beach maintains that an adequate orientation program minimizes the likelihood of rule violations, grievances, and misunderstandings; fosters feelings of belonging and acceptance; and promotes enthusiasm and morale.

SPECIAL ORIENTATION NEEDS

The previous discussion has addressed the needs of the new employee in a health care agency. There are, however, three types of employees with special orientation needs: (1) the new nurse accepting her first job after graduation from nursing school, (2) the novice nurse manager, and (3) the experienced nurse who enters a totally new area of nursing. Helping to meet these employees' special needs by providing an appropriately tailored orientation will help to ensure a positive outcome to their employment. Following is a discussion of the orientation needs of each type.

The New Nurse

Kramer (1974) described special fears and difficulty in adapting to the work setting that are common to new graduate nurses. Kramer called this phenomenon *reality shock* and stated that it occurs as a result of the conflict between a new graduate's expectations of the nursing role and the reality of the actual role in the work setting. Most of Kramer's work centered around hospital settings, since that is where most new graduates are employed.

Much of Kramer's work is substantiated by other researchers who have studied professionals in their first year of employment (Becker, 1952; Corwin, 1961; Sarta, 1972; Wacker, 1979). Cherniss (1980) stated that no one is immune to a loss of idealism and commitment in response to stress in the work place, but it is in the first year of employment that the greatest change in attitude and behavior takes place.

Following the publication of Kramer's work, many hospitals began to look at methods they could use in their orientation programs that would alleviate some of the shock of entering the real world of nursing. Some hospitals developed a prolonged orientation period for new graduates that lasts from 6 weeks to 6 months. This extended orientation, called an *internship*, contrasts sharply with the routine 1- to 2-week orientation that is normal for other employees. During this time the graduate nurse is usually assigned to work with a *preceptor*, an experienced nurse who can both provide emotional support and be a strong clinical role model. During the internship the new nurse gradually takes on a patient assignment that equals that of the preceptor.

Some hospitals have discontinued such internship programs due to their expense but have continued with the preceptor concept of teaming a new graduate with another nurse. May

(1980) suggests that, in addition to providing orientation and socialization for new graduates, a preceptorship provides recognition to preceptors for demonstrated excellence in their nursing practice. Although internships appear to be one answer in reducing reality shock, such programs are not without hazards. *Practices* (1984) identified the following advantages and disadvantages of such a program:

ADVANTAGES

1. The quality of patient care is increased, as the intern has an opportunity to learn how to do more effective nursing assessments and interventions.
2. The intern is exposed to contrasting schools of thought about nursing.
3. Peer relationships with the staff are enhanced.
4. The intern is less likely to receive conflicting information when paired with a preceptor.
5. The duplication of information that occurs when more than one staff person is teaching is reduced.
6. The self-confidence of the intern is increased.

DISADVANTAGES

1. Internships may assist new graduate nurses in coping with reality, but they do not attempt to fix the underlying problem of the gap between academia and the work setting.
2. An internship may further delay new graduates' adjustment to reality.
3. Some internships attempt to rotate nurses through too many specialty units in too short a time period.
4. In programs in which the preceptor and the intern have a prolonged formal relationship (more than 1 year), the intern may become overly dependent on the preceptor.

Many of the potential hazards of internship and/or preceptor programs can be overcome by (1) careful selection of the preceptors, (2) selection only of preceptors who have a strong desire to be role models, (3) preparation of preceptors for their role through formal classes in adult learning and other social/learning concepts, and (4) close monitoring by experienced staff development or supervisory personnel of the preceptor and new graduate to ensure that the relationship continues to be beneficial and growth producing for both parties.

New Managers

Probably no aspect of an employee's work life has as great an influence on productivity and retention as does the quality of supervision exhibited by his or her immediate supervisor. Unfortunately, the orientation of new managers in many areas of business is a neglected part of staff development.

According to Beach (1980), there is growing recognition that good managers do not emerge from the work force without a great deal of conscious planning on the part of the organization. The management development program should be ongoing and should be implemented prior to the individual's appointment to a management position. The planning and administration of a management development program is discussed in detail in Chapter 17. Therefore, the discussion here will be limited to the type of support and orientation new managers should receive during the first few months in their new positions.

Orientation to the management position by the outgoing manager should be relatively short. The previous manager should usually spend no longer than 1 week working directly with the new manager. This is especially true if the new manager is familiar with the organization. If the new manager has been recruited from outside the organization, the orientation period may need to be extended. The justification for a short orientation by the outgoing manager is that it allows the newly appointed manager to quickly gain control of the unit and establish his or her own management style.

Frequently, a new manager will be appointed to a management position that is vacant or to a newly created position. In either case, there will be no one readily available to orient the new manager to the position. It is very important that the new manager's immediate superior appoint someone to orient the new manager. This could be a manager from another unit, the manager's supervisor, or someone else from the unit who is familiar with the duties and role of the manager.

The orientation of a new manager should not cease following the short period spent in introductions to the various tasks of the job. Every new manager needs guidance and direction, continued orientation, and development during the first year in this new role. This kind of direction comes from several sources in the organization, specifically:

1. *The new manager's immediate superior.* Again, as in the orientation of the new manager, this could be the unit supervisor if the new manager is a charge nurse, or it could be the chief nursing executive if the new manager is a unit supervisor. The immediate superior should have regularly planned and scheduled sessions with the new manager to continue the ongoing orientation process of the management role.

2. *A group of the new manager's peers.* There should be some type of management group in the organization that the new manager can consult with during the orientation period. These individuals should be identified to the new manager, who should be encouraged to use them as resources.

3. *A mentor.* New managers who are truly fortunate will have someone in the organization as a mentor. A full discussion of mentors and their role in leadership development, retention, and productivity appears in the following chapter.

The Experienced Nurse in a New Position

Another transition for the registered nurse occurs when experienced nurses decide to make a lateral transfer within the same organization, take other positions that are a great deal different from their previous roles, or take similar positions in other organizations. These nurses have particular needs during orientation that arise from the following:

1. *Transition from expert to novice.* This is a very difficult role transition. Many nurses transfer or change jobs because they no longer find their present jobs challenging, but this makes it necessary for them to assume a learning role in their new environments. The employees assigned to orient them in the new positions should be aware of the difficulties these nurses will experience. A sample orientation schedule for the experienced nurse is shown in Tool 12-2. The transferred employees' lack of knowledge in the new area should never be belittled, and, whenever possible, the special expertise they bring from their former work areas should be acknowledged and utilized.

Tool 12-2   Sample Two-Week Orientation Schedule for Experienced Nurses

WEEK 1
Day 1, Monday:

8:00–10:00 a.m.	Welcome by Personnel Department: Employee handbooks distributed and discussed
10:00–10:30	Coffee and fruit served and welcome by Staff Development Department
10:30–12:00	General orientation by Staff Development Department
12:00–12:30	Tour of the organization
12:30–1:30	Lunch
1:30–3:00	Fire and safety films, and body mechanics demonstration
3:00–4:00	Afternoon tea and introduction to each unit supervisor
Day 2, Tuesday:	Report to individual units
8:00–10:00 a.m.	Time with unit supervisor and introduction to assigned preceptor
10:00–10:30	Coffee with preceptor
10:30–12:00	General orientation of policies and procedures
12:00–12:30	Lunch
12:30–4:30	CPR recertification
Day 3 Wednesday:	Assigned all day to unit with preceptor
Day 4, Thursday:	Assigned all day to unit with preceptor
Day 5, Friday:	Morning with preceptor, afternoon with supervisor, and staff development for wrap-up

WEEK 2

Monday to Wednesday:	Work with preceptor on shift and unit assigned, gradually assuming greater responsibilities
Thursday:	Assign 80% of normal assignment with assistance and supervision from preceptor
Friday:	Carry normal workload; have at least a 30-minute meeting with immediate supervisor to discuss progress

2. *Transition from familiar to the unfamiliar.* In the old surroundings the employee knew everyone and where everything was located. In the new position the employee not only will be learning new job skills, but also will be in an unfamiliar environment.

Managers of departments that receive frequent transfers, such as a critical care unit, should prepare a special orientation for experienced nurses transferring to the department. In addition to providing necessary staff development content, these orientation programs should be focused around efforts to promote the self-esteem of new nurses as they are learning the necessary skills for their new role.

Orientation and induction provide the manager and the organization with an opportunity to build loyalty and team spirit. This is the time to instill employees with pride in the organization and the unit. This type of affective learning becomes the foundation for subsequent increased retention and productivity.

KEY CONCEPTS CHAPTER 12

1. A well-prepared and executed orientation program is a proven way to educate new employees about the desired behaviors and expected goals of the organization.
2. The induction of new employees should include all the activities that educate employees about the company.
3. A well-written employee handbook is part of the induction process.
4. There are many acceptable types of orientation structure.
5. It is preferable that various individuals assist with the orientation process, but a new employee's immediate supervisor must take an active role.
6. Research has shown that the orientation process is a successful method to prevent burnout.
7. Some individuals need special orientations; these groups include new graduates, new managers, and experienced nurses in new roles.

REFERENCES

Bastien, S., Glennon, P., and Stein, A., Orientation: Off Toward a nurse's 'personal best', *"Nursing Management* 17(10):64, 1987.

Beach, D.S., *Personnel: The Management of People at Work*, Fourth Edition, Macmillan, New York, 1980.

Becker, H.S., "The Career of the Chicago Public School Teacher," *American Journal of Sociology*, 57:470–477, 1952.

Cherniss, G., *Professional Burnout in Human Services Organizations*, Praeger, New York, 1980.

Corwin, R., "The Professional Employee: A Study of Conflict in Nursing Roles," *American Journal of Sociology*, 66:604–615, 1961.

Holle, M.L., and Blatchley, M.E., *Introduction to Leadership and Management in Nursing*, Second Edition, Wadsworth Health Sciences Division, Monterey, CA, 1987.

Kramer, M., *Reality Shock*, C.V. Mosby, St. Louis, 1974.

May, L., "Clinical Preceptors for New Nurses," *AJN*, 80:1824, 1980.

Practices, Nurses Reference Library, Nursing '84 Books, Springhouse Corporation, Springhouse, PA, 1984, p. 333–336.

Sarta, B.P.V., *Job Satisfaction of Individuals Working with the Mentally Retarded*, PhD Dissertation, Yale University, 1972.

Sovie, M.D., Fostering Professional Nursing Careers in Hospitals: The Role of Staff Development," *JONA*, 12:5, 1982.

Tucker, P.T., "Recruiting nurses with an extern program," *Nursing Management*, 18(5):90–94, 1987.

Wacker, S.W., *Job Stress and Attitude Change in Teachers, Lawyers, Social Workers and Nurses*, Phd Dissertation, University of Michigan, 1979.

ADDITIONAL READINGS

Andrews, C.A., "Orientation: Graduates' Perceptions of Initiation," *Nursing Management*, 18(11):110, 1987.

Charron, D.C., "Save the New Graduate," *Nursing Management*, 13:45, 1982.

Dear, M.R., et al., "Evaluating a Hospital Nursing Internship," *JONA*, 12:16, 1982.

Marquis, B.L., and Huston, C.J., *Decision Making for Nurses: 101 Case Studies*, J.B. Lippincott, Philadelphia, 1980.

Sullivan, E.J., and Decker, P., *Effective Management in Nursing*, Addison-Wesley, Menlo Park, CA, 1985.

13
The Socialization/ Resocialization Process

THE INDOCTRINATION content listed in Tool 12-1 indicates that the employee should develop a sense of belonging as the last step in the indoctrination process. This belonging concept is often referred to as the *socialization function* of indoctrination. Orientation in itself is usually not an adequate mechanism to ensure that new employees are properly socialized into the organization. Since the proper socialization of employees impacts so greatly on retention, a separate chapter is devoted to this phase of indoctrination.

Much has been written about the importance of socializing new members into their professional roles (Cherniss, 1980; Kramer, 1974; Schmalenberg and Kramer, 1979). Research has also documented the importance of this process in the prevention of burnout and the promotion of retention. However, there has been less research into the special resocialization needs of nurses as they change roles throughout their professional careers.

It is not only the novice professional for whom socialization into the organization is critical. Adequate socialization of all types of new employees has been shown to reduce attrition (Cherniss, 1980). Beach (1980) maintains that it is during the socialization phase of indoctrination that employees need to be instilled with high morale and enthusiasm for the organization. Employers should use the indoctrination process as a time to socialize the new employee into an employee mold so that there is a good fit between the employee and the organization.

Socialization differs from orientation because it involves little structured information. Rather, it is a sharing of the values and attitudes of the organization by the use of role models, myths, and legends. Kramer and Schmalenberg (1988) state that one of the major roles of leaders in magnet hospitals is to generate enthusiasm in every worker. The ability to instill and clarify the value system of the organization to new employees is a part of the socialization process that creates the team approach found in excellent organizations (Kramer and Schmalenberg, 1988).

This chapter will assist the manager in understanding the socialization process and how role expectations are learned. The use of role models, mentors, and managers in carrying out the socialization of employees will be discussed. A role assessment tool to assist the manager in determining employee socialization needs is included.

THE SOCIALIZATION PROCESS

There is no one theory of socialization. Among sociologists, the phenomenon of socialization has generally focused on role theory, according to which we learn the behaviors that accompany each role via two simultaneously occurring processes. One process, referred to as an *interactional process*, involves both groups and significant others in a social context. The other, a *learning process*, includes such mechanisms as role playing, identification, modeling, operate learning, instruction, observation, imitation, trial and error, and role negotiation (Hardy and Conway, 1978).

Unfortunately, this well-researched phenomenon has been sadly neglected in formal indoctrination programs, although the proper socialization of individuals is critical to any retention program. Marlene Kramer's research is well known and has been used as a foundation for new graduate intern programs, but there has been little attention paid to the resocialization needs of other employees (Hinshaw, 1986). Resocialization occurs (1) when new graduates leave the educational socialization process of nursing school and enter the work world; (2) when the experienced nurse changes work settings, moving either within the organization or to a new organization; and (3) when the nurse undertakes new roles.

Brim (1966) states that resocialization would be more effective if efforts were made to determine why individuals have difficulty with it. He maintains that there are usually three areas of difficulty: (1) *ignorance of the particular role prescriptions and expectations*, (2) *inability to meet role demands*, and (3) *deficiencies in motivation*. Some employees have little difficulty with the process of resocialization, but most experience some stress when there is role change (Hardy and Conway, 1988). Tool 13-1 is a role assessment questionnaire that can be given to employees to assess how well they perceive their roles. Therefore, the remainder of this chapter will focus on how organizations can plan in advance to ease the stress of resocialization by the conscious use of appropriate interventions.

CLARIFYING ROLE EXPECTATIONS

Role expectations can be clarified by the use of role models, preceptors, and mentors. While all three utilize both social interaction and educational processes to clarify roles, each has a different focus and uses different mechanisms. All have an appropriate place in the socialization of employees.

1. *Role models*. Role models serve as examples of experienced employees that are performing their roles adequately. The relationship between new employees and role models is a passive one; employees see that role models are skilled and attempt to emulate them, but the role models do not actively seek this emulation. One of the exciting aspects of role models is their cumulative effect. The greater the number of excellent role models available for new employees to emulate, the greater are the possibilities for new employees to perform well. This concept has been borne out by Kramer and Schmalenberg's recent research on excellence in hospitals (Kramer and Schmalenberg, 1988).

2. *Preceptors*. While the educational function of role models is passive, that of preceptors is active and purposeful. Preceptors

(Text continued on p. 229)

Tool 13-1 Role Assessment for New Employees

HOW WELL DO YOU PERCEIVE YOUR ROLE?

DIRECTIONS: This is a role assessment for new employees that will help your manager and you determine how well you are being socialized into your role at this hospital. Please answer the questions to the best of your ability. We will use the results of this assessment to help you in mastering any area where you indicate you might need assistance.

The first set of questions have to do with how well you understand your job expectations and the organization's goals. Place a circle around the rank position that most clearly defines how you feel. Remember that "strongly agree" is on the left and "strongly disagree" is on the right.

1. I have a clear understanding of my job duties.

1	2	3	4	5
strongly agree			strongly disagree	

2. I have a clear understanding of the amount of work expected.

1	2	3	4	5

3. I know how much authority and latitude I have in my job.

1	2	3	4	5

4. I know what my charge nurse and supervisor expect of me.

1	2	3	4	5

5. I have a clear understanding of the goals of the hospital and my unit.

1	2	3	4	5

6. I have a clear understanding of nursing department policies.

1	2	3	4	5

The next set of questions solicits answers regarding how much conflict you are experiencing in your new role.

7. I am experiencing pressure from my supervisor.

1	2	3	4	5

8. I am experiencing some pressure from my coworkers.

1	2	3	4	5

9. I am experiencing pressure from patients and relatives.

1	2	3	4	5

10. I am experiencing pressure because of the way I am performing my job.

1	2	3	4	5

11. I am experiencing pressure because of the way I feel about how I am meeting patients' needs.

1	2	3	4	5

12. I am experiencing pressure because of value conflict.

1	2	3	4	5

13. I am experiencing pressure due to doctors' expectations.

1	2	3	4	5

The next set of questions determines if you feel your perceptions of how you do your job match those of other people.

14. My supervisor agrees with me on how I should do my job.

1	2	3	4	5

15. Other unit staff agree with me on how I should do my job.

1	2	3	4	5

16. My patients agree with me on how I should do my job.

1	2	3	4	5

The next set of questions determines how you feel you are meeting the demands of the job.

17. I am able to keep up with the work activity in my job.

1	2	3	4	5

18. I am able to delegate and coordinate my activities well.

1	2	3	4	5

19. I am able to find on-the-job time to incorporate current developments into my job, i.e., reading memos, looking up new procedures, and keeping abreast.

1	2	3	4	5

20. I am able to function in a manner that ensures safe practice and meets the standards of my profession.

1	2	3	4	5

Interpretation of the role assessment sheet: The nursing manager and employee should meet and discuss areas of concern to either party. In areas of role ambiguity, which is assessed in the first set of questions, the manager should attempt to clarify the job description and unit expectations. In areas of role conflict or role overload, the manager should assist the new employee in setting priorities and in clarifying values.

should serve as both role models and educators in the clarification of role expectations. Preceptors need to have an adequate knowledge of adult learning theory if they are to fulfill their role in the socialization process. Careful selection of preceptors will assist the organization in role clarification.

3. *Mentors.* Mentors take an even greater role in education as a basis of role clarification. Not every nurse will be fortunate enough to have a mentor each time he or she is resocialized. Most nurses are lucky if they have one or two mentors throughout their careers. May and associates (1982) define mentoring as "an intense relationship calling for a high degree of involvement between a novice in a discipline and a person who is knowledgeable and wise in that area." Madison (1984) has documented the value of mentors in the socialization process. Mentors serve a particularly useful role in the socialization of nurses to the manager role (Marquis and Huston, 1987).

ASSISTANCE IN MEETING ROLE DEMANDS

Wheeler (1966) feels that there are two distinct areas in which individuals need assistance in meeting role demands. The first is with the specific skills and requirements for the role, and the second is with the status behavior that accompanies each role. What Wheeler terms *status behavior*, Linton refers to as the *values and attitudes component* of any given role (Linton, 1945). There are various means that organizations may utilize to assist employees in meeting role demands.

1. *Meeting knowledge and skill requirements.* In order to assist employees in meeting the demands of the job, managers need to determine what those needs are. This requires more than just asking employees, or giving them some sort of skills check list or test. It requires careful observation by managers and preceptors so that deficiencies are identified and corrected before they become a handicap to employees' socialization into the organization. When such deficiencies are not corrected early, other employees often create a climate of nonacceptance that prevents assimilation and socialization from occurring.

2. *Assisting in the development of values and attitudes.* Both Hinshaw and Kramer have completed much research in the area of values and attitudes and their relationship to the socialization and resocialization of nurses in the work place. Both agree that values and attitudes may be a source of conflict as nurses learn new roles but that there are various methods organizations can employ that will assist new employees in meeting this requirement of socialization (Hinshaw, 1986; Kramer, 1974). Among the strategies they suggest are (1) the use of role models, (2) providing a safe climate for new employees to ventilate their frustrations with value conflicts, (3) clarifying differing nurse role expectations that are held by physicians, patients, and other staff, and (4) assisting new employees in developing strategies to cope with and resolve value and attitude conflicts (Hinshaw, 1986; Kramer, 1974).

MOTIVATIONAL DEFICIENCIES

Brim suggests that if difficulties in resocialization occur as a result of motivational deficiencies, a planned program of reorientation to the defined goals that uses rewards and punishment should be instituted (Brim, 1966). Although sanctions—the bestowing of rewards and punishment—occur at many levels during employee socialization, they are rarely carried out in a systematic and planned manner. Yet many employees learn very quickly what type of behavior is rewarded in an organization. Does getting off duty on time or excellent patient care receive the greatest number of reward sanctions? This is one area where managers need to become consciously aware of how their behavior and values impact on the socialization of new employees.

1. *Use of positive sanctions.* Positive sanctions can be employed as an interactional or educational process of socialization. If deliberately planned, as Brim suggests, they become educational in nature. However, through the group process, or reference group, sanctions are used in the social interaction process to socialize new employees. The reference group sets norms of behavior and then employs sanctions to ensure that new members adopt the group norms before they are accepted into the group. This informal use of sanctions is an extremely powerful tool used for socialization and resocialization in the work place. Managers should become cognizant of what role behaviors they reward and

should observe their staff to see what behaviors of new employees are being rewarded by senior employees.

2. *Use of negative sanctions.* Punishment, like rewards, may be viewed as a means of providing learners with cues that enable them to consciously evaluate their performances and then to modify behavior where necessary. In order for either type of sanction to be effective, it must result in the role learner's internalizing the values of the organization. Negative sanctions are often employed in very subtle and covert ways. Making fun of a new graduate's awkwardness with certain skills, or belittling the desire of a new employee to use nursing care plans, are very effective ways to use negative sanctions to mold behavior to group norms. The nursing manager should be aware of what the group norms are and should be observant of sanctions that are used by the group to make newcomers conform. This is not to say that negative sanctions should not be used. New employees should be told when their behavior is not an acceptable part of the role they have been employed to fulfill.

EMPLOYEES WITH SPECIAL PROBLEMS IN RESOCIALIZATION

The three types of employees with special orientation needs discussed previously are the same employees that have difficulty with resocialization, namely, (1) new graduate nurses in their first jobs, (2) experienced nurses changing positions laterally, and (3) nurses in new roles, such as the new nurse manager or the new nurse educator. The term *resocialization* is used here, rather than the term *socialization*, because all of these employees have been socialized to the nursing role, either in school or in another position. It is often more difficult to resocialize individuals than to initially socialize them to a role, because resocialization requires that they give up some values and attitudes. Examples are the practical nurse who becomes a professional nurse or the critical care nurse who becomes a hospice nurse.

The New Nurse Graduate

1. *Special needs of the new nurse graduate.* Schmalenberg and Kramer suggest that there are four phases of role transition from student nurse to staff nurse: the honeymoon phase, shock, recovery, and resolution. They maintain that there is cultural conflict because values in the school and work

subcultures differ (Schmalenberg and Kramer, 1979). There is little difficulty with the first phase, as long as the novice nurse is sincerely welcomed into the work place. However, during the second phase, the novice often has great difficulty after discovering that many nursing school values are not work place values. Usually the new graduate will be appropriately resocialized if the manager and the organization take certain actions during the recovery and resolution phases.

2. *Interventions to assist the new graduate with resocialization.* Organizations use several mechanisms to ease the role transition of new graduates. Kramer suggests that anticipatory socialization be carried out in educational settings to prepare new nurses for the inevitable shock of reality (Kramer, 1974). However, organizations should not assume that such anticipatory socialization has occurred. Therefore, they should build into their orientation programs opportunities for sharing and clarifying values and attitudes about the nursing role. Use of the group process is an excellent mechanism to promote sharing. Additionally, the nurse manager should be on the alert for signs and symptoms of the shock phase of role transition and should intervene by listening to new graduates and assisting them in coping with the real world. Some of the new nurses' values should be supported and encouraged so that there is a blending of work and school values. Some authorities in role stress suggest that new professionals need to understand that the process they are experiencing is universal and not limited to nurses. For example, Cherniss (1980) has found role transition difficulty in all the helping professions. Providing some type of class on role transition might be another helpful mechanism to assist new graduates in resocialization.

The Experienced Nurse

1. *Special needs of the experienced nurse in resocialization.* The special needs of this new employee are often overlooked, since many organizations are unaware that this individual needs special attention. Hardy and Conway (1988) maintain that organizations rarely address the socialization problems that occur in changes in jobs, position, or status. They suggest that transition into new jobs would be associated with less role strain if programs were designed to facilitate role modification and role expansion. A staff nurse who moves from a medical floor to labor and delivery does not know what the new group's norms are, is unsure

of the expected values and behaviors, and goes from being an expert to being a novice. All of these create a great deal of role strain. This same type of role stress occurs when experienced nurses move from one organization to another. Nurses often sense a feeling of powerlessness during these role transitions, which may be evidenced by their anger and frustration as they seek to become socialized into a different role.

2. *Interventions to assist the experienced nurse in resocialization.* Hardy and Conway (1988) state that programs should be designed to assist the nurse with the role transition of position change. They suggest that these programs not only provide an orientation to the new position but also address specific values and behaviors necessary for the new roles. The values and attitudes expected in a hospice nursing role may be very different from those expected in a trauma nurse. Managers should not assume that experienced nurses are aware of the expected role attitudes. The excellent companies identified by Peters and Waterman have leaders who take responsibility for shaping the values of new employees. By instilling and clarifying the values of an organization in its new members, managers are able to create a homogeneous staff who work as a team (Peters and Waterman, 1982).

Employees adopting new values often experience role strain, because acceptance of the new values may involve giving up former values. Nurse managers need to support employees during this period of resocialization into a new role. Often very negative sanctions are employed by members of the reference group. For example, saying things like, "Well, we don't believe in doing that here," can make new, but experienced, employees feel as though the values held in their other nursing roles were bad values. Therefore, the manager should make efforts to see that formerly held values are not belittled.

The Nurse with Role Status Change

1. *Resocialization needs of nurses in role status change.* Although nurses undergoing a change in status have similar resocialization needs, there are some variations. These nurses often experience guilt as they leave the bedside for other nursing roles. When employees and physicians see a nurse manager or a nurse educator assuming the role of care giver, they often make disparaging remarks, such as, "Oh, you're working as a real nurse today." This tends to reinforce the nurse's value conflict in her new role.

Nurses moving into positions of increased responsibility also experience the role stress created by role ambiguity and role overload. Role ambiguity describes the stress that occurs when job expectations are unclear. Role overload occurs when the demands of the role are excessive. Scalzi (1988) demonstrated that role overload is a major job stressor for nurse managers, but she also maintained that all of these stresses make the role transition of nurses moving into higher status positions difficult.

2. *Mechanisms to assist with resocialization in role status change.* In all resocialization, the use of role models, preceptors, and mentors is helpful, but in this particular role change, the use of mentors to facilitate resocialization is invaluable. Individuals lucky enough to find mentors as they move into roles with increased responsibilities and status will find that their resocialization into the new roles will be much smoother, for the mentor, as no other, is able to instill the values and attitudes that accompany each role. In describing her mentor, one writer states, "I would have become a nurse without her, but never would I have sought the professionalism, the degree of compassion, the depth of humor, the height of empathy that are set as guidelines for me by the conduct of my mentor" (Schorr, 1979).

The second most valuable mechanism that organizations use to assist in this type of resocialization is a clear understanding of role expectations. As nurses move into increased status positions, their job descriptions tend to become increasingly vague. Therefore, clarifying job roles becomes an important tool in the resocialization process.

Resocialization is a complex process directed at the acquisition of appropriate attitudes, cognitions, emotions, values, motivations, skills, knowledge, and social patterns necessary to cope with the social and professional environment (Hardy and Conway, 1988). Resocialization differs from and has a greater impact than either induction or orientation on resulting productivity and retention.

KEY CONCEPTS CHAPTER 13

1. Socialization into roles occurs with all roles we occupy and is a normal sociological process.

2. The two methods used to socialize others are social interaction and education.

3. Socialization is a neglected area of the indoctrination process.

4. Role models, preceptors, and mentors all play important roles in the socialization of employees.

5. Most types of role transition create some stress during socialization and resocialization.

6. Difficulties with resocialization are usually centered around unclear role expectations, inability to meet job demands, or deficiencies in motivation.

7. There are many effective interventions nurse managers may utilize to assist employees during the resocialization process.

REFERENCES

Beach, D.S., *Personnel: The Management of People at Work*, Fourth Edition, Macmillan, New York, 1980.

Brim, O.G., Jr., "Socialization Through the Life Cycle," in Brim, O.G., Jr., and Wheeler, S. (eds.), *Socialization After Childhood: Two Essays*, Wiley, New York, 1966.

Cherniss, C., *Professional Burnout In Human Service Organizations*, Praeger, New York, 1980.

Hardy, M.E., and Conway, M.E., *Role Theory: Perspectives for Health Professionals*, Second Edition, Apple-Century-Crofts, New York, 1988.

Hinshaw, A.S., "Socialization and Resocialization for Professional Nursing Practice," in Hein, E.C., and Nicholson, M.J. (eds.), *Contemporary Leadership Behavior: Selected Readings*, Second Edition, Little, Brown and Company, Boston, 1986.

Kramer, M., *Reality Shock: Why Nurses Leave Nursing*, C.V. Mosby, St. Louis, 1974.

Kramer, M. and Schmalenberg, C., "Magnet Hospitals: Part II," *JONA*, 18(2):11–19, 1988.

Linton, R. *The Cultural Background of Personality*, Appleton-Century-Crofts, New York, 1945.

Madison, J., *A Study To Determine Nurse Administrators' Perceptions of the Mentoring Relationship and its Effect on their Professional Lives*, unpublished Masters Thesis, University of Minn., 1984.

Marquis, B.L., and Huston, C.J., *Decision Making in Nursing Management: 101 Case Studies*, J.B. Lippincott, Philadelphia, 1987.

May, K.M., Meleis, A.I., Winstead-Fry, P., "Mentorship for Scholarliness: Opportunities and Dilemmas," *Nursing Outlook*, Jan.:22–28, 1982.

Peters, T.J., and Waterman, R.H., Jr., *In Search of Excellence*, Harper and Row, New York, 1982.

Scalzi, C.C., "Role Stress and Coping Strategies of Nurse Executives," *JONA*, 18(3):34–38, 1988.
Schmalenberg, C., and Kramer, M., *Coping with Reality Shock*, Nursing Resources, Wakefield, MA, 1979.
Schorr, T.M., "Mentor Remembered," *AJN*, 79:12, 1979.
Wheeler, S., "The Structure of Formally Organized Socialization Settings," in Brim, O.G., Jr., and Wheeler, S. (eds.), *Socialization After Childhood: Two Essays*, Wiley, New York, 1966.

ADDITIONAL READINGS

Rice, J., "Transition from Staff Nurse to Head Nurse: A Personal Experience," *Nursing Management*, 19(4):25–27, 1988.
Throwe, A.N., and Fought, S.G., "Landmarks in the Socialization Process from RN to BSN," *Nurse Educator*, 12(6):34–36, 1987.

• UNIT SIX
Developing Optimal Performance in Human Resources

THE POSITIONS individuals hold in organizations and the work they perform are the basis for the establishment of their identities. Work gives meaning and focus to our lives and provides an opportunity for satisfying our desires for recognition and achievement.

Employees, therefore, view the organization's promotion of their professional growth and development as evidence that the organization is interested in them as individuals, and not just workers. It is the organization that profits the most as a result of the growth and development of employees.

Employers holding high expectations of their employees will be rewarded by high productivity, providing the following conditions are met:

1. Employees must understand clearly what those expectations are.

2. Employees must be told frequently how well they are meeting those expectations.

3. Employees must receive frequent encouragement and support.

4. Employees must be given training and education to assist them in meeting the expectations.

5. The organization must show that it is willing to invest time and energy in employees' personal careers.

This unit covers the growth and development functions of an organization, with emphasis on the responsibility of the manager for those functions. One such responsibility is accurate assessment of performance and frequent communication of that assessment to employees. Another area of responsibility discussed is team building through encouragement and support. Strategies and interventions for fulfilling the management functions of coaching, performance appraisal, education and training, and career development are included.

The alert and effective manager accurately assesses each employee's present capabilities, strengths, and weaknesses and then uses a systematic plan for growth and development. Showing employees that the organization has faith in their potential to achieve is a proven method of increasing productivity and retention.

If individuals are viewed as responsible, helpful, and trustworthy, then managers will lead by being supportive and by creating opportunities for growth, self-control, and personal responsibility. While it may be true that people seldom change their core personalities, it has been demonstrated that under the right environment most individuals can grow and learn. It is a responsibility of organizations to supply that environment.

14

Performance Appraisal: Tool Selection and Data Gathering

INDIVIDUALS ARE continually appraising others. We form opinions of others in all aspects of our lives. Although people use these judgments of others as a guide in selecting a dentist or someone to repair their cars, such judgments are rarely arrived at in a systematic manner.

Organizations also continually make judgments about their employees – about their contributions to the organization, and about their abilities to carry out the responsibilities of their job. Because the opinions and judgments of supervisors in organizations are used for far-reaching decisions regarding the work life of employees, it is necessary that these opinions and judgments be arrived at in a formalized and systematic manner. The use of a formal system of performance review will reduce the subjectivity of the appraisal.

Marquis and Huston (1987) state that no action of the manager is as personalized as appraising the work performance of others. Because our work is an important part of our identity, we are very sensitive to others' opinions about how we perform our work. It is for this very reason that performance appraisal is one of the greatest tools an organization has to develop and motivate staff. When used correctly, performance appraisal can increase retention and productivity. In the hands of an inept or inexperienced manager, however, the appraisal process may discourage and demotivate staff.

The more professional an employee is, such as the professional nurse, the more sensitive the evaluation process becomes. The skilled manager becomes proficient in using the formalized system of performance appraisal to increase the productivity of professional staff. Beach (1980) maintains that the difference between an indifferent and a formalized appraisal system is that in a formalized system managers are encouraged to constantly observe their staff in order to provide adequately for their training and development, and in an indifferent system they are not so encouraged. Therefore, in an indifferent system, employees' training and development are not individually planned.

This chapter will focus on the motivational factors inherent in performance appraisal and how the appraisal can be used to determine developmental needs of staff. Types of appraisal tools will be discussed, including positive and negative aspects of each. There will be an emphasis on how data should be gathered so that it is fair and accurate. The process for the implementation of management by objectives and peer review will be delineated. Various appraisal tools will be included, including samples of MBO (Management by Objectives) that would be effective in increasing the productivity of staff nurses.

USING THE PERFORMANCE APPRAISAL TO MOTIVATE EMPLOYEES

Although systematic employee appraisals have been used in management since the 1920s, it was only in the 1950s that much interest was directed toward the use of the appraisal as a tool to promote employee growth. In a discussion of trends in performance appraisal, Beach (1980) states that the present focus is on the appraisal of the professional worker and the manager rather than the hourly paid worker. Beach elaborates by stating that hourly workers are frequently locked into merit increases through union contracts, making the performance appraisal less effective as a motivational tool.

However, others maintain that even when pay raises are automatic, the appropriately used performance appraisal can still be a tool to increase productivity (Case, 1983; Clark, 1982; Loraine, 1982). The performance appraisal becomes a useless waste of management time if it is merely an exercise to satisfy regulations and does not result in employee growth.

The evolution of performance appraisals can be demonstrated by a review of changing terminology. At one time the appraisal was called a *merit rating* and was tied fairly closely to salary increases. In the more recent past it was frequently termed a *performance evaluation*, but because the term *evaluation* implies that a personal value is being placed on the performance review, that term has come into disuse. Some organizations continue to use both of the above terms or use other terms, such as *effectiveness report* or *service rating*. Most health care organizations have come to use the term *performance appraisal*, which is felt to imply an appraisal of how well someone is performing the duties of the job as delineated by the job description.

An important point to consider, if the appraisal is to have a positive outcome, is how the employee views the appraisal. If employees feel that appraisals are based on their job descriptions, rather than on whether the appraiser approves of them as persons, they are more likely to view appraisals as having relevance. Management research has shown that various factors influence whether the appraisal ultimately results in increased motivation and productivity. The effectiveness of the appraisal is influenced by the following:

1. Employees must feel that appraisals are based on a standard that all employees are held accountable to. This standard must be communicated clearly to employees when they are hired. The standard may be a job description or individual goals set by each employee on a regular basis, as in management by objectives (MBO). MBO is discussed later in this chapter.

2. Employees should have some input into the development of the standard or goals against which their performance is judged. This is *imperative* for the professional employee. Nurses must have some input into the development of their job descriptions, since this is the standard against which their performance will be assessed.

3. Employees must know in advance what happens if they do not meet the standards of performance outlined in their job descriptions.

4. Employees need to be aware of how information will be obtained to determine their performances. Marquis and Huston (1987) maintain that the appraisal tends to be more accurate if various sources and kinds of information are solicited. Examples of sources would be peers, co-workers, nursing care plans, patients, and personal observations. Employees need to be told which sources will be used and how such information will be weighed.

5. Appraisers should be those who directly supervise the employees. For example, the charge nurse who works directly with the staff nurse should be involved in the appraisal process and interview. It is appropriate, and advisable in most instances, for the head nurse and/or supervisor also to be involved. However, it is most important for employees to feel that the individuals doing the major portion of the appraisals are people who have actually observed their work and not people who have never personally observed them performing in their professional roles.

6. Performance appraisals are most likely to have positive outcomes if the appraisers are looked upon with trust and professional respect. This increases the chance that employees will view appraisals as fair and accurate assessments of their work performance.

STRATEGIES TO ENSURE ACCURACY AND FAIRNESS

If appraisals are viewed as valuable and valid by employees, they can have many positive results. Information obtained during performance appraisals can be used to develop employees' potentials, to assist employees in overcoming difficulties they may have in fulfilling their roles, to point out strengths of employees that they may not be aware of, and to assist employees in setting goals for the future. Since the outcomes of inaccurate and unfair appraisals are all negative and demotivating, it is critical that managers employ strategies that increase the likelihood that appraisals will be fair and accurate. Although there will always be some subjectivity in any performance appraisal, the following suggestions will assist managers in arriving at more objective assessments:

1. *Appraisers should develop an awareness of their own biases and prejudices.* This helps them guard against allowing subjective attitudes and values to influence their appraisals.

2. *Consultation should be sought frequently.* Another manager should be consulted not only when there is a question

about personal bias, but in many other situations as well. For example, it is important that new managers solicit assistance and consultation as they first begin to complete performance appraisals. Even experienced managers should seek consultation when employees are having great difficulty in fulfilling the duties of the job.

3. *Data should be gathered appropriately.* Many different sources should be used in gathering data regarding employee performance; in addition, the information should cover the entire time period of the appraisal. Frequently, managers gather data and observe employees only just prior to completing appraisals. This gives an inaccurate picture of the job performance. All employees have periods during which they are less productive and motivated than usual, so data should be gathered systematically and regularly.

4. *Information should be written down and not trusted to memory.* Managers should make a habit of making written notations regarding their observations, comments by others, and their periodical reviews of charts and nursing care plans.

5. *Collected assessment should contain positive examples of growth and achievement as well as areas of needed development.* Nothing delights employees more than discovering that their immediate supervisors know of their growth and accomplishments and can cite specific instances in which good clinical judgment was used. Too frequently the collected data concentrates on negative aspects of performance.

6. *The appraiser needs to guard against the three common pitfalls of assessment: the "halo" effect, the "horns" effect, and the "central tendency."* The "halo" effect occurs when the appraiser lets one or two positive aspects of the assessment, or a positive behavior of the employee, unduly influence all other aspects of the employee's performance. The "horns" effect occurs when the appraiser allows some negative aspects of the employee's performance to influence the assessment to such an extent that many other levels of job performance are not accurately recorded. The manager who falls into the "central tendency" trap is hesitant to risk true assessment and therefore rates all employees as average. These types of appraiser behaviors lead employees to discount all of the assessment of their work performance.

7. *Some effort must be made to include employees' own self-appraisals of their work as part of the performance review process.* Self-appraisal may be performed in several appropriate ways. Employees can be instructed to come to the appraisal interview with some informal thoughts regarding

their performances, or they can work with the manager in completing joint assessments. One advantage of management by objectives is the manner in which it involves employees in assessment of their work performances and in goal setting.

TYPES OF PERFORMANCE APPRAISALS

Since the 1920s a wide variety of appraisal tools have been developed. At various times in the history of personnel management, certain types of tools or review techniques have been popular. Presently, the Joint Commission of Accreditation of Hospitals (JCAH) advocates that the performance review be based, in some manner, on the employee's job description. Although the best-designed tool cannot overcome the difficulties created by inaccurate and unfair data collection, the proper use of a well-designed appraisal tool will assist the manager in having positive appraisal outcomes. Still, many effective managers are able to produce great results through performance appraisals even though the appraisal forms they use are poorly designed. It is important that employees be involved in the development and design of performance appraisal instruments. Following is a brief overview of some of the appraisal tools used in health care institutions.

Rating Scales

A rating scale is a method of rating an individual against a set standard, which may consist of the job dimensions, desired behaviors, or personal traits. The rating scale is probably the most widely used of the many available appraisal methods.

Trait rating scales. Rating personal traits and behaviors is the oldest type of rating scale, but because these types of rating scales are subject to central tendency, halo, and horns effect errors, they are not used as often today as they were in the past. The place of traditional rating scales has been taken by two newer rating methods: the job dimension scale and the behavior-anchored rating scale (Table 14-1).

Job dimension scale. This technique requires that a rating scale be constructed for each job. The rating factors are taken from the context of the written job description. Although job

Table 14-1.   Sample of a Trait Rating Scale

Job Knowledge

Serious gaps in essential knowledge	Satisfactory knowledge of routine	Adequately informed on job phases	Good knowledge of all phases of job	Excellent understanding of the job
1	2	3	4	5

Judgment

Decisions are often wrong on issues	Makes some errors	Good decisions made often	Sound and logical thinker	Makes good complex decisions
1	2	3	4	5

Attitude

Resents suggestions, no enthusiasm	Apathetic but cooperative	Satisfactory cooperation of new ideas	Cooperates and accepts new ideas	Helpful and enthusiastic
1	2	3	4	5

Table 14-2.   Sample Job Dimension Rating Scale for Industrial Nurse

Job Dimension	*Rating*				
Renders first aid and treats job-related injuries and illnesses	5	4	3	2	1
Holds fitness classes for workers	5	4	3	2	1
Teaches health and nutrition classes	5	4	3	2	1
Performs yearly physicals on workers	5	4	3	2	1
Keeps equipment in good working order and maintains inventory	5	4	3	2	1
Keeps appropriate records	5	4	3	2	1
Dispenses medication and treatment for minor injuries	5	4	3	2	1

5 = excellent; 4 = good; 3 = satisfactory; 2 = fair, and 1 = poor.

dimension scales have some of the same weaknesses as the trait scales, they do focus on the requirements of the job rather than on such ambiguous terms as quantity of work (Table 14-2).

Behaviorally Anchored Rating Scales. This technique, commonly abbreviated *BARS*, is quite new and has only recently been used as a rating technique in the health care industry. BARS overcomes some of the weaknesses of other rating systems and therefore shows considerable promise.

Like the job dimension scale, the BARS technique requires that a separate rating form be developed for each job and that the employees in specific positions work with management to delineate key areas of responsibility. However, in BARS many specific examples for each area of responsibility are defined, and these examples are given various degrees of importance on a numbered scale from 1 to 9. It is less important that the highest ranked example of a job dimension is being met than that a lower ranked example is not. Table 14-3 shows the BARS for the job dimension of supervising staff for a nurse manager. Other job dimensions that would need accompanying BARS would be communicating information, handling conflict, meeting deadlines, providing resources, diagnosing unit problems, and developing future strategies and plans.

The greatest disadvantage to BARS is the amount of time it requires for implementation. However, it is an excellent tool because it focuses on specific behaviors and allows employees to know exactly what is expected of them.

Although all rating tools are prone to the usual rating weaknesses and interpersonal bias, they do have some advantages. Although they must still be individualized to each organization, tools purchased from form companies reduce the number of expensive human hours spent developing them. Tool 14-1 is an example of combined trait and job dimensional rating scale for a staff nurse. Rating scales also force the rater to look at more than one dimension of work performance, which serves to eliminate some bias.

Interpersonal Comparisons

There are several types of interpersonal comparisons, but all use the same approach. Here the emphasis is on comparing employees with one another rather than looking at specific job dimensions or traits. Supervisors are asked to rank their employees in one of three ways. In *alternative ranking* the supervisor selects the best and weakest employees first and then continues to select the poorest and best until all have been ranked. In the *paired-comparison ranking*, each employee is ranked against every other employee.

A slight variation on the above, the *forced distribution ranking*, is designed to keep supervisors from ranking their employees so that they are clustered at either end of the scale. They are forced to rank employees in a pattern that conforms to a normal frequency distribution curve. There are few advantages to this appraisal method. It is a fairly simple technique, but it is based on questionable reasoning. Its many disadvantages have resulted in its disuse in today's enlightened management science.

Table 14-3. Sample BARS Rating Scale*

	9-
	Could be expected to act as a mentor for one or more nurses
	8-
Could be expected to give the unit personnel confidence and a strong sense of responsibility by delegating important jobs to them	
	7-
	Could be expected to *never* fail to conduct monthly conferences with the staff
	6-
Could be expected to exhibit courtesy and respect toward all the staff on the unit	
	5-
	Could be expected to remind the staff to be prompt in answering lights and to be responsive to family needs
	4-
Could be expected to be critical of organizational policies in front of the staff, thereby risking the development of poor attitudes	
	3-
	Could be expected to insist that someone come to work even though they were ill
	2-
Could be expected to go back on promises made to staff members	
	1-
	Could be expected to make promises to employees that were against company policy

*The job dimension being rated is *supervision*; the position is Nursing Unit Manager.

Check List

There are two types of check lists. The most frequently used type comprises a large number of behavioral statements that represent behaviors desired on a job. Each of these behavior statements has a weighted score attached to it. Each employee then receives an overall score for the performance appraisal. Often merit raises are tied to the total point score; that is, employees need to reach a certain point score in order to receive an increase in pay.

The second type of check list requires that the supervisor select an undesirable as well as a desirable behavior for each

Tool 14-1   Sample Trait and Job Dimension
Rating Scale Appraisal Form

Name _____

Rating Period _____
       From   To

Job Title _____

Dept. Area _____

Reason For Evaluation

3 Months Employment	□
6 Months Employment	□
Annual Evaluation	□
Terminal Evaluation	□
Other	□

Employee Eligible For: Rec.
                               Yes No

□ Permanent Status on _____ □ □
□ Step Increase from
    Step ____ to ____ on _____ □ □

Rate EACH FACTOR according to the scale below. Make comments as necessary in the space provided and continue on separate sheet if needed. Comments are required for all ratings except satisfactory.

Unacceptable: Must re-evaluate in 3 months; if no improvement found, formal action is to be taken.
Needs Improvement: Areas where the employee needs to improve
Satisfactory: Areas where the employee is performing adequately
Excels: Areas where the employee has shown excellence; this category must be documented with objective criteria.

R A T I N G

ALL NURSING EMPLOYEES	Unacceptable	Needs Improvement	Satisfactory	Excels	COMMENTS
1. *Priority Setting* Demonstrates the ability to do the most important work first, and if workload is heavy, never eliminates vital work.					
2. *Nursing Judgment* Demonstrates good nursing judgment in observation and reporting pertinent information.					
3. *Interpersonal Relationships* Demonstrates tact, compassion, and consideration to other employees, patients, and families.					
4. *Competence* Works safely and competently within job description.					
5. *Evidence of Continued Education* Attendance at in-service classes, workshops, reading material, lectures, CPR certification, etc.					
6. *Attendance* On duty on time when scheduled.					
7. *Dependability* Reports safety hazards, patients' conditions, and follows through.					

R A T I N G

ALL REGISTERED NURSES	Unacceptable	Needs Improvement	Satisfactory	Excels	COMMENTS To be documented by chart, audit, observed reports, nursing care plans, histories, and referrals.
1. Nursing assessment and appropriate action taking.					
2. Provides for continuity of care					
3. Communication skills					
4. Teaching skills					
ALL RNs ABOVE STAFF II LEADERSHIP FACTORS					COMMENTS
1. Role model					
2. Promotes growth and development in staff: delegates, staff free to attend meetings and in-service, gives goal-directed evaluations.					
3. Capable of long- and short-range planning.					
4. Prompt and appropriate action taking to solve problems.					
5. Follows through					
6. Has developed appropriate counseling techniques					

employee. Both desirable and undesirable behaviors have quantitative values, and the employee again ends up with a total point score that is used for making certain employment decisions.

The former type of check list, often called a *weighted scale*, is used much more frequently than the latter type. A major weakness of both methods is that there are no set standards of performance and specific components of behavior are not addressed. However, check lists do focus on a variety of job-related behaviors and avoid some of the bias inherent in a number of the trait rating scales.

Essay

This method of appraisal is often referred to as the *free-form review*. The appraiser describes, in narrative form, the strengths of the employee and the areas in which improvement or growth is needed. Although this method can be totally unstructured, it usually calls for certain items to be addressed. Tool 14-2 provides an example of an essay appraisal form using specific criteria. A major strength of this technique is that it forces the appraiser to focus on positive aspects of the employee's performance. However,

---

**Tool 14-2   Sample Appraisal Tool: A Portion of an
Essay Appraisal Form for a Staff Nurse**

EXPECTATIONS OF A STAFF NURSE

I. Maintains a safe and cooperative work environment.
  A. Utilizes additional help as necessary when ambulating or transferring patients.
  B. Keeps patient rooms neat and free of obstacles.
  C. Functions efficiently during fire and disaster drills.
  D. Provides for patient privacy.
  E. Identifies interpatient conflicts and if possible arranges for improved environment.
  F. Gives assistance to co-workers willingly.
  G. Is pleasant to patients and co-workers.
  H. Directs critical evaluation of situation to proper person.

II. Reports and records observations of patient's condition.
  A Observes and reports significant changes in patient's condition to Team Leader and when requested to other members of the medical team.
  B. Participates actively in team conferences.
  C. Records accurately, completely and neatly observations of patient's condition.

III. Participates in teaching co-workers.
  A. Aids in orientation of new personnel on the nursing unit.
  B. Willingly demonstrates and explains policies, procedures, techniques, nursing care and ward routine to co-workers.
  C. Participates actively in ward conferences.

IV. Operates and cares for equipment.
  A. Operates equipment necessary for patient care on her unit.
  B. Asks questions about equipment she's not familiar with.
  C. Reports non-functioning equipment.
  D. Maintains equipment by proper cleaning while in use and terminal cleaning when discontinued.

---

it undoubtedly also leaves a great deal of room for supervisor bias.

Many organizations are combining various types of appraisals in order to improve the quality of their review processes. Since the essay method requires no exhaustive development, it can quickly be adapted as an adjunct to any type of structured format. The organization can thereby decrease bias and focus on employee strengths.

Self-Appraisal

There are both advantages and disadvantages to using self-appraisal as a method of performance review. Marquis and Huston (1987) maintain that introspection and self-appraisal result in growth for individuals who are mature and self-aware. However, even mature individuals require feedback and validation of their performances.

Some employees may look upon their annual performance reviews as a time when they receive positive feedback from their supervisors. This is especially true if they receive infrequent praise on a day-to-day basis. Asking these employees to write their own performance appraisals would probably be seen as negative rather than positive.

Since studies have shown that employees tend to rate themselves lower in performance than their supervisors do (Lefton, 1977), it is probably unwise to have employees' self-evaluations be the only performance appraisals that are made. However, there is ample evidence that the self-appraisal, when used in conjunction with an organizational appraisal, is an excellent method to promote further development of employees (Maier, 1976). It is for this reason that MBO is such an excellent tool for assessing individual employee progress, since it incorporates the assessments of both the employee and the organization.

Management by Objectives

Drucker's MBO concepts have already been discussed; therefore, the focus here will be on how these concepts are used as an effective performance appraisal method, rather than as a planning technique or organizational philosophy.

The MBO method is tailor-made for the performance appraisal of managers and autonomous professionals (Beach, 1980). It is infrequently used in the health care setting, yet it is an excellent method to appraise the performance of the registered nurse in a manner that promotes growth in the individual and excellence in nursing. McGregor (1960) has probably best delineated how the important features of MBO can be used effectively in performance appraisal. The following steps guide the employee and supervisor in their roles:

1. The employee and supervisor meet and agree on the principal duties and responsibilities of the employee's job. (The job description serves as a guide only; other things may also be included.)

2. The employee sets his or her own short-term goals and targets in cooperation with the supervisor or manager. The manager helps guide the process so that it relates to the duties of the position.

3. Both parties agree on what criteria will be used for measuring and evaluating whether the goals have been met.

4. On a regular basis, but more than once a year, the two get together to discuss progress. At these meetings some modification can be made if agreed on by both parties.

5. The role of the manager is supportive. The manager tries to help the employee reach his or her goals by coaching and counseling.

6. During the appraisal process, the manager judges whether the goals have been met by the employee.

7. The entire process focuses on outcomes and results, and not on personal traits.

Beach (1980) states that one of the many advantages of MBO is that employees set their own goals, giving them a vested interest in meeting those goals. Additionally, defensive feelings are minimized and a spirit of team work prevails. In MBO the focus is on the controllable present and future rather than on the uncontrollable past (Beach, 1980).

There are also disadvantages to MBO as a performance appraisal method. Highly directive and authoritarian managers find it difficult to lead employees in this manner. Also, marginal employees frequently attempt to set easily attainable goals.

However, research has shown that MBO is a very effective tool when used correctly, especially when it is used as a total management system, rather than only as a method of performance appraisal (Carroll and Tosi, 1973; Meyer et al., 1965). Table 14-4 is an example of the use of MBO, and Tool 14-3 is an example of the use of nursing service objectives as an appraisal tool.

Table 14-4. Sample Use of MBO in a Performance Appraisal

It is time for Nancy Irwin's annual performance appraisal. Nancy is an RN on a post-surgical unit, dealing with complex trauma patients requiring high-level nursing intensity. You are the evening charge nurse and have worked with Nancy for the 2 years since she has been out of nursing school. Last year, in addition to the regular 1–5 rating scale of job expectation, all the charge nurses added a MBO component to the performance appraisal form. Each employee developed five goals, in collaboration with the charge nurse, that were supposed to have been carried out over a 1-year period.

In reviewing Nancy's performance, you use several sources, examine your written notes, look at her charting, etc., and your conclusion is that she has strengths and weaknesses, but overall, she is a better-than-average nurse. You feel she has not grown a lot in the past 6 months. This observation is confirmed when you review her objectives from last year and find the following goals and assessment of accomplishments:

Objective	*Result*
1. Personally will conduct a mini-inservice or patient care conference 2 times a month during the next 12 months	Met goal first 2 months; last 10 months conducted only six conferences
2. Will attend five educational classes related to work area; at least two of these will be outside the agency	Attended one surgical nursing wound conference in the city and one in house (a conference on TPN)
3. Will become an active member of a nursing committee in the hospital	Has become an active member of the Policy and Procedure Committee and attends meetings on a regular basis
4. Reduce number of late arrivals at work by 50% (from 24 to 12)	First 3 months: no late arrivals Second 3 months: 3 late arrivals Third 3 months: 6 late arrivals Last 3 months: 6 late arrivals
5. Ensure that all parties discharged have discharge instruction slips and instructions documented in the chart	Incidental notes show that Nancy still frequently forgets to document these nursing actions.

From Marquis, B., and Huston, C.J., *Management Decision Making For Nurses: 101 Case Studies*, J.B. Lippincott, Philadelphia, 1987.

Peer Review

The concept of collegial evaluation of nursing practice is closely related to the maintenance of professional standards. When the monitoring and assessment of performance is carried out by peers rather than by supervisors, it is referred to as *peer review*. Although the prevailing practice in most organizations is to have managers evaluate the performance of employees, there is much to be said for the practice of peer review.

Tool 14-3   Sample Appraisal Form Using Nursing Service Objectives

STAFF NURSE PERFORMANCE EVALUATION

Name:_____ Unit:_____ Date:_____

Position:_____ Length of time in position:_____

Using the Evaluation Supplement and Guide as needed, please comment on the manner in, and the extent to which, the staff nurse is achieving the objectives of the Hospital Nursing Services.

1. Assists the patient to meet the needs of daily living.

2. Develops productive interdepartmental and interprofessional working relationships.

3. Contributes to student education by practicing quality nursing care.

4. Provides nursing personnel with opportunities for individual growth and development in the practice of nursing.

5. Includes patients and their families in decisions regarding care.

6. Promotes an atmosphere within the nursing services where creative ideas may be expressed.

7. Continually evaluates methods of nursing practice for areas of improvement.

8. Uses results of nursing evaluation to effect change in nursing practice.

Evaluation Summary

PERFORMANCE EVALUATION:
  A. Principal strengths:

  B. Principal difficulties:

  C. Improvement demonstrated in performance:

  D. Counseling plan for improvement: (May be completed during conference)

RECOMMENDATIONS:
  A. Consider for promotion:
  B. Continue in present position:
  C. Unsatisfactory in present position:

EMPLOYEE'S COMMENTS:

Employee   Evaluator

Date   Title

                                      Supervisor

SUPERVISOR'S COMMENTS:

It is most likely that the view a supervisor receives of employees is not complete unless some type of peer review is included in the gathered data. Peer review, when implemented properly, provides employees with valuable feedback, which promotes employee growth. Research has demonstrated that peer review is a valid tool for accurately assessing the performance of employees (Lewin and Zwany, 1976; Roadman, 1964). Peer ratings are widely used by colleges and universities, and by physicians, but they have not been widely used by business and industry.

Marquis and Huston (1987) maintain that health care organizations have been slow to adopt peer review for the following reasons:

1. Poor orientation of staff to the peer review method. Peer review is viewed as very threatening when not enough time is spent orienting employees to the peer review process or providing necessary support throughout the process.

2. Peers feel uncomfortable sharing feedback with people they work closely with, so they omit needed suggestions for improving colleagues' performance. Thus, the review becomes more advocacy than evaluation.

3. Peer review is viewed by many as more time consuming than traditional superior/subordinate performance appraisals.

4. Because much socialization takes place in the work place, friendships develop that often result in inflated evaluations, or interpersonal conflict may result in unfair appraisals.

5. Because peer review shifts the authority away from the management hierarchy, the insecure manager may feel threatened.

Peer review has its shortcomings, as evidenced by the unjustified tenure of some university teachers or the failure of physicians to adequately maintain quality control among members of their profession. Additionally, peer review involves much risk-taking, is time consuming, and requires a great deal of energy.

However, Sliefert (1985) has put forth a strong argument for placing the responsibility for quality control in the hands of the profession. If performance appraisal of the professional nurse is viewed as a type of quality control, it becomes apparent that the nursing profession must have some input into it.

Peer review can be carried out in several ways. The process may require the reviewer to share the results with only the reviewee, or the results may be shared with the reviewee's supervisor and the reviewee. The results may or may not be used for personnel decisions. The number of observations, the number of reviewers, the qualifications and classifications of peer reviewers, and the review procedure will need to be developed for each organization.

However, if peer review is to be successful, the organization needs first to overcome some inherent difficulties:

1. Peer review appraisal tools must reflect the standards to be measured, based on the job description.
2. Staff must receive a thorough orientation to the process prior to its implementation. The role of the manager should be clearly defined.
3. Ongoing support, resources, and information must be made available to the staff during the process.
4. Data for peer review needs to be obtained from agreed on sources (e.g., observations, charts, patient care plans, etc.).
5. It must be decided whether information that is anonymous will be allowed. This is controversial and needs to be addressed in the procedure.
6. Decisions must be reached on whether the peer review will affect personnel decisions, and if so, in what manner.

Peer review has the potential to increase the accuracy of performance appraisal and is especially useful in determining the performance of the professional nurse. The use of peer review in nursing should continue to increase as nursing increases its autonomy and professional status.

EFFECTIVE USE OF APPRAISAL DATA

This chapter has provided the manager with some valuable information on gathering data for a performance appraisal that will result in increased productivity and motivation. However, the most accurate and thorough appraisal will fail to produce growth in the employee unless the information is used appropriately. Many managers fail to conduct an appraisal interview that results in positive outcomes. Secondly, many organizations view performance appraisal interviews as a time to instruct employees on what they are doing wrong. McGregor (1957) stated that this approach to the appraisal interview comes close to violating an individual's integrity.

The next chapter will provide managers with some insight into the use of performance appraisal information as a means to stimulate employee growth and development and for long-term career planning. Additionally, the reader will be provided with approaches and solutions to appraisal interview problems.

KEY CONCEPTS CHAPTER 14

1. Employee performance appraisal is a sensitive and important part of the management process and requires much skill.

2. When accurate and appropriate appraisal assessments are performed, the outcomes can be very positive.

3. Performance appraisals are used to determine how well employees are performing, using the job description as a standard measurement.

4. There are many different types of appraisal tools. While some appraisal tools are better designed than others, all have advantages and disadvantages.

5. It is essential that employees be involved in the appraisal process and that they view appraisals as accurate and fair.

6. Management by objectives has proven to be a method that increases productivity and commitment in employees.

7. Peer review, although infrequently utilized in the appraisal process, has much potential for developing professional accountability.

REFERENCES

Beach, D., *Personnel: The Management of People at Work*, Fourth Edition, Macmillan, New York, 1980.

Carroll, S.J., Jr., and Tosi, H.L., *Management by Objectives: Applications and Research*, Macmillan, New York, 1973.

Case, B.B., "Moving Your Staff Toward Excellent Performance," *Nursing Management* 11:45, 1983.

Clark, M.D., "Performance Appraisal," *Nursing Management*, 13:27, 1982.

Lefton, R.E., et al., *Effective Motivation Through Personnel Appraisal*, John Wiley and Sons, New York, 1977.

Lewin, A. Y., and Zwany, A., "Peer Nominations: A Model. Literature Critique and a Paradigm for Research," *Psychology Today* 29:3, 1976.

Loraine, K., "Work Evaluations: Are They Effective?" *Nursing Management*, 13:44, 1982.

McGregor, D., *The Human Side of Enterprise*, McGraw-Hill, New York, 1960.

McGregor, D., "An Uneasy Look at Performance Appraisal," *Harvard Business Review*, 35:3, 1957.

Maier, N.R.F., *The Appraisal Interview: Three Basic Approaches*, University Associates, LaJolla, CA, 1976.

Marquis, B.L., and Huston, C.J., *Decision Making for Nurses: 101 Case Studies*, J.B. Lippincott, Philadelphia, 1987.

Meyer, H., Keye, E., and French, T., "Split Roles in Performance Appraisal," *Harvard Business Review*, 43(1):123–129, 1965.

Roadman, H.E., "An Industrial Use of Peer Ratings," *Journal of Applied Psychology*, 48(4):211–214, 1964.

Sliefert, N., "Quality Control: Professional or Institutional Responsibility?" in McClosky, Jr., and Grace, H. (eds.), *Current Issues in Nursing*, Second Edition, C.V. Mosby Company, St. Louis, 1985.

ADDITIONAL READINGS

Dickson, B., "Maintaining Anonymity in Peer Evaluation," *Supervisor Nurse* 10:21, 1979.

O'Loughin, E.L., Kaulbach, D., "Peer Review: A Perspective for Performance Appraisal," *JONA*, 11:22, 1981.

15

Coaching: During the Appraisal Interview and as a Management Function

THE EFFORT that has been applied to gathering accurate and appropriate appraisal data will be useless unless the appraisal interview in which the information is shared is carried out in an effective manner. The word *coaching* has become a popular contemporary term used to convey the spirit of the supervisor's role in the appraisal interview. Coaching is not limited to the appraisal interview, but should occur as a regular part of the supervisor's job functions.

Coaching is one of the most important aspects of staff development and is perhaps the most difficult role for the supervisor to master. Coaching is an effective strategy for increasing retention and motivation. A good coach develops both individuals and the team. Individual needs and interests must be considered, while at the same time all members must be molded together to make a team effort.

This chapter will address the setting of the appraisal interview, the necessary preparation, the interview itself, and the post-interview follow-up. Additionally, coaching techniques will be discussed, including both short-term and long-term coaching needs. Specific examples of coaching strategies for use with marginal employees, overwhelmed employees, and motivated employees are given. Tools included in this chapter are an example of a form to be used to document the appraisal interview, a sample of an appraisal interview using management by objectives (MBO), and a form to assist in the planning of long-term coaching.

DIFFICULTIES WITH APPRAISAL INTERVIEWS

Managers often dislike the appraisal interview more than they dislike the actual data gathering for the performance appraisal. Beach (1980) suggests that one of the reasons supervisors find this job function so distasteful is due to their own past experiences having their performance evaluated. McGregor (1957) supports this view, stating that in the past approaches to the appraisal interview have focused on judging and criticizing the personal worth of the employee.

Since both parties in the appraisal process tend to become anxious prior to the interview, it is not surprising that the appraisal interview remains an emotionally charged event. For many employees this event is also traumatizing. Since the nursing manager is dealing with adults whose emotional reactions are based on many previous appraisal interviews, not much can be done to completely eliminate the emotional climate of the interview. However, the supervisor can manage it in such a manner that individuals will not be traumatized further.

Nearly everyone agrees that performance appraisals are necessary and beneficial both to the organization and to the individuals involved. Some research, however, indicates that how the information from the performance appraisal is shared has an impact on later performance. Excessive criticism has been found to have a negative effect on later goal attainment (Meyer et al., 1965). The interview appraiser must make sure that there is no threat to the individual's self-esteem, because this will prevent the development of a meaningful and constructive relationship between the manager and employee. For growth to occur in the work place, it is necessary for a constructive relationship to exist.

OVERCOMING APPRAISAL INTERVIEW DIFFICULTIES

Feedback is perhaps the greatest tool a manager has for changing behavior, but to be effective the feedback must be given in an appropriate manner (Marquis and Huston, 1987). The performance appraisal is most likely to result in increased productivity and retention if certain conditions are met before, during, and following the interview. The following guidelines are suggested:

Before the Interview

1. Make sure the conditions mentioned in the preceding chapter have been met (i.e., the employee knows the standards by which his or her work will be evaluated and has a copy of the appraisal form).
2. Select an appropriate time for the appraisal conference. Do not select a time when the employee has just had a traumatic personal event or a time when the employee is too busy at work to take the time necessary for a meaningful conference.
3. Give the employee advance notice of the scheduled appraisal conference (2–3 days) so he or she can prepare mentally and emotionally for the interview.
4. The manager should also be prepared mentally and emotionally for the conference. If something should happen to interfere with the manager's readiness, the interview should be rescheduled.
5. Adequate uninterrupted time should be scheduled for the interview, and it should be held in a private, quiet, and comfortable place.
6. The seating arrangement should reflect collegiality rather than power. Having the individual seated across a large desk from the appraiser denotes power/status position, but placing the chairs side by side denotes equal status.

During the Interview

1. The employee should be greeted warmly and should be shown that the organization has a sincere interest in his or her future growth.
2. Throughout the conference the manager should utilize the coaching techniques that will be discussed later in this chapter.

3. The conference should begin on a pleasant informal note.

4. The employee should be asked to comment on his or her progress since the last performance appraisal.

5. The appraisal conference should contain few surprises. The effective supervisor will be coaching and communicating informally with staff on a continuous basis, so there should be little new information at an appraisal conference.

6. Occasionally an appraisal will reveal several problems that are either new or long-standing. When this occurs the employee should not be overwhelmed at the conference. If there are many problems to be addressed, select only a few major ones.

7. The conference should be conducted in a nondirective and participatory manner. Frequent input from the employee should be solicited throughout the interview. The employee's performance, not personal characteristics, must be the focus of the conference.

8. Be prepared with explicit examples of the employee's performance, being liberal with positive examples and sparing with examples of poor performance. Examples of poor performance should be brought up only if the employee has a great deal of difficulty with self-awareness and requests a specific example of a problem area in performance.

9. Never threaten, intimidate, or use status in any manner.

10. This is the time for the manager to show the employee that he or she is aware of the employee's uniqueness, special interests, and valuable contributions to the unit. Remember that nearly all employees make some special contribution to the work place.

11. Make every effort to ensure that there are no interruptions during the conference.

12. Make an effort to use terms and language that are clearly understood and carry the same meaning for both of you. Words that carry a negative connotation should be avoided. Do not talk down to the employee or use language that is inappropriate for the employee's level of education.

13. Goal setting for further growth or for improvement in performance should be reached by mutual involvement, including a decision on how goals will be accomplished, how goals will be evaluated, and what support is necessary for the employee to reach these mutually agreed-upon goals. An example of the use of MBO in setting agreed-upon goals and their subsequent evaluation is shown in Tool 15-1.

Tool 15-1 Example of Management-by-Objectives Post-Appraisal Interview

In the preceding chapter an example of management-by-objective (MBO) goals was given. In that example, the manager found, in reviewing the previously set goals, that only some of the goals had been successfully met. The reader is asked to refer back to that example in order to prepare for the post-appraisal interview.

There are several things important in reviewing the goals. First it appears that Nancy is a person who needs reminders. She had functioned well in Objective #3 because she received monthly reminders of the meetings, and because she worked with a group of people, she was able to make a real contribution to this committee.

The similarities among the other four objectives are that they all required Nancy to (1) work alone to accomplish them and (2) there were no built-in reminders. Rather than using this performance appraisal to criticize, the charge nurse should spend his or her energy in developing a plan to ensure Nancy's success in the following months. Nothing is as depressing or demotivating to an employee as failure.

The following plan concentrates only on the MBO portion of Nancy's performance appraisal and does not focus on the rating scale of job performance.

PLAN

PRIOR TO INTERVIEW	RATIONALE
1. Ask Nancy to review her objectives from last year and to come prepared to discuss them.	1. Gives employee opportunity for self problem solving and personal introspection.
2. Set a convenient time for you and Nancy and allow adequate time and privacy.	2. Shows interest in and respect for employee.

AT INTERVIEW	RATIONALE
1. Begin by complimenting Nancy on Objective #4. Ask her about her work on the committee, what procedures she is working on, etc.	1. Shows interest in and support of employee.
2. Review each of the other four objectives and ask for Nancy's input. Withhold any advice or criticism at this point.	2. Allows the employee to make own judgments about performance.

3. Ask Nancy if she sees a pattern.

3. Guides employee into own problem solving.

4. Tell Nancy that MBO often works better if objectives are reviewed on a more timely basis and ask how she feels about this.

4. This is an offer to assist the employee in improved performance and is not a punitive measure. Allows employee to have input.

5. Suggest that Nancy keep her unmet four objectives and add one new objective for the one that she met.

5. Employees should be encouraged to meet objectives, unless they were stated poorly or were unrealistic.

6. Work with Nancy in developing a reminder or check-point system that will assist her in meeting her objectives.

6. Again, this is helping the employee succeed. Don't just tell employees they should do better; show them how.

7. Do not sympathize with or excuse Nancy for not meeting her objectives.

7. The focus should remain on growth and not on the status quo.

8. End on a note of encouragement and support. "Nancy—I know that you are capable of meeting these objectives."

8. Employees often live up to their manager's expectations of them, and if those expectations are for growth, then the chances are greater that growth will occur.

---

14. Always plan on being available for the employee to return to discuss the appraisal review further. Employees frequently need to return for elaboration if their conferences did not go well or if they received unexpected new information. This is especially true for new employees.

Following the Interview

1. Both the manager and the employee need to sign the appraisal form to document that the conference has been held and that the employee received the information contained in the appraisal. This does not mean that the employee is agreeing to the information in the appraisal; it merely means that the employee has read the appraisal. An example of such a form is shown in Tool 15-2. There should be a place for comments by both the manager and the employee.

2. The interview should end on a pleasant note.

3. The manager should document what mutual goals for further development have been agreed on by both parties. The documentation should include target dates for accomplishment, and necessary support needed, and when goals are to be reviewed. This documentation is often part of the appraisal form.

Tool 15-2   Sample Cover Sheet for Performance Appraisal Form

---

Performance appraisal for:

Name: _____

Unit: _____

Prepared by: _____

Reason: _____
              (Merit, terminal, end of probation, general reviews)

Date of evaluation conference:_____

> Comments by employee.
>
>
>
>
>
>   Employee's signature: _____
> (Signature of employee denotes that the evaluation has been read. It
> *does not* signify acceptance and/or agreement. Space is provided for
> any comments employee wishes to make.)

> Comments by evaluator:
> (These comments are to be written at the time of the evaluation
> conference and in the presence of the employee.)
>
>
>
>
>
> _____   _____   _____
> Employee's signature   Date   Evaluator's signature

4. If the interview reveals specific long-term coaching needs, the manager should develop a method of follow through to ensure that such coaching takes place. The long-term coaching form in Tool 15-3 could be modified for this purpose.

COACHING

Quick (1985) maintains that coaching falls into one of two types: short-term, which is problem-centered coaching; and long-term, which may or may not involve a problem. The problem may be work centered rather that performance centered. Quick maintains that coaching is not counseling; counseling occurs as one of the last steps that a manager takes to correct a performance deficiency.

Peters and Austin (1985), however, feel that counseling is a form of coaching. They state that the five roles of a manager coach are (1) educating, (2) sponsoring, (3) coaching, (4) counseling, and (5) confronting. Examples of various types of coaching will be presented in this chapter.

Rather than debate what is, or what is not, appropriately termed *coaching*, it is more important to have the reader understand the impact coaching can have on an organization. The following three quotations from the coaching chapter in *A Passion for Excellence* (Peters and Austin, 1985) clarify the coaching role in human resource management:

There is no magic: only people who find and nurture champions, dramatize company goals and direction, build skills and teams, spread irresistible enthusiasm. They are cheerleaders, coaches storytellers and wanderers. They encourage, excite, teach, listen, facilitate. Their actions are consistent. Only brute consistency breeds believability: they say people are special and they treat them that way—always. You know they take their priorities seriously because they live them clearly and visibly: they walk the talk. (page 324)

Coaching is face-to-face leadership that pulls together people from diverse backgrounds, talents, experiences, and interests, encourages them to step up to responsibility and continued achievement, and treats them as full-scale partners and contributors. Coaching is not about memorizing or devising the perfect game plan. It is about really paying attention to people—really

Tool 15-3   Sample Long-Term Coaching Form

Name of employee _____

Name of supervisor _____

Date _____ Date of last coaching interview_____

1. What new challenges and responsibilities could be given to this employee that would utilize his or her special talents?

   _____

   _____

   _____

2. What events happening in the organization do you foresee impacting on this employee? (Examples would be plans to go to an all-RN staff, changing the mode of patient care delivery, an increased emphasis on credentialing by the new CEO of the nursing division, changing the medication system, changing the ratio of nonprofessionals to professionals for nursing staffing, etc.)

   _____

   _____

   _____

3. How should the employee be preparing to meet new or changing expectations?

   _____

   _____

   _____

4. What are specific suggestions and guidance for the future that you can give this employee? (Examples would be taking specific courses to prepare for a change, urging the employee to take an advanced degree, considering changing shifts, urging the employee to seek challenges outside of your unit, suggesting that the employee apply for the next management opening, etc.)

   _____

   _____

   _____

5. What specific organizational resources can you offer the employee?

_____

_____

_____

6. What new information regarding long-term plans, aspirations, and potential of this employee have the perusal of the personnel record, your observations, and this interview given you?

_____

_____

_____

7. Do the organizational and professional career plans held by the individual match your vision of his or her future? If not how do they differ?

_____

_____

8. What developmental and professional growth has taken place since the last coaching session?

_____

_____

9. Date of next coaching interview _____

believing in them, really caring about them, really involving them. (page 325)

A former IBMer stresses the point: "Coaching isn't always noisy and obvious. The best coach I ever had used to come around and ask, 'How's such and such going?' or 'What do you think the customer wants?' Those questions were perfectly aimed. I'd leave those little meetings believing I'd come up with the answers. Only later did I realize that he directed my attention with those questions of his, used them as rudders, to steer me in a certain direction. He never once came out and told me what to do; he led me there and made me feel like I'd figured it out on my own. He was never impatient or too busy to listen. But I think what I appreciated about him the most was that he never asked me to do something I didn't have the ability to do, even if I didn't realize it.

He knew me well enough to judge my reach; that was his credibility. If he had put me in situations where I failed, I would have doubted his ability as a coach more than mine as a player. I knew he wanted me to succeed and that we could count on each other. After talking to him I felt empowered." (page 362)

While the coaching that takes place during a performance appraisal interview is always planned, much of day-to-day coaching is unplanned. This is perhaps the reason that coaching is such a difficult technique for a manager to master. The manager must be constantly on guard for the opportunity to advance an employee's effectiveness and skills through the timely use of coaching.

Perhaps the best way to explain coaching is to think of it as helping the other reach an optimum decision. The emphasis is always on assisting the employee in recognizing greater options, in clarifying statements, and in encouraging the employee to grow. Coaching is not solving an employee's problems, but in helping the employee see how to reach his or her own solutions to problems.

Short-Term Coaching

Short-term coaching may involve (1) a problem that results because of a performance deficiency, (2) a difficulty that one employee has with a peer or a subordinate, or (3) a problem related to work. When it is possible, the supervisor should take time to plan prior to the coaching interview, and this is an absolute must if it involves an employee criticism. However, many opportunities for excellent coaching would be missed if the manager were unable to coach spontaneously. The following scenario is an example of short-term coaching with an employee who is in a new role, with the supervisor acting as teacher/coach.

PAUL'S COMPLAINT

Paul is the 3–11 charge nurse on a surgical floor. One day he comes to work a few minutes early, as he occasionally does, so that he can chat with his supervisor, Mary, prior to taking a patient report. Mary usually is in her office around this time, and Paul enjoys talking over some of his work-related management problems with her, as he is fairly new in the charge nurse role, having been appointed 3 months ago. Today he asks Mary if she can spare a minute to discuss a personnel problem he is having. The following conversation takes place:

> *Paul*:   Sally is becoming a real problem to me. She is taking long break times and has not followed through on several medication order changes lately.
>
> *Mary*:   What do you mean by "long breaks" and not following through?
>
> *Paul*:   In the last 2 months she has taken an extra 15 minutes for dinner 3 nights a week and has missed changes in medication orders 8 times.
>
> *Mary*:   Have you spoken to Sally?
>
> *Paul*:   Yes, and she said she has been an RN on this floor for 4 years and no one has ever criticized her before. I checked her personnel record and there is no mention of those particular problems, but, on the other hand, her performance appraisals have only been mediocre.
>
> *Mary*:   What is your recommendation regarding Sally?
>
> *Paul*:   I could tell her that I won't tolerate her extended dinner breaks and her poor work performance?
>
> *Mary*:   What are you prepared to do if her performance does not improve?
>
> *Paul*:   I could give her a written warning notice, and eventually fire her if her work remains below standard.
>
> *Mary*:   Well, that is one option. What are some other options available to you? Do you think Sally really understands your expectations? Do you feel she might resent you?
>
> *Paul*:   I suppose I ought to sit down with Sally and explain exactly what my expectations are. Since my appointment to charge nurse, I've talked with all the new nurses as they have come on shift, but I just assumed the old timers knew what was expected on this unit. I've been a little anxious about my new role. I never thought about her resenting my position.
>
> *Mary*:   I think that is a good first option. Maybe Sally interpreted your not talking with her, as you did all the new nurses, as a rejection. After you have another talk with her let me know how things are going.

ANALYSIS

Here the supervisor coaches Paul toward a more appropriate option as a first choice in solving this problem. Though Mary's choice of questions and guidance assisted Paul, she never "took over" or directed Paul, but instead let him find his own better solution. As a result of this conversation, Paul had a series of individual meetings with all the staff on his shift and shared with them his expectations and enlisted their assistance in his efforts to have the shift run smoothly. Although he began to see an improvement in Sally's work performance, he realized she was a marginal employee and that she would take a great deal of coaching. He reported back to Mary and outlined his plans for improving Sally's performance further. Mary complimented Paul on his handling of the problem.

The Marginal Employee

People become marginal employees for various reasons. Jernigan (1988) suggests the following may result in performance deficiencies: (1) burnout, (2) boredom, (3) job dissatisfaction, (4) resentment of the need to work for economic reasons, (5) personal problems, (6) drug or alcohol abuse, (7) knowledge deficits, (8) inability to learn, (9) emotional disturbances, and (10) failing health.

Regardless of the reason for unsatisfactory work performance, frequent coaching is often effective in increasing the productivity of the marginal employee. The coaching might take the form of counseling, or even confronting, the employee, but there should also be the inclusion of frequent spontaneous coaching that is encouraging and supportive of the employee's efforts to improve performance.

The Manager as Counselor/Coach

The key role for the manager in the counseling role is to listen and not to meddle or practice psychiatric therapy. Peters and Austin (1985) maintain that when counseling is needed, it is often delayed. When counseling is necessary, it should be performed as soon as there is evidence that a problem exists. Secondly, in contrast to coaching done at the performance appraisal, there should be *little advance notice* for performance deficiency coaching. Since most employees know when they are not doing well, giving them long advance notice of a scheduled conference produces unnecessary stress for them (Peters and Austin, 1985).

Counseling should never be punitive. The aim of the counseling session is to let employees know that you, as the manager, want people to do well and that you are interested in them and are encouraging them to try harder.

When the coaching involves a deficiency in performance, there is less spontaneity and more need for planning. Sullivan and Decker (1985) maintain that before entering the coaching session, the manager needs to spend at least a few minutes preparing for the interaction, and that during the session the manager needs to follow the behaviors outlined in Table 15-1. The following scenario is an example of a performance deficiency coaching session.

BETH'S PHONE CALLS

Beth is a nurse on the day shift and a relatively new mother. Mary, the supervisor, has recently become aware that Beth is making and receiving quite a number of personal phone calls on duty. This has resulted in interruptions to Beth's work and has increased her overtime. Mary has the following coaching session with Beth, which is held in Mary's office.

Mary: You have been making and receiving a considerable number of personal phone calls. This concerns me because it is interrupting your work and your patient care and has resulted in some need for overtime. Could you tell me why this problem is occurring?

Beth: I'm just so worried about my baby. I hate leaving her. I guess I'm just a worried new mother. I know I've been on the phone a lot lately.

Mary: You are aware of the policy on personal phone calls and know that this could affect your performance appraisal?

Beth: Yes I know that. I'll try to do better.

Mary: Can you think of some ways to solve the problem?

Beth: Well, I suppose I could try to just call on my breaks and ask my sitter to call me only if there is an urgent problem.

Mary: Do you have a qualified sitter?

Beth: Oh, yes. I spent weeks researching the right person.

Mary: Has the baby experienced a lot of illness or other problems?

Beth: No, she's doing very well. I really will try to not get phone calls on duty or make them.

Mary: Since this problem has never occurred before, I am sure you will correct it, but why don't we have a follow-up chat in 2 weeks to see how things are going?

Table 15-1. Steps in Performance Deficiency Coaching

1. State the problem in behavioral terms. Begin the session by focusing immediately on the problem. Make sure the individual is not attacked.
2. Ascertain that the employee understands how the problem is tied to the functioning of the organization.
3. Make sure the employee understands the personal consequences of the problem.
4. Ask for input from the employee on why the problem is occurring.
5. Ask the employee for suggestions on solving the problem. If possible, lead the employee to greater self-awareness about the problem.
6. Agree on the steps each of you will take to solve the problem. Write them down.
7. Agree on a follow-up procedure and date.

ANALYSIS

In keeping with most recommendations on coaching for performance deficiencies, this session lasted only a few minutes. However, the manager was able to accomplish all the goals of a good coaching session, which are:

1. Focus on the problem.
2. Have the employee take responsibility for solving the problem.
3. Show genuine interest in the employee and in the employee's ability to solve his or her own problems.

When Counseling Fails

Sometimes managers are unsuccessful in their efforts to educate by coaching or counseling. An employee, for whatever reason, is unable to improve performance. If this occurs, the manager must assume the role of a confronting coach and deal with the problem by bringing to the employee's attention the consequences of unacceptable performance.

Confrontation is a last resort, but it is an alternative that is occasionally necessary. In confrontation the employee needs to be told exactly what will happen if performance does not improve. Confrontation is the last step before disciplinary action. If confrontation is necessary, it should not be delayed. Following confrontation the employee should be given time to improve performance. There must be follow through, with disciplinary action if unsatisfactory work performance continues. The steps in disciplinary action are discussed in Chapter 21.

Coaching the Well-Motivated Employee

Managers often fall into the trap of spending so much time dealing with employees who have performance deficiencies that they neglect coaching well-motivated employees. The following scenario is an example of the type of coaching of motivated employees that leads to increased retention and productivity:

JOAN'S REQUEST

Joan is a new nurse on the unit but has had much experience in other agencies. Mary calls Joan into her office to compliment her on how quickly she has learned the unit routine and how well she is functioning in her role.

> *Mary*: I'm really pleased with your work, Joan. It's nice to have you join our team.
>
> *Joan*: Thank you. I really like the staff, and the doctors here are really great. But I feel badly when I miss the doctors' visits, especially when I need to talk with them about a patient problem—something that really doesn't warrant a phone call, just a need to discuss patient progress or something.
>
> *Mary*: Have you tried telling the unit secretary the names of the doctors you need to see, so she can locate you when they make rounds, or leaving a note on the patient's chart?
>
> *Joan*: Yes, I've tried both those things, and they do work sometimes. But the unit clerk is often not at the station and misses the doctors, and it is time consuming to make out notes to place on the charts. Also, sometimes doctors read the notes, and then they go and see the patient but forget to see me or to take care of the problem.
>
> *Mary*: Do you have any suggestions?
>
> *Joan*: Yes, I do. At one hospital where I worked there was a large board posted with the names of the patients and their physicians and the nurses assigned to the patients that shift. There was also a section labeled, "nurse needs to see doctor." The unit secretary kept the board up to date, and each shift after patient rounds the nurses checked what doctors they needed to talk with. Because it was so visible, the entire unit really worked to see that none of the doctors left the unit until they had taken care of all the problems. Even the doctors thought it was great.
>
> *Mary*: Would you be willing to follow through on this, get some more information on cost, where to order, and make a formal

presentation to the staff? You would need to get good support from the unit secretaries, as it would mean some additional work for them.

Joan: I've thought about that, and I think I can bring them around. I'd really like to start working on this.

Mary: Why don't you check back with me after you have all your information gathered? I'd like you to role play your presentation to me before presenting it to the staff. I'd also like to check the cost before the final approval.

ANALYSIS

What started out as a routine session on positive reinforcement ended in a situation that will provide Joan with a stretching experience and an opportunity for growth. Instead of Mary taking over Joan's idea, she has given Joan encouragement and permission to go ahead with the project. Mary has given Joan the responsibility for the preparatory work, and at the same time, has set up a further coaching session. Mary has also discovered a talent in Joan that she might be able to use in the future. Mary should make a note of this coaching session to add to Joan's long-term coaching file.

Long-Term Coaching

Quick (1985) maintains that long-term coaching is the major step in building an effective team. Since team building is such an excellent strategy to increase productivity and retention, it is necessary that all managers become proficient in coaching. Good coaches have some of the same attributes as mentors but coaching is less intense and is not limited to one or a few subordinates. The effective supervisor makes sure that at least one coaching session is held with each employee annually, in addition to any coaching that may occur during the appraisal interview.

This is not to say that no coaching should occur during the performance appraisal interview; on the contrary. But due to the high emotion present at that time, it is necessary to plan additional coaching at less stressful times. Coaching should be a continuous process, and frequently is a spontaneous and ongoing part of the experienced manager's repertoire. However, long-term coaching is often left to chance, especially with the novice manager. Tool 15-3 is an example of a long-term coaching record form that managers can use to plot the progress of their coaching efforts.

Quick (1985) feels that effective coaching has several specific components. These components are discussed in the following three phases:

1. *Gathering data.* One of the best ways to gather data about employees is to observe their behavior. When managers spend time observing employees, they are able to determine who has good communication skills, who is well organized, who is able to use effective negotiating skills, and who works collaboratively.

   Other sources of data are employees' past work experiences, past performance appraisals, and past educational experiences. What academic qualifications and what credentials do they hold? Most of this information can be obtained from the personnel files.

   Lastly, employees themselves are an excellent source of information that can assist the manager in the long-term coaching interview. All these sources of data should be reviewed before the coaching interview.

2. *What is possible.* As part of the coaching interview planning, the manager should assess the department for possible changes in the future, for openings or transfers, and for potential challenges and opportunities. The manager should anticipate what types of needs lie ahead, what projects are planned, and what staffing and budget changes will occur.

   After a careful assessment of the future, the manager should consider the strengths of the various staff members. How can the manager help them become better prepared to take advantage of the future? Who needs to be encouraged to return to school, to get credentials, or to take special courses?

   Do some employees need to be encouraged to transfer to another more challenging position, to be given more responsibility on their present unit, or to move to another shift? Many of these questions will be explored further in Chapter 16 on career development. Career development is part of any coaching session.

3. *The coaching interview.* The goals of the long-term coaching interview are to help employees increase their effectiveness, see where potential is in the organization, and advance their knowledge, skills, and experience. Many of the techniques and guidelines listed in the post-appraisal interview are also useful in the coaching interview. It is important

that you not intimidate employees as you question them about their future and their goals.

There is no standard procedure for conducting the coaching interview. The main emphasis should be on employee growth and development. Whenever appropriate, the manager can assist employees in exploring future options. This type of career planning will be discussed in more detail in the next chapter. Coaching sessions give the manager a chance to discover potential future managers, employees who in subsequent coaching sessions should be groomed for a future managerial role.

Both the performance appraisal interview and the coaching session are wonderful opportunities to assist employees in the growth and development necessary for expanded roles and responsibility. One of the major roles of the manager is the development of subordinate staff. This interest of the manager in the future of individual employees plays a vital role in retention and productivity.

KEY CONCEPTS CHAPTER 15

1. Unless the appraisal interview is carried out in an appropriate and effective manner, the performance appraisal data will be useless.

2. Due to past experiences, most performance appraisal interviews are highly charged emotional events.

3. Showing a genuine interest in the employee's performance growth and seeking the employee's input at the interview will result in a positive outcome of the appraisal process.

4. The performance appraisal should be signed to show that feedback has been given to the employee.

5. Coaching is an effective way to help employees reach their potential and should be an ongoing function of all managers.

6. Short-term coaching occurs as a result of day-to-day observations and interactions between the supervisor and the employee.

7. Long-term coaching is a planned intervention on the part of the manager that results in the professional growth and development of subordinates.

8. Short-term coaching in the form of counseling is an effective method for correcting performance deficiencies.

9. When employees do not improve performance, there is a need to confront them with the consequences of continued unsatisfactory performance.

REFERENCES

Beach, D. *Personnel: The Management of People at Work*, Fourth Edition, Macmillan, New York, 1980.

Jernigan, D.K., *Human Resource Management in Nursing*, Appleton & Lange, East Norwalk, CT, 1988.

McGregor, D., "An Uneasy Look at Performance Appraisal," *Harvard Business Review*, 35(3):89–94, 1957.

Marquis, B., and Huston, C.J., *Management Decision Making for Nurses: 101 Case Studies*, J.B. Lippincott, Philadelphia, 1987.

Meyer, H.H., Keye, E., and French, J.R.P., Jr., "Split Roles in Performance Appraisal," *Harvard Business Review*, 43(1):123–129, 1965.

Peters, T., and Austin, N., *A Passion for Excellence*, Random House, New York, 1985.

Quick, T.L., *The Manager's Motivation Deskbook*, Ronald Press for John Wiley and Sons, New York, 1985.

Sullivan, E.J., and Decker, P.J., *Effective Management in Nursing*, Addison-Wesley, Menlo Park, CA, 1985.

ADDITIONAL READINGS

Billings, C.V., "Employment Setting Barriers to Professional Actualization in Nursing," *Nursing Management*, 18(11):69–71, 1987.

Brief, A.P., "Developing a Usable Performance System," *JONA*, 9:7, 1979.

Case, B.B., "Moving Your Staff Toward Excellent Performance," *Nursing Management*, 14:45, 1983.

Ganong, J., and Ganong, W., *Performance Appraisal for Productivity: The Nurse Manager's Handbook*, Aspen Systems, Gaithersburg, MD, 1983.

Maier, N.R.F., *The Appraisal Interview: Three Basic Approaches*, University Associates, La Jolla, CA, 1976.

Oberg, W., "Make Performance Appraisal Relevant," *Harvard Business Review*, 50(1):61–67, 1972.

Rosen, A., "Performance Appraisal Interviewing Evaluated by Proximal Observers," *Nursing Research*, 16:32, 1972.

Smith, J., "Managing Employee Performance," *Nursing Management*, 13:4, 1982.

Thompson, P.H., and Dalton, G.W., "Performance Appraisal: Manager Beware," *Harvard Business Review*, 48:149, 1970.

Wellbank, H.L., Hall, D.T., Morgan, M.A., and Hammer, W.C., Planning Job Progression For Effective Career Development and Human Resource Management," *Personnel*, 55(2):54–64, 1978.

16
Career Development, Transfers, Promotions, and Stress Management

UNTIL THE 1970s organizations did little to help employees plan and develop their careers. The emphasis in management was on the needs of the organization rather than the needs of the employees. Recently, however, career development has taken on new importance due to equal employment opportunity and the desire of more men and women in the work place to focus on career advancement when selecting a position. The impact of career development programs as a positive force in successful businesses has been well documented in studies by Ouchi (1981), Peters and Waterman (1982) and Kramer and Schmalenberg (1988).

Unfortunately, much of the career planning effort has centered around management development rather than activities that would promote growth in nonmanagement employees. Since over 80% of the employees in an organization are nonmanagement, it is imperative that attention also be paid to their career development.

Career development discussions in this chapter will focus primarily on (1) appropriate management interventions that become evident as a result of long-term coaching, (2) the personal responsibility for career planning that managers need to encourage and promote in their employees, (3) the appropriate use of lateral and downward transfers, (4) identification and selection of employees for promotion, and (5) identification of, and interventions for, temporarily overwhelmed employees.

Included in tools for implementation are a career planning guide, a career management assessment tool, a guide to assess an organization's career development program, and a stress assessment tool. Tables present the responsibilities of individuals and managers in career development and a typical career sequence for a professional nurse.

JUSTIFICATIONS FOR CAREER DEVELOPMENT

The most obvious justification for an organization to include career development as part of its management functions is the impact such a program has on retention. White (1988) reported that 47% of employees would quit their jobs if there were no opportunity for advancement. Marquis and Huston (1988), however, feel that nurses have not traditionally had a career focus and suggest that most nurses look on nursing as a job and not a career. Therefore, these figures might not hold true for nurse retention. Beach (1980) does include retention in the following list of justifications for a career development program:

1. *Reduces employee attrition.* Career development influences turnover of those ambitious employees who would otherwise be frustrated and seek other jobs because of lack of job advancement.

2. *Provides equal employment opportunity.* Minorities and women will have a better opportunity to move up in an organization if they are identified and developed early in their careers.

3. *Improves utilization of personnel.* When employees are kept in jobs they have outgrown, they often have reduced productivity. People have a better performance when they are placed in jobs they like, that fit them, and that provide challenges.

4. *Improves quality of work life.* Nurses, especially young ones, have a greater desire today to control their own careers.

They are less willing to settle for any role or position that comes their way and want greater job satisfaction and more career options.

5. *Improves competitiveness of the organization.* Highly educated professionals often give preference to organizations that have a good record of career development. In the current nursing shortage, a recognized program of career development can be the deciding factor for young professionals selecting a position.

6. *Avoids obsolescence and builds new skills.* Due to the rapid changes in the health care industry, especially in the areas of consumer demands and technology, employees may find that their skills have become obsolete. A successful career development program begins to retrain employees proactively, providing them with the necessary skills to remain current in their fields and therefore valuable to the organization.

A CAREER DEVELOPMENT PROGRAM

Before organizations can plan a successful career development program, they need to understand the normal career stages of individuals, since people require different types of development in different stages of their careers.

Van Maanen and Schein (1977) described four successive career stages. A majority of their population was male; the stages in a predominantly female occupation might differ slightly. The four career stages are:

1. *Exploration.* This occurs during early years as educational choices are made. With nurses it is often during their senior year in college that beginning career goals are formulated.

2. *Early establishment.* This is the early part of the professional career, as individuals seek their first jobs, are successfully hired, and begin working. Not only do individuals often experience reality shock at this time, but they also must often take the least desired positions and shift assignments.

   Once individuals have been in their first jobs for several months, the second phase of the early career stage occurs. During this phase of the early career, individuals find out whether they are succeeding in the organization. If they are not succeeding, they may be terminated or may obtain remedial education. During this stage most individuals will become competent, begin to feel good about their chosen careers, and often form a commitment to both the organization and the profession.

The final phase of the early career stage occurs as individuals internalize their competence and worth in their chosen fields. This is often referred to as the *granting of tenure phase*.

3. *Career maintenance.* There are two phases to this stage. In the first phase, which occurs mid-career, individuals become proficient, and many become experts. They receive more important work assignments and are at their maximum productivity. It is often at this stage in a nursing career when nurses feel very good about their work. However, if continued stretching and challenges are not given at this stage, individuals will become bored or look outside the organization for further advancement. This is frequently the time when nurses seek transfers to a new clinical area within the organization or even leave nursing. Individuals often move upward rapidly in an organization or in their career during this period.

During the second phase, which occurs late in careers, job assignments usually reflect the judgment, wisdom, and broad perspective of veterans in the profession. Many enjoy teaching at this stage. Problems often occur during this time if individuals feel that their past contributions to the field are not appreciated. Many also feel threatened by younger, more recently trained, professionals, especially if the latter are aggressive and better educated. At some point during this period, individuals must begin to adjust ambitions and dreams to what is realistic and possible to accomplish in the remaining years left in the career lifetime.

4. *Career decline.* This is the stage when retirement plans begin and individuals learn to accept a reduced role in their professions. It is often a time for a renewed interest in community, family, and friendships.

It is important to note that while there is some correlation between age and career stage, there are also many variances. For example, many women enter nursing in mid-life, and other women frequently interrupt their careers for childrearing. The differences in male and female career patterns were well documented in Sheehy's research (1974) regarding differences in the ages of men and women in various stages of their careers. As more women delay childbearing, the future may reveal greater similarities in male and female career stages.

In addition to having a knowledge of career stages, managers need to have an understanding of the components of career development and the delineation of personal and organizational responsibility. Beach (1980) suggests that career development is both the planning and the implementation of the plans. The latter can be accomplished through education, training, job search and acquisition, and work experience. There are two areas of responsibility for career development, personal and organizational, which are shown in Table 16-1 and discussed below:

Career planning is that subset of career development that is the responsibility of the individual. It includes evaluating one's strengths and weaknesses, setting goals, examining career opportunities, preparing in advance for potential opportunities, and using appropriate developmental activities. Although career planning is a personal responsibility, sensitive managers and progressive organizations can assist employees in career planning through the use of long-term coaching, as described in the previous chapter. The use of various career planning guides can also be useful in developing career responsibility in individuals. Managers should encourage the use of such tools and make them available to their staff.

Career management is the subset of career development that focuses on the responsibilities of the organization. Management decides such things as career paths and career ladders. It attempts to match position openings with appropriate individuals. There is a need to accurately assess the performance and potential of employees and to offer career guidance, education, and training.

Career Planning

Vestal (1987) maintains that career planning is (1) an ongoing process, (2) conscious and deliberate, and (3) much more difficult than it sounds. Vestal suggests that career planning is made easier when a career map is created to assist in the development of a long-term master plan. Various personnel experts have developed career assessment tools and other planning tools to assist individuals in planning their careers. Whatever assistance individuals use in developing career plans, the steps outlined in Table 16-1 should be incorporated. An example of such a career map is shown in Tool 16-1. Although career planning is the responsibility of the individual, managers should

Table 16-1.   The Components of Career Development

Career Planning	Career Management
Self-assessment of interests, skills strengths, weaknesses, and values	Integrate individual employee needs with organizational needs
Determine goals	Establish, design, communicate, and implement career paths
Assess the organization for opportunities	
	Disseminate career information
Assess opportunities outside the organization	Post and communicate all job openings
	Provide work experience for development
Develop strategies	
Implement plans	Provide training and education
Evaluate plans	Give support and encouragement
Reassessment and add new plans as necessary, at least biannually	Develop new personnel policies as necessary

guide their employees in this endeavor through the coaching techniques outlined in Chapter 15. Many novice professionals, as well as most young people, often neglect to plan long-term career activities (Marquis and Huston, 1988; Vestal, 1987).

Career Management

In addition to encouraging individuals to develop long-term career goals, managers and organizations have additional responsibilities if a career development program is to be successful. Many of the organizational responsibilities outlined in Table 16-1 have been discussed elsewhere in this book and therefore will be only briefly mentioned here.

1. *Integration of needs.* This type of planning is essential. The personnel department, the nursing division, nursing units, and the education department must work and plan together if the goal of matching job openings with the skills and talents of present employees is to be met.

2. *Career paths.* Career paths not only must be developed, they must also be communicated to the staff and implemented consistently. One of the often cited contributory causes of the present nursing shortage is the lack of adequately compensated career paths in nursing (Weisman, 1982). Although career ladders of various types have been present for some time, they are still not widely utilized. This problem is not unique to nursing; according to Beach (1980), most organizations do not have systematically designed career paths in place. Tool 16-2 is an assessment tool for managers

Tool 16-1   A Career Planning Guide for a Professional Nurse

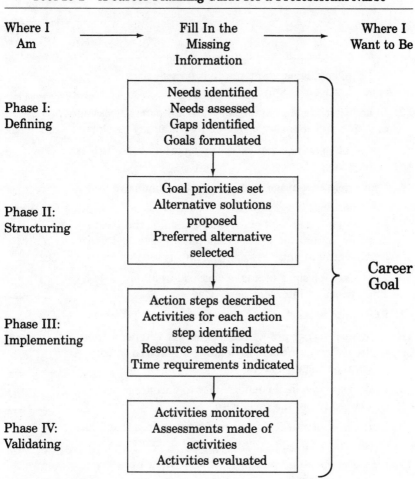

| Where I Am | ⟶ | Fill In the Missing Information | ⟶ | Where I Want to Be |

		Needs identified		
Phase I:		Needs assessed		
Defining		Gaps identified		
		Goals formulated		

		Goal priorities set		
Phase II:		Alternative solutions		
Structuring		proposed		
		Preferred alternative		
		selected		Career Goal

		Action steps described		
Phase III:		Activities for each action		
Implementing		step identified		
		Resource needs indicated		
		Time requirements indicated		

		Activities monitored		
Phase IV:		Assessments made of		
Validating		activities		
		Activities evaluated		

to use to ascertain how effective they are in the area of career management.

Even when health care organizations do design and utilize a career structure within an organization, there is no follow-through once the nurse leaves the organization. For example, a nurse at the level of Clinical Nurse III in one hospital loses that status when he or she leaves the organization.

Tool 16-2   Career Management Assessment Guide

	Yes	No
1. I provide my employees with stretching experiences and challenging assignments that provide learning opportunities.	—	—
2. In addition to performance appraisals I plan at least one coaching and/or career discussion with all my employees.	—	—
3. I post job openings and career opportunity literature as appropriate.	—	—
4. I routinely encourage continuing education, advanced degrees, and nonlocal seminars.	—	—
5. I keep in mind special experiences, such as the assignment for committee work, or special projects that will provide growth and development for my employees.	—	—
6. I am alert for signs of stress overload in all my employees and intervene as needed.	—	—
7. I facilitate requested transfers as quickly as possible.	—	—
8. I anticipate what promotional openings will be possible in the future and coach my staff to be able to be competitive for such positions.	—	—
9. I take every available opportunity to encourage my employees to pursue excellence.	—	—
10. In the last year at least one of the employees that I have developed has sought and obtained a promotion.	—	—
11. I counsel my employees immediately when I observe poor performance.	—	—
12. I make a genuine effort to share my talented staff so that the entire organization benefits.	—	—
13. I let my staff know when they are doing well.	—	—
14. When there is an inservice program being given, I try to free up my staff so they can attend.	—	—
15. I am on the alert for signs of boredom in my staff and, if necessary, encourage them to seek a more challenging position, even when this means a transfer from my department.	—	—

16. I personally attend educational programs so that I am a
role model in support of lifelong learning.   ___ ___

17. My employees know that I believe in them.   ___ ___

18. I know my employees well and am cognizant of personal
circumstances that could lead to stress.   ___ ___

19. I delay change in my department when I am aware that
the staff are experiencing stress from other sources.   ___ ___

20. I encourage all my staff to develop both short-term
and long-term career goals.   ___ ___

One of the most exciting career structures presently
being implemented is that designed by the Royal Australian
Nursing Federation (RANF). The RANF has successfully
negotiated this career structure throughout Australia's
public and private hospitals. This means that nurses can
move throughout Australia and retain their status; for
example, if a nurse has reached level III, the nurse can
maintain that status when going to another hospital. The
system adopted by the RANF incorporates some of the
Japanese philosophy of moving individuals slowly through
an organization (Ouchi, 1981). The RANF career structure
is summarized in Table 16-2.

A career path should be designed so that each successive
job in the path contains additional responsibilities and
duties but is also related to previous jobs and utilizes
previous skills. It is important that once career paths are
established they be communicated effectively to all the
concerned staff. It should be made very clear what employees must do to be advanced in a particular pathway.

3. *Dissemination of career information.* The education department, personnel department, and unit manager all have
some responsibility in sharing such information. Care
should be taken that employees are not encouraged to
pursue unrealistic goals.

4. *Posting of job openings.* Although this is usually the responsibility of the personnel department, managers should communicate this information, even when it means that one of
the unit staff may transfer to another area. If managers do

Table 16-2.   Royal Australian Nursing Federation Career Structure

Level I Registered Nurse			
Level II: Staff Developmental Nurse	Clinical Nurse	Area Manager	Research Nurse
Level III: Staff Developmental Educator	Clinical Nurse/Specialist	Nursing Manager	Nursing Researcher
Level IV: Nursing Staff Developmental Coordinator	Clinical Nursing Corrdinator	Nursing Management Coordinator	Research Coordinator
Level V Director of Nursing			

Explanation:
The entry-level position of registered nurse requires from 2 to 7 years, depending upon educational level, before advancement can be made to Level II. The level I position has six pay increments. At the end of the registered nurse tenure, nurses decide if they want an educational development path, a clinical path, an administrative path, or a research path. Each path has three levels. At level IV in each path, the nurse has reached the level of coordinator.

a good job coaching, they will know which staff need to be encouraged to apply for openings and who is ready for more responsibility and challenges.

5. *Employee assessment.* One of the benefits of a good appraisal system is the information it gives managers on the performance, potential, and abilities of all staff members. Using the techniques of long-term coaching will also give managers insight into employees on their unit so that they can provide appropriate career counseling.

6. *Challenging assignments.* Planned work experience is one of the most powerful career development tools. This includes jobs that temporarily stretch employees to their maximum skills, temporary projects, assignments to committees, shift rotations, assignments to different units or shift charge duties, and so on.

7. *Support and encouragement.* Many managers hoard their subordinates' talent. Because good subordinates make a manager's job easier, managers are often reluctant to encourage their excellent subordinates to move up the corporate ladder or to seek other more challenging experiences, which would result in those employees' leaving the managers' span of control. Effective managers look beyond their immediate units or departments and consider the needs of the entire organization; they recognize and share talent.

8. *Policy development.* When an active program of career development is pursued, it is often found that certain personnel policies and procedures are impeding the success of the

program. When this occurs, the various members of the organization should re-examine their policies and make necessary changes.

9. *Education and training.* Due to the impact of education and training on career development and retention, a separate chapter (Chapter 17) has been devoted to this subject.

TRANSFERS

A transfer may be defined as a reassignment to another job within the organization. In a strict business sense of the word, a transfer usually implies similar pay, status, and responsibility. Because of the variety of positions available for nurses in any health care organization, coupled with the lack of sufficient upper-level positions available, two different terms have come into use. A *lateral transfer* is one as defined above, as exemplified by a staff nurse moving to another unit within a hospital. A *downward transfer* occurs when someone takes a position within the organization that is below that person's previous level. This frequently happens in hospitals, as when a charge nurse decides she wants to learn another nursing specialty and steps down from her supervisory position on a medical-surgical unit to become a staff nurse in labor and delivery.

Vestal (1987) suggests that it is in the interest of nurses to consider a downward transfer, since it often increases their chances of long-term career success. For example, a nurse decides that she would like to have a position in cardiac rehabilitation and determines that most of the cardiac rehabilitation staff are hired out of the hospital cardiac care unit (CCU). Although she has had previous experience in a CCU, she has not held that position in this organization; presently, she is an evening charge nurse on a surgical unit. She decides to request a downward transfer to the CCU on the day shift, as this will give her current experience in a CCU and exposure to the cardiac rehabilitation supervisor. In this example, a downward transfer increases the likelihood that the nurse's long-term goal will be realized.

Downward transfers should also be considered when nurses are experiencing periods of stress or role overload. Self-aware nurses will often request or initiate such transfers by themselves.

However, in some circumstances the manager may need to intervene. This type of transfer will be further explored later in this chapter as an appropriate management intervention in cases of temporary overwhelming stress.

Another type of transfer often occurs late in a career. Managers often assist valuable employees who want a reduced role in locating a position that will utilize their talents and still allow them a degree of status. These *accommodating transfers* often allow someone to receive a similar salary as before but with a reduction in energy expenditure. For example, a long-time employee might be made ombudsman, a status position that could use the employee's expertise and knowledge of the organization and would not be very physically demanding.

Inappropriate Transfers

One deterrent to successful career development is the inappropriate transfer. Some managers solve unit personnel problems by transferring difficult employees to other, unsuspecting departments. Such transfers decrease productivity. It is also unfair to employees to continually move them around an organization because they have a poor work performance that various managers have been unable to correct.

This is not to say that employees who do not "fit" in one department won't do well in a different environment. It is not uncommon for an employee to start off poorly in one department but improve in a new department or unit. Prior to such a transfer, however, it is important that both of the managers and the employee speak candidly with each other regarding the employee's capabilities and the managers' expectations. All types of transfers should be individually evaluated for appropriateness.

PROMOTIONS

Promotions are reassignments of individuals to positions of higher rank. It is normal for promotions to include pay raises. Additionally, most promotions include increased status, title changes, more authority, and greater responsibility. Because of the importance our society places on promotions, it is necessary for promotions to follow certain guidelines to ensure that the promotional process is fair.

Promotion as a Planned Event

Many organizations do not develop a planned program of promotion. Position openings are often posted and filled in a hasty manner, with little thought of long-term organizational or employee goals. In order for this not to occur, the following should be determined in advance:

1. *Recruitment from without or within.* There are obvious advantages and disadvantages to each decision. Weisman (1982) puts forth an excellent argument for recruitment from within. Weisman's research revealed that one of the few things that make a significant difference in nurses' degree of dissatisfaction is incentives for long-term careers. She suggests that a career development program that promotes from within is the key to nursing retention.

   One advantage to recruiting from outside the organization, mentioned in Chapter 9, is that outsiders bring in new ideas. Regardless of what the organization decides, the policy should be consistently followed, and it should be communicated to the employees. Some companies recruit from within first, recruiting from outside the organization only if they are unable to fill the position from within.

2. *Establishment of a method of selection and criteria to be used.* Employees should know in advance what the selection criteria are and what type of selection method is to be used. Some hospitals use an interview panel as a selection method to promote all employees beyond the level of charge nurse. Decisions regarding both method and criteria for selection should be justified. Additionally, employees need to know what place seniority will have in the selection criteria.

3. *Identification of a pool of candidates.* When promotions are planned, the management team will identify a pool of candidates who are prepared to seek higher level positions. A word of caution must be given regarding the zeal with which managers urge subordinates to seek promotions. The manager's role here is to identify and prepare such a pool. It is not the role of the manager to urge employees to seek a position in a way that would lead employees to think that the job is theirs or to unduly influence them in their decision to seek such a job. When employees actively seek

promotions, they are making a commitment to do well in a new position. When someone pushes them into such a position, the necessary commitment to put forth the energy to do the job well may be lacking. For many reasons employees may not feel ready to move into a new position.

4. *Handling of rejected candidates.* All employees who have applied for the promotion and have been rejected must be notified prior to notification of the selected candidate. This is simply common courtesy. Care must be taken to tell candidates of their nonselection in a manner that is not demotivating. Applicants should be thanked for making the effort to apply and, when appropriate, be encouraged to apply for future openings. Sometimes employees should be told what deficiencies kept them from getting the position. For instance, employees should be told if they lack some educational component or work experience that would make them a stronger competitor for future promotions. This can be an effective way of encouraging career development.

5. *Handling of employee releases.* Knowledge that the best candidate for the position is in a vital other role should not influence decisions regarding promotions. It is always difficult for managers to release employees so they can accept other positions. Policies regarding the length of time that a manager can delay releasing an employee should be written and communicated.

Some managers are so good at developing their employees that they frequently become frustrated. They seem to be constantly losing their developed staff to other departments. Higher level management needs to reward such managers by recognizing their effectiveness in career development and by setting release policies that ease the hardship on such managers.

STRESS REDUCTION AS PART OF CAREER MANAGEMENT

Stress in the work place, especially in health care organizations, is common. Although stress is not inherently bad and can frequently be motivating, too much stress reduces productivity. Since it is recommended that career management techniques include providing employees with some types of stress, such as that created by stretching and challenging assignments, it is necessary for managers to recognize the appropriateness of induced stress. It is also important for managers to be cognizant of aspects of stress overload that may interfere with career development.

Selye (1976) maintains that stress occurs regardless of whether the stressor is positive or negative. Therefore, such things as pay raises and promotions may be as stressful as work overload. Sullivan and Decker (1985) suggest that stress for health care personnel falls into the following four categories:

1. *Task-based stress.* This is work-overload stress. It may occur because (1) the employee has been given an unrealistic amount of work to complete, (2) the employee lacks preparation or experience to handle the tasks, (3) the employee lacks time management or organizational skills, or (4) the employee lacks sufficient information regarding the assignment.

   In order for career development to be effective, employees must feel good about their abilities to accomplish their work. The manager, therefore, needs to determine why an employee is experiencing work overload and take steps to utilize appropriate strategies to correct the cause of the stress. Among other things, this might include education and training, time management assistance, improved assignment communication, restructuring of the work, or reassignment of work.

2. *Role-based stress.* This category of stress occurs as a result of role overload, role ambiguity, and role conflict. These types of role stress, discussed in Chapter 13, occur frequently in newly transferred employees, promoted employees, new graduates, and newly hired personnel. The employee experiencing multiple roles, especially new roles, will often experience role overload. The new mother in the coaching scenario in Chapter 15 provides an example of role stress.

   Career management techniques for dealing with role stress include clearly written job descriptions and clearly communicated job expectations. Additionally, managers should be aware that when employees are experiencing overwhelming stress from either new or too many roles, it is usually unwise to add to their role overload. For example, it would be inappropriate to transfer or promote the new mother while she was experiencing role stress created by role overload.

3. *Institution-based stress.* This stress is created as a result of institutional norms, conditions, and expectations that conflict with the employee's needs. Examples would be staffing and assignment policies that were in conflict with the views of the employee.

When employees are properly selected and indoctrinated, this type of stress is less likely to occur. Keeping communications open can help reduce this type of stress. Care should be taken to recognize such stress and not to promote or transfer employees experiencing such conflict, as this would only create more stress.

4. *Person-based stress.* This stress occurs when there is incongruence between employees' performance expectations and their perceptions of their actual performances. An example might be the excellent clinician who is promoted to a management role. The employee expects to do well but becomes very disappointed in her own performance. It is a self-imposed stress.

Persons who are subject to this sort of stress often have a pattern of creating unrealistic expectations for themselves and are often perfectionists. There is little that can be done to prevent person-based stress from occurring, since it tends to be a long-standing, repeated behavior. Sometimes young professionals can be assisted in setting more realistic goals and expectations. Encouraging a support network is also helpful. Managers should help these individuals set realistic short-term and long-term career goals.

Stress Overload

As part of career management, managers should be able to recognize symptoms of stress. Among the early warning signs are (1) undue or prolonged anxiety, (2) abrupt changes in mood and behavior, (3) depression, (4) perfectionism, and (5) physical illness. Tool 16-3 will assist managers in stress recognition.

Cherniss (1980) suggests that institutions have some responsibility both in recognizing employee stress and in intervening to reduce that stress. Among Cherniss's suggested interventions are: (1) staff development and education; (2) orientation programs; (3) a periodic "burnout" checkup (such as a questionnaire) performed by someone who has no formal authority over the employee, such as someone from a stress referral center or from the personnel or industrial health department; (4) individual counseling, by the manager when appropriate and by others when the difficulties are not job related or require a professional counselor; (5) staff support groups; (6) job restructuring; (7) modification of the workload; (8) increases in the

---

Tool 16-3   Tool for Recognizing Stress Overload in Employees

---

Evidence of a number of the following behaviors may be indicative of increased stress in an employee, especially when the behaviors are recent and not part of the employee's normal pattern of behavior:

1. Appears hard-driving and competitive.
2. Exhibits excessively perfectionistic behavior.
3. Eats quickly and/or takes short breaks.
4. Has outbreaks of inappropriate emotion, such as flashes of anger, depression, irritability.
5. Is frequently absent from work for minor illnesses.
6. Is frequently late for work.
7. Has a reduced attention span.
8. Complains of sleeplessness, headaches, and stomachaches.
9. Becomes impatient with others.
10. Jiggles knee or taps foot or fingers frequently.
11. Complains frequently of feeling tired.
12. Has had a noticeable weight loss or weight gain.
13. Interrupts other people's speech.
14. Appears excessively pessimistic and frequently indecisive.
15. Appears distant and withdrawn.

---

amount and type of feedback regarding job performance; (9) reduction of social isolation; and (10) reduction of the employee's full-time hours to part-time schedules.

In addition to implementing Cherniss's suggestions, managers should recognize that in all career decisions it is the employee who must, and should, decide when he or she is ready to pursue promotions, return to school, or take on greater responsibility. Success and stress are both perceived by every individual in a different manner.

The Psychologically Impaired Employee

When stress overload is persistent, rather than temporary, it requires different interventions. The consistently or severely stressed individual may present the same symptoms as the chemically impaired employee. Just as in the dealing with the chemically impaired employee (Chapter 23), the manager's role is not to diagnose the cause of the problem but rather to focus on how the employee's problems are affecting work performance. The overly stressed employee who becomes psychologically impaired and jeopardizes patient safety should be removed from the work setting, confronted with the impairment, and referred for professional counseling and guidance.

Successful career management should result in positive career development, alleviate burnout, reduce attrition, and promote productivity. Tool 16-4 is an organizational check list for assessing career development programs. There is little doubt that a well-designed career development program increases retention and productivity.

Although career development programs benefit all employees, as well as the organization, for the professional nurse there is an added bonus. When professional nurses have the opportunity to experience expert career development, their commitment to the profession increases.

KEY CONCEPTS CHAPTER 16

1. There are many outcomes of a career development program that justify its implementation, including the reduction of attrition, better utilization of personnel, increased recruitment, promotion of equal opportunity, and prevention of obsolescent skills.

2. Career stage sequencing should assist the manager in career management.

3. Career development programs consist of a set of personal responsibilities called *career planning* and a set of management responsibilities called *career management*.

4. Young people often need to be encouraged to make long-term career plans.

5. Designing career paths is an important part of organizational career management.

Tool 16-4 Assessing an Organization's Career Development Program

	Yes	No
1. There is a tuition-reimbursement program in place in this organization.	—	—
2. Recruitment for promotions below top-level management will be sought from within first.	—	—
3. Employees know that top-level management positions will be recruited from without as well as within.	—	—
4. Selection criteria and method for selection is posted with every job position.	—	—
5. There is a written policy regarding how transfers are to be handled.	—	—
6. Individuals not selected for a promotion are notified either prior to, or at the same time as, the individual selected for the position.	—	—
7. There is an ongoing acceptable education and training program in this organization that is adequately funded.	—	—
8. Career development is a function of management that is encouraged in this organization.	—	—
9. As individuals reach the end of their careers, this organization attempts to accommodate their needs.	—	—
10. When signs are present that unit or department staff are unusually stressed, efforts are made to discover the cause and take appropriate interventions.	—	—
11. Part-time positions to meet the needs of our employees are adequate.	—	—
12. Budgeted monies are in place to cover the cost of occasional nonlocal workshops.	—	—
13. An ongoing management development program is producing well-qualified managers.	—	—
14. There are professional resources available for stress counseling for employees working in high-stress areas.	—	—
15. I have high expectations for my employees, but they are well communicated and obtainable.	—	—
16. Employees who demonstrate excellence are well rewarded.	—	—
17. The organization pays the cost of fees for certification exams for registered nurses.	—	—

6. Managers should plan specific interventions that promote growth and development in each of their subordinates.

7. Transfers, when used appropriately, are often an effective way to provide career development.

8. Policies regarding promotion should be in writing and should be communicated to all employees.

9. Recruitment from within has been shown to have a positive effect on employee satisfaction.

10. Recognition of, and interventions in, employee stress overload is a part of career management.

11. There are numerous management interventions that organizations and managers should utilitize to reduce work stress.

REFERENCES

Beach, D.S., *Personnel: The Management of People at Work*, Fourth Edition, Macmillan, New York, 1980.

Cherniss, C., *Professional Burnout In Human Service Organizations*, Praeger, New York, 1980.

Kramer, M., and Schmalenberg, C., "Magnet Hospitals: Institutions of Excellence Part I," *JONA*, 18 (1):11–19, 1988.

Marquis, B., and Huston, C.J., "Ten Behaviors and Attitudes Necessary for Nurses to Overcome Powerlessness," *Nursing Connections*, 1 (2):39–47, 1988.

Ouchi, W.C., *Theory Z: How American Business Can Meet the Japanese Challenge*, Addison-Wesley, Reading, MA, 1981.

Peters, T.J., and Waterman, R.H., Jr., *In Search Of Excellence*, Harper and Row, New York, 1982.

Royal Australian Nursing Federation, Western Australia RANF, Professional Officer H. Attrill, Perth, W.A., Australia, Feb. 1987.

Selye, H., *The Stress of Life*, McGraw-Hill, New York, 1976.

Sheehy, G., *Passages*, E.P. Dutton, New York, 1974.

Sullivan E.J., and Decker, P.J., *Effective Management In Nursing*, Addison-Wesley, Menlo Park, CA, 1985.

Van Maanen, J., and Schein, E.H., "Career Development," in Hackman, J.R., and Suttle, J.L., *Improving Life At Work*, Good Year Publishing, Santa Monica, CA, 1977.

Vestal, K.W., *Management Concepts For The New Nurse*, J.B. Lippincott, Philadelphia, 1987.

Weisman, C.S., "Recruit From Within: Hospital Nurse Retention in the 1980s," *JONA*, 12 (5):18–22, 1982.

White, D.K., "Few People Quit Jobs Over Money," *San Francisco Chronicle*, June 23, 1988.

ADDITIONAL READINGS

Alt, J.M., and Houston, G.R., *Nursing Career Ladders: A Practical Manual*, Aspen Systems, Rockville, MD, 1986.

Cohen, A., "Career Advancement Ladder – Morale and Productivity Builder," *Hospital Topics*, 63 (3):2–3, 1984.

Sanford, R.C., "Clinical Ladders: Do They Serve Their Purpose?" *JONA*, 17 (5):34–37, 1987.

17
Education, Training, and Management Development

A QUALITY education department is a requirement for any modern health care organization. This is true for many reasons: the specialization in health care, the complexity of modern technology, and the rapid changes in our scientific knowledge base. Education departments in health care organizations share the responsibility for all staff development activities with department managers and the personnel department.

Education and training, the two components of staff development that take place after an employee's indoctrination, may occur either within or outside the organization. Both have a great impact on productivity and, to a lesser extent, on retention.

The concept of education and training is relatively new in modern business and health care organizations. It was only during World War II that a systematic program of education and training became a part of business and industrial management functions. In the beginning, the staff development emphasis was on orientation and inservice training. In the last 20 years, however, other forms of education have become commonplace in health care organizations. Management development, certification classes,

and continuing education courses to meet relicensure requirements are now a part of many staff development programs.

This chapter will discuss the differences between training
and education and the responsibilities of the education department and managers in staff development. The difficulties occurring as a result of the staff (advisory) position of most education
departments will be discussed, and suggestions will be given on
how these difficulties can be overcome. Learning theories and
their implications for trainers and educators will be reviewed.
Principles of adult learning, as well as adult teaching techniques, will be included. Tools in this chapter include a needs
assessment tool, recommended content for a management development course, and an evaluation guide for a cost analysis of
specific educational programs.

TRAINING VERSUS EDUCATION

The pendulum tends to swing back and forth regarding who has
responsibility for a department's education and training. At one
time this was a responsibility shared by managers and inservice
education, but in the 1970s education departments enlarged,
and supervisors and managers willingly relinquished their education and training responsibilities. The difficulties arising
from this centralized system of staff development was briefly
discussed in Unit 5.

Currently, most organizations decentralize the responsibility
of orientation and/or staff development to include the first-level
manager. This has occurred primarily as a result of fiscal concerns, although other things, such as the need to socialize new
employees at the unit level, have also contributed to the changes.
There are, however, some difficulties associated with decentralized
staff development (Gillies, 1982). One of these difficulties results
from the conflict caused by the role ambiguity that is always
created whenever two people share responsibility. It sometimes
lessens role ambiguity when staff development personnel and managers delineate the differences between training and education.

Training may be defined as an organized method of ensuring
that people have knowledge and skills for a specific purpose. This
means acquiring the necessary skills to perform the duties of the
job. It is expected that the new skills learned will be used to

increase productivity and/or create a better product. It is obvious from this definition that all managers, at all levels, must assume some responsibility for the training of the employees they supervise.

Education is much broader in scope than training. Whereas training has an immediate use, education is designed to develop the individual. Recognizing educational needs and encouraging educational pursuits is the responsibility of the supervisor. However, unless managers have expertise in a particular area and knowledge in adult learning principles and theories of teaching and learning, they would not normally be responsible for the formal education of employees. Managers may appropriately be requested to give a formal class, if they are qualified to do so, but this would not be a regular job function.

RESPONSIBILITIES OF THE EDUCATION DEPARTMENT

Most education departments are in a staff position on the organization chart. Marquis and Huston (1987) identified several difficulties that may occur with staff positions. Since staff positions are advisory, they do not carry with them line authority. This means that education personnel have no authority over those for whom they are providing education programs. Likewise, managers have no authority over the education department, as that department is directly responsible to top-level management.

Most health care personnel departments feel they should have considerable input into the education department. Then there is the decision of who is to educate other health care staff who also have educational needs, such as physicians, respiratory therapists, and pharmacists. Should the education department coordinate all education activities? Should the education department provide orientation for all employees? Who should be responsible for employee induction activities: the personnel or the education department? These questions reveal the complexity of the education department's responsibilities.

Clearly, if education and training activities are to be successful, the authority and responsibility for all components of these activities must be clearly delineated in writing and communicated to all concerned.

Other difficulties arising out of the shared responsibility of managers, personnel staff, and educators for the indoctrination, education, and training of personnel are (1) a frequent lack of cost-effectiveness evaluation and (2) accountability for quality control.

The following are suggestions to overcome the difficulties inherent in the current system of shared authority:

1. The nursing division CEO must ensure that all parties involved in the indoctrination, education, and training of nursing staff understand and carry out their responsibilities in that process.

2. If the nursing division CEO is not directly responsible for the education and training department (in large institutions authority for this department may reside in a nonnursing vice president), the nursing division must be allowed a great deal of input into the formulation of policies and the delineation of duties.

3. Some type of advisory committee, with representatives from top-, middle- and first-level management, from staff development, and from personnel, should be formed. Employees representing all categories of workers receiving training and/or education should be part of this committee.

4. Accountability for various parts of the staff development program must be clearly communicated.

5. Some method of determining the cost and benefits of various types of programs should be utilized.

THEORIES OF LEARNING

Since all levels of management teach employees as a normal part of their role, it is important that managers be familiar with theories of learning. Knowledge and utilization of teaching/learning principles enable trainers to change employee behavior, which is the goal of all employee training.

Readiness to Learn

Many people confuse readiness to learn with motivation to learn. *Readiness* refers to both the maturational and experiential factors in the learner's background that influence learning. *Maturation* means that the learner has completed the necessary prerequisites for the next stage of learning. The prerequisites could be behaviors or prior learning. *Experiential factors* are skills previously acquired that are necessary for the next stage of learning.

Learners should be assessed to determine whether the necessary prerequisites have been met before the next stage of learning begins. Furthermore, learning should occur in sequential patterns that build on each other. Many training programs fail because prerequisite skills and knowledge are not considered.

Motivation to Learn

Many of the motivational theories discussed in the chapter on motivation apply to learning motivation. Such things as expected benefits and reinforcement theory have specific applications to learning.

If learners are informed in advance regarding resulting benefits of learning specific knowledge and adopting new behaviors, they will be more likely to be motivated to attend the training sessions *and* learn. Telling employees *why* and *how* specific educational or training programs will personally benefit them is a vital role of the manager in staff development.

Reinforcement is also important. A learner's first attempts are often unsuccessful. The best preceptors are wonderful reinforcers. Once the behavior or skill is learned, it needs continued reinforcement until it becomes internalized. Managers should influence the maintenance of new learning through rewards and benefits on the job.

Task Learning

Learning theory research (Wexley and Latham, 1981) has shown that the learning of a complex task is facilitated when the task is broken down into parts, beginning with the simplest and continuing to the most difficult. It is necessary, however, to combine part learning with whole learning. When learning motor skills, spaced practice is more effective than massed practice. When learning tasks, overlearning has also been shown to be effective.

Task-learning research has been especially helpful in teaching health care workers, since much of the learning involves tasks and motor skills. Trainers teaching tasks should remember to (1) teach complex tasks in steps, (2) teach in frequent short sessions, and (3) teach repeatedly until the task can be performed automatically.

Transfer of Learning

The goal of training is for new learning to be used in the work setting. In order for this to occur, Ellis (1965) has made several suggestions. There should be as much similarity as possible between the training context and the job. Adequate practice is mandatory, and overlearning is recommended. The training should include a variety of different situations so that the knowledge is generalized. Whenever possible, important features or steps in a process should be identified. Lastly, the learner must understand the basic principles underlying the tasks and how a variety of situations will modify how the task is accomplished.

Transfer of learning principles has many implications for the trainer. One of the reasons many inservice training sessions fail to transfer classroom learning to the bedside is poor follow-through on these suggestions. Learning in the classroom will not be transferred unless there is adequate practice in a simulated or real situation and unless there is an adequate understanding of theoretical principles.

Social Learning Theory

Social learning theory builds on reinforcement theory with respect to motivation to learn; it also has many of the same components as the theories of socialization discussed in previous chapters. Bandura (1977) suggests that individuals learn most behaviors by direct experience and by observation. Behaviors are retained or not retained based on positive and negative rewards.

In social learning theory, four separate processes are involved. First, individuals become knowledgeable as a result of the direct experience of the effects of their actions. Second, knowledge is frequently obtained through vicarious experiences (e.g., observing the effects of someone else's actions). Third, individuals learn from the judgments of others, especially when vicarious experience is limited. Lastly, after individuals use the knowledge obtained from the prior three sources, they can evaluate the soundness of their own reasoning through both inductive and deductive logic. Social learning theory also acknowledges that anticipation of reinforcement influences what is observed and what goes unnoticed (Bandura, 1977). Figure 17-1 depicts the social learning theory process.

Not everyone agrees about the degree to which social learning affects behavior. Some educators, however, believe that certain types of learning occur best when social learning theories are utilized. For example, Marquis and Huston (1987) believe that leadership is best taught within a social context, and they therefore recommend that leadership and management be taught by the case study approach.

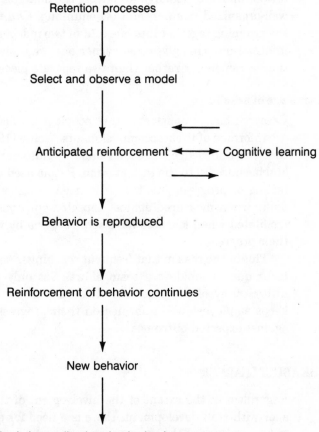

Retention processes

↓

Select and observe a model

↓

Anticipated reinforcement ←→ Cognitive learning

↓

Behavior is reproduced

↓

Reinforcement of behavior continues

↓

New behavior

↓

Behavior is internalized and attitude change occurs

FIGURE 17-1. *The social learning theory process*

Social learning theory is also demonstrated by the effectiveness of role models, preceptors, and mentors. Because the cognitive process is very much a part of social learning, observational learning will be more effective if the learner is informed in advance of the benefits of adopting a role model's behavior.

Span of Memory

The effectiveness of training and inservice programs depends to some extent on the ability of the participants to retain information. Many factors have been found to increase memory span.

Among effective strategies are (1) the chance for repeated rehearsal, (2) grouping items to be learned (3–4 for oral presentations and 4–6 visually), (3) having the material presented in a well-organized manner, and (4) chunking. *Chunking* refers to the grouping together into one unit of two independent pieces of information. This gives the learner one large piece of information to remember rather than two separate pieces.

Knowledge of Results

Research has demonstrated that people learn faster when they are informed of their accomplishments. Wolfle (1951) concluded that the knowledge of results must be automatic, immediate, and meaningful to the task at hand. People need to experience a feeling of progress, but they also need to know how they are doing when measured against expected outcomes. Learning is facilitated when learners have some criteria by which to judge their progress.

This is one reason that frequent coaching is such an effective technique in molding a team effort. Not only does coaching utilize many of the processes of social learning theory, it also keeps employees well informed on their progress as measured against expected outcomes.

THE ADULT LEARNER

Regardless of the extent of the involvement of the nurse manager with staff development, there is a need for every manager to be cognizant of the uniqueness and special needs of the adult learner. Knowles (1970) was the first to develop the concept of androgogy, or adult learning, as distinct from pedagogy, or child

Table 17-1. Pedagogy vs. Androgogy—Basic Differences

Pedagogy	Androgogy
• Learner is dependent	• Learner is self-directed
• Learner needs external rewards and punishment	• Learner is internally motivated
• Learner's experience is unimportant or limited	• Learner's experiences are valued and varied
• Subject centered	• Task or problem centered
• Teacher directed	• Self-directed

learning. Table 17-1 summarizes the basic differences between the two categories. Adult learners are mature, self-directed individuals who have learned a great deal from life experiences and are focused on solving problems that exist in their immediate environment.

Adult learning theory has contributed a great deal to the manner in which adults are taught. By understanding the assets the adult learner brings to the classroom and the obstacles that might interfere with adult learning, trainers and educators are able to create an effective learning environment. Table 17-2 depicts obstacles and assets to adult learning, and Table 17-3 shows how child and adult learning environments should differ.

According to Sullivan and Decker (1985), Knowles's studies have the following implications for use by trainers and educators:

1. A climate of openness and respect will assist in the identification of what the adult learner wants and needs to learn.

2. Adults enjoy taking part in and planning their learning experiences.

3. Adults should be involved in the evaluation of their progress.

4. Experiential techniques work best with adults.

5. Mistakes are opportunities for adult learning.

6. If the value of the adult's past experience is rejected, the adult will feel rejected.

7. Adult readiness to learn is greatest at the point at which the adult recognizes a need to know (e.g., in response to a problem).

8. Adults need the opportunity to apply what they have learned very quickly following the learning.

9. Assessment of need is imperative in adult learning.

Table 17-2.   Obstacles to and Assets for Learning in the Adult

Obstacles to Learning	Assets for Learning
• Institutional barriers	• High motivation
• Time	• Self-directed
• Self-confidence	• Proven learner
• Situational obstacles	• Knowledge/experience reservoir
• Family reaction	• Special individual assets
• Special individual obstacles	

Table 17-3.   Pedagogy vs. Androgogy—The Learning Environment

Pedagogy	Androgogy
• Climate is authoritative	• Climate is relaxed and informal
• Competition is encouraged	• Collaboration is encouraged
• Teacher sets goals	• Teacher and class set goals
• Decisions made by teacher	• Decisions by teacher and students
• Lecture by teacher	• Process activities and inquiry projects by students
• Evaluation by teacher	• Evaluation by teacher, self, and peers

Needs Assessment for Adult Learning

Managers may or may not be involved in the implementation of educational programs, but they are responsible for identification of learning needs. Marquis and Huston (1987) suggest that managers often do not perform this function well. Chatham's studies (1977) corroborate this assumption. Chatham identified major differences in the ranking priority of needs for continuing education between nursing managers and staff nurses.

Organizations often implement training programs because such programs are faddish and have been advertised and marketed well. Educational programs are expensive and should not be undertaken unless a demonstrated need exists. Educational resources should be justifiable. Tool 17-1 is an educational justification guide.

In addition to a rationale for education programs, the use of an assessment plan will be helpful in meeting learner needs. Langford (1981) suggests the following systematic plan:

1. Identify the desired knowledge or skills the staff should have.

2. Identify the present level of knowledge or skills.

3. Determine the deficit of desired knowledge and skills.

4. Identify the resources available to meet the needs.

Tool 17-1   Assessment and Plan for Needed Education and Training

---

Prepared by: _____ Unit:_____
Identified need:_____

Methods used to assess need (explain in detail and be specific):_____

(Acceptable examples are incident reports, patient complaints, physician complaints, poor nursing judgment induced complications, or delayed discharge, etc. Staff request is acceptable only if 30% of the staff feel this is a need.)

Estimated cost of education and training program to meet identified need (include paid employee time):_____

Mandatory or optional education and training (if optional, approximately how many staff will attend):_____

Expected outcome of program:_____

How is outcome to be evaluated?_____

What is the degree of knowledge deficit?_____

Who is to teach this program?_____

Date_____

Copy to Nursing Administration and Staff Development Office

---

    5. Make maximum use of the available resources.

    6. Evaluate and test outcomes after use of the resources.

EVALUATION OF STAFF DEVELOPMENT ACTIVITIES

Because staff development involves the participation of many departments, it is difficult to effectively control. It is very easy for the personnel department, middle-level managers, and the education department to "pass the buck" among each other for accountability regarding staff development activities.

Evaluation of staff development consists of more than merely having class participants fill out an evaluation form at the end of the class session, signing an employee handbook form, or assigning a preceptor for each new employee. Evaluation of the three components of staff development (indoctrination, training, and education) should include the following:

1. *The learner's reaction.* How did the learner perceive the orientation, the class, the training and/or the preceptor?

2. *The behavior change.* What behavior change occurred as a result of the learning? Was there transfer of learning? Testing someone at the end of a training or educational program does not confirm that the learning changed behavior. There needs to be some method of follow-up to observe whether behavior change occurred.

3. *Organizational impact.* Although it is often difficult to measure how staff development activities affect the organization, efforts should be made to do so. Quality of care, number of medication errors, number of accidents, quality of clinical judgment, amount of turnover, and productivity can all be measured to determine the impact of staff development activities on the organization.

4. *Cost effectiveness.* All staff development activities should be quantified in some manner. This is perhaps the most neglected aspect of accountability in staff development. Tool 17-2 is an example of a cost effectiveness tool. A thorough review of cost analysis is beyond the scope of this book; however, Cascio (1982) is an excellent source for reviewing techniques to calculate human resource outcomes in terms of dollars.

MANAGEMENT DEVELOPMENT

Management development is a *planned* system of training and developing individuals so that they acquire the skills, insights, and attitudes to effectively manage people and to do the work to be performed within the organization. Marquis (1988) reported that the quality of supervision has a great impact on retention. It follows, therefore, that it is cost effective for organizations to have in place a planned program of management development.

Tool 17-2 Cost Analysis of Education and Training Activity

Staff development activity_____
Does this fulfill a legal requirement?_____
Describe all resources used with identifiable cost

1. Employee time _____
2. Trainer or educator time _____
3. Training facilities _____
4. Meals/coffee/snacks _____
5. Teaching materials _____
6. Duplicating _____
7. Line employee time _____
8. Other _____
9. Other _____
   Total Cost:_____

Total identifiable benefits (examples are reduced absenteeism, less patient falls, etc.)

1.
2.
3.
4.
   Total Savings:_____
Intangible cost_____
Consequences of not acting_____
Other considerations_____

There are three fundamental characteristics in any successful management development program. First, the program must begin at, and be supported by, top-level administration. Second, the program must be planned and systematically implemented. Lastly, the program must include both a means of developing appropriate attitudes through social learning theory and adequate management theoretical content.

Support by Top Management

Support by management should occur in two ways. First, top-level management must do more than bear the cost of management development classes. Research suggests that management training has little effect on the quality of supervision unless managers are allowed to apply their new knowledge (Wagel, 1977). Therefore, for such programs to be effective, the organization must be willing to practice a management style itself that incorporates sound management principles.

Second, training outcomes will be improved if the CEO of the nursing division takes an active part in planning and developing the program. Whenever possible, the top nursing administrator should teach some of the classes and, at the very least, make sure that the program supports top management philosophy.

Planned and Systematically Implemented

Just as nurses are required to be certified in critical care before they accept a position in a critical care unit, so too should managers be involved in a management development program *before* their appointment to management positions. Potential managers should be identified and groomed early. The first step in this process is an appraisal of the present management team and an analysis of possible future needs.

The second step is the establishment of a training and development program. This would require decisions regarding such questions as: (1) How often should the formal management course be offered? (2) Should outside educators be involved, or should it be taught by inhouse staff? (3) Who should be involved in teaching the didactic portion? (4) Should there be two levels of classes, one for first-level and one for middle-level managers? (5) Should management development courses be open to all, or should individuals be recommended by someone from management? (6) In addition to formal course content, what other methods should be used to develop managers? Other appropriate training methods are job rotation through an understudy system of pairing a potential manager with a supervisor and management coaching.

Inclusion of Social Learning Activities

Management development will not be successful unless there are ample opportunities for learners to try out new skills. Providing potential managers with didactic management theory alone inadequately prepares them for the attitudes, skills, and insights necessary for effective management.

Stevens (1982) suggests case studies as an excellent technique for teaching management decision making and insight. This technique, and other teaching techniques, appropriately employ social learning theory strategies. Management games, certain types of transactional analysis, and sensitivity training are also effective in changing attitudes and increasing self-awareness.

As in all types of education and staff development, there should be periodic evaluation of the management development program, including a cost analysis and quality of outcomes. Tool 17-3 lists the suggested content and organization of a management course.

As this chapter has demonstrated, the impact of education and training activities on productivity and retention can not be overemphasized. Most organizations are aware of the need for education and training programs and have responded to that need by creating some type of education department.

However, these same organizations often do not follow through appropriately to determine how effective such departments are. There is a need, therefore, to ensure that all such activities be evaluated for quality control, impact on the institution, and cost effectiveness. This is true regardless of whether the education and training activity is carried out by the manager, the preceptor, the personnel department, or the education department.

KEY CONCEPTS CHAPTER 17

1. Training and education are both important parts of staff development.

2. Managers and education department staff have a shared responsibility for education and training.

3. It is important that duties, responsibility, and accountability for all staff development activities be well delineated and communicated to all concerned.

Tool 17-3   Suggested Content for a Management Development Course

---

I. Required for All Levels of Management
   A. The organization
      1. History of the organization
      2. Organizational mission and philosophy
      3. The future of the organization
      4. Financial outlook—present and future
   B. The management process
      1. Planning
         a. Philosophy, goals, and objectives of the nursing division
         b. Fiscal planning in this organization; responsibility of level managers for budgetary planning
         c. Planned change theories and goal setting
      2. Organizing
         a. Organizational theories
         b. Organizational structure and principles
         c. Organization for delivery of patient care
      3. Staffing
         a. Recruitment, selection, and interviewing
         b. Staffing and scheduling
         c. Delineation of staff-development responsibilities
      4. Directing
         a. Time-management skills
         b. Organizational communication
         c. Management of conflict
         d. Facilitating collaboration
         e. Negotiation techniques
         f. Dealing with unions
      5. Control
         a. Fiscal control
         b. Quality control
         c. Subordinate performance appraisal
         d. Professional and peer control
         e. Discipline and limit setting
         f. Legislative controls in nursing and health care
   C. Human relations
      1. Power, authority, and influence
      2. Working with groups
         a. Committees
      3. Management and leadership
         a. Styles of leadership
         b. Contingency theories

    4. Human behavior
       a. Theories of motivation
       b. Attitudes
  D. Social, economic, and ethical considerations
     1. Ethics
        a. Professional ethics
        b. Business ethics
        c. Personal ethics
     2. Social
        a. Community relations
        b. Consumer responsibility
     3. Economics
        a. Competition
        b. Government controls
  E. Personal skills
     1. Communication
        a. Speaking skills
        b. Writing skills
        c. Conducting meetings
        d. Listening skills
     2. Interpersonal skills

II. Advanced Management Development Content Would Include
  A. Management information systems
  B. Methods analysis and work measurements
  C. Marketing
  D. Advanced financial management
  E. Advanced personnel management
  F. Research and statistics
  G. Risk management

---

4. There are many theories of learning and principles of teaching that should be considered if staff development activities are to be successful.

5. Planning of educational programs for adult learners should include a consideration of the learners' unique learning needs and the assets they bring to the learning process.

6. It is important to determine deficits in knowledge and skills prior to beginning any training or education activity.

7. Training and education activities require economic justification.

8. All staff development activities should be evaluated retrospectively for quality control and fiscal accountability.

9. Management development must be planned and supported by top-level management if it is to be successful.

10. If appropriate management attitudes and insight are goals of a management development program, social learning techniques need to be part of the teaching strategies utilized.

REFERENCES

Bandura, A., *Social Learning Theory*, Prentice-Hall, Englewood Cliffs, NJ, 1977.

Cascio, W.F., *Social Learning Theory*, Prentice-Hall, Englewood Cliffs, NJ, 1982.

Chatham, M., "Discrepancies in Learning Needs Assessments: Whose Needs Are Being Assessed?" *Journal of Continuing Education in Nursing*, 10(5), 1979.

Ellis, H.C., *The Transfer of Learning*, Macmillan, New York, 1965.

Gillies, D.A., *Nursing Management, A Systems Approach*, Philadelphia, W.B. Saunders, 1982.

Knowles, M., *The Modern Practice of Adult Education: Androgogy Versus Pedagogy*, Association Press, New York, 1970.

Langford, T., *Managing and Being Managed*, Prentice-Hall, Englewood Cliffs, NJ, 1981.

Marquis, B., "Attrition: The Effectiveness of Retention Activities," *JONA* 18(3):25–29, 1988.

Marquis, B., and Huston, C.J., *Management Decision Making For Nurses: 101 Case Studies*, J.B. Lippincott, Philadelphia, 1987.

Stevens, B., *Educating The Nurse Manager*, Aspen Publications, Germantown, MD, 1982.

Sullivan, E.J., and Decker, P.J., *Effective Management in Nursing*, Addison-Wesley, Menlo Park, CA, 1985.

Wagel, W.H., "Consensus: Evaluating Management Development and Training Programs," *Personnel*, 54(3):4–10, 1977.

Wexley, K.N., and Latham, G.P., *Developing and Training Human Resources in Organizations*, Scott, Foresman, Glenview, IL, 1981.

Wolfle, D., "Training," in Stevens, S.S. (ed.), *Handbook of Experimental Psychology*, John Wiley and Sons, New York, 1951.

ADDITIONAL READINGS

Mooney, V.A., Diver, B., and Schnackel, A.A., "Developing a Cost-Effective Clinical Preceptor Program," *JONA*, 18(1):31–36, 1988.

Tarnow, K., "Working with Adult Learners," *Nurse Educator* 4(5): 34, 1982.

Taylor, B., and Lippitt, G.L. (eds.), *Management Development and Training Handbook*, McGraw-Hill, New York, 1975.

Verduim, J., Miller, H., and Greer, C., *Adults Teaching Adults*, Learning Concepts, Austin, TX, 1977.

· UNIT SEVEN
Management of Human Behavior for Increased Productivity and Retention

A TEN-YEAR study by Marquis (1988) determined that most organizations accept high attrition levels as inevitable. It is almost as if organizations either deny or do not recognize the power they hold to influence human behavior. Organizations must begin to recognize the impact they can have in creating a work environment that maximizes employee satisfaction and results in desired behaviors. In fact, the satisfaction or dissatisfaction employees experience as a result of their work is directly related to the quality of the environment in which they are expected to work. The organization that can create a positive work environment that is satisfying, nurturing, and growth producing provides an environment that results in increased employee retention and productivity.

Unit 7 examines factors that are necessary in the creation of such an environment. These factors include maximal development of leaders and managers in the organization, and the awareness and replication of behaviors, attitudes, and practices within the organization that motivate employees or keep them from becoming dissatisfied.

For example, it is generally accepted that the success of the organization is a direct reflection of the quality of the employees that work there. Organizations that assume they are powerless to affect that quality do not seek to further develop and refine managerial and leadership talent in the organization. Thus, a vital opportunity to affect human behavior through optimal leadership and management is lost.

Another example is the organization that assumes that, because motivation must come from within the individual, little can be done to influence worker morale and motivation. In fact, just the opposite is true. The organizational climate can reinforce intrinsic motivational factors or it can demoralize and demotivate. Productive employees can become even more productive, or demotivated employees can stagnate. The role that organizations play in the management of human behavior is a direct reflection of the climate they build and foster.

REFERENCES

Marquis, B., "Attrition: The Effectiveness of Retention Activities," *JONA* 18(3): 25–29, 1988.

18
Developing Effective Leadership and Management

ALTHOUGH THE terms *leadership* and *management* are used synonymously by many people, they are very different. Leadership is the art of getting work done through others acting willingly. Leaders do not have to have an assigned position or formal authority to do this; group members can be motivated to achieve goals by voluntarily following a leader's direction. These goals may be organizational goals or they may be group goals. They may even be leader goals, but followers frequently become so aligned with leader values that it is difficult to separate them. Because interpersonal relationships are the key element in a leader/follower relationship, leaders lose their assumed authority and stop being leaders when their followers choose not to follow.

Evidence strongly suggests that (1) required leadership traits depend on the situation, (2) leadership is a relationship existing among people in a social setting, and (3) someone who becomes a leader in one setting may not necessarily do so in another situation (Stogdill, 1948). Although there is no one personality type common to all leaders, leaders generally have greater intelligence then their followers. Likewise, they are perceptive, possess social sensitivity, and are aware of the values, feelings, problems, and goals of individuals (DiVincenti, 1972). Tool 18-1 is a personal check list for assessing leadership effectiveness.

Management is the formal manipulation of people, the environment, money, time, and other resources to reach organizational goals. In contrast to leaders, managers have formal or legitimate authority to direct the actions of their followers by virtue of their positions or titles within the organization. Individuals may follow the directions of the managers because of their authority and not as a result of choice. The manager loses this authority outside of the work environment.

Management is manifested on more of a cognitive level than leadership. While leadership is inductive, management is deductive, in that general knowledge of organizational theory and process is learned and can be applied to particular events (Kern et al., 1987). Management also can be equated with efficiency, as it entails accomplishing tasks in the most efficient manner. Leaders inspire others to do a task, but there is less internalized responsibility to see that the job is done in the most effective manner (Kern et al., 1987).

Organizations need *both* good leaders and good managers. Leaders are required in situations in which personal dynamics are more important than the task to be accomplished. Managers are needed when a mission is clearly defined and there are rigid timelines or methods of accomplishing the task. In nursing, where the work is accomplished by working with people, leadership is a necessary qualification of managers (Beyers and Phillips, 1979). Some individuals are both good leaders and good managers, but often this is not the case. Becoming a good leader or manager is not a passive process. It requires active teaching and development of human resources. Some individuals incorrectly argue that leadership characteristics are an inborn part of personality and therefore cannot be taught; to the contrary, these characteristics *can* be nurtured and developed more formally by the organization.

Chapter 3 discussed the characteristics of effective supervision as they impact on the employee. Chapter 18 will focus on the process of developing effective leaders and managers within the organization. Different leadership and management styles will be presented and contingency leadership, which is defined as the need for leaders to vary their leadership style in response to

Tool 18-1 Leadership Effectiveness — A Personal Check List

Directions: Think of a current situation you are involved in that requires leadership skills. Analyze your current actions in terms of the items on this check list.

	Very much	Somewhat	Not at all

A. *Goals*
1. Have you identified:
   Your personal goals?
   Group members' personal goals?
   Group goals?
   Environmental (such as organization and community) goals?
2. Are your goals congruent with the group's goals?
3. Do you identify with the group, for example, use "we" instead of "I" and "you"?
4. Do members of the group see you as identifying with the group?
5. Have you clearly and specifically stated the group's goals including the:
   People involved?
   Target?
   Outcome?

B. *Knowledge and skills*
1. Do you have more knowledge and skill than the rest of the group?
2. Do you feel confident with your knowledge and skill in this situation?
3. Are you able to speak to the group on their level?
4. Have you identified the needs and motives of people in your group?
5. Have you identified the sources of power and authority in the situation?
6. Have you critically analyzed the situation including the leader, co-actor(s), and environment?
7. Have you kept an open mind about the situation?

C. *Self-awareness*
1. Do you know what your own needs are?
2. Do you know what you expect to gain from this situation?
3. Are you able to empathize with people in the group?
4. Do you see yourself as a leader?

D. *Communication*
1. Do you know what channels of communication are usually used?
   Are you using them?

	Very much	Somewhat	Not at all
2. Is there an adequate flow of information?			
3. Have you created any new channels of communication?			
4. Are your communications open and direct?			
5. Do you attend to and respond to (listen actively to) what others are saying?			
6. Have you checked out your perceptions of the situation with the people involved?			
7. Do you see and point out connections (links) between the statements of different people?			

E. *Energy*

	Very much	Somewhat	Not at all
1. Are you interested in the work of the group?			
2. Have you shared your interest and enthusiasm with the group?			
3. Do you really believe what you say to the group?			
4. Do you have enough energy for the task?			

F. *Action*

	Very much	Somewhat	Not at all
1. Have you planned how to get the job done?			
2. Have you organized the work efficiently?			
3. Do you share your ideas with others?			
4. Do you call the group together often enough?			
5. Have you defined your nursing role and communicated it to the group?			
6. Do you use the authority you have?			
Do you delegate it?			
Have you tried to increase it?			
7. Have you mobilized support systems?			
8. Are you willing to take risks?			
9. Do you confront when it is needed?			
10. Do you initiate action when it is needed?			
Without delay?			
11. Do you seek feedback?			
Informally?			
Formally?			
12. Do you provide feedback?			
Informally?			
Formally?			
13. Have you tried to improve your leadership ability?			

Analysis: This guide is intended to help leaders become self-aware about their personal leadership strengths as well as areas that need improvement. Items that are marked "very much" tend to be leadership strengths. Items that are marked "somewhat" are strengths that can be improved even more. Items that are marked "not at all" should be evaluated carefully by the leader, as the absence of these behaviors may have a significant negative impact on leadership effectiveness.

From Tappen, R., "Components of Effective Leadership," *Nursing Leadership, Concepts and Practice*, p. 94. F.A. Davis, Philadelphia, 1983.

the individual worker and the environment, will be stressed. Necessary components of a management development program, as well as roles assumed by nursing managers, will be discussed. Lastly, this chapter will examine the need for an organizational fit between the expectations of the manager and the organization. Tools for implementation include a personal check list for leadership effectiveness and a check list for assessing management development programs.

LEADERSHIP STYLES

Organizational theorists have identified three primary and distinct patterns of leadership behavior, called *leadership styles*. These leadership styles reflect how managers use interpersonal behaviors in influencing the accomplishment of goals on their units (Sullivan and Decker, 1988). These three styles are authoritarian, democratic, and laissez-faire and are described by Marquis and Huston (1987):

1. *Authoritarian or autocratic*. The authoritarian leader demonstrates aggressive dominance by making all decisions in the work environment. Worker input is not sought, and all workers are expected to follow the decisions of the autocratic leader. Clear, direct, and detailed orders are given to employees regarding the work to be accomplished. In this type of environment, worker productivity may be high, but creativity, motivation, and self-esteem are generally low. Authoritarian leaders are more concerned with the task to be accomplished than worker satisfaction.

   Authoritarian leadership is appropriate in situations in which decisions must be made quickly or in which the leader has information or expertise that group members do not. For example, a nurse certified in critical care would be expected to use an authoritarian style of leadership in a cardiac arrest situation on a medical surgical unit.

2. *Democratic or participative*. The democratic leader is "people centered" and encourages group governance. Group members are actively encouraged to participate in decision-making either by providing input into decisions made by the leader (consultive) or by group decision-making (participative). This leadership style requires that the leader believe that employees are goal directed and that

their contribution to the work environment is valuable. Democratic leadership may be less productive and more time consuming than authoritarian leadership, but it also results in greater motivation and self-esteem of the group members.

An example of democratic leadership is the use of team conferences for care planning. The democratic leader may also ask the staff to actively participate in short- and long-term strategic planning at the unit level.

3. *Laissez-faire or permissive.* Laissez-faire leaders are passive and deliberately abstain from directing their staffs. These leaders allow group members to determine their own individual goals and relinquish decision-making power to the group. The role of the laissez-faire leader in the group is solely as moderator or facilitator. Laissez-faire leadership is appropriate in situations that require brainstorming or in which group conflict should be resolved among group members themselves. It is not appropriate when it is used because the manager is weak, feels too threatened to exercise authority, or does not wish to offend subordinates. Generally, laissez-faire leadership results in low productivity, except in cases in which individuals are highly motivated to work independently or in groups that are highly motivated.

All three of these basic leadership styles have been described in the purest sense. In reality, most managers fall on a continuum somewhere in between the descriptions that have been provided. Managers also find that the leadership style they utilize is not constant. This variation in leadership style in response to individual workers and the environment is called *contingency leadership*.

CONTINGENCY LEADERSHIP

Tannenbaum and Schmidt (1973) were among the first theorists to suggest that managers should be capable of using various leadership styles and that the primary determinants of the appropriate leadership style should be the situation itself, the abilities of the manager, and the abilities of the group members. Fielder (1967) agreed that no single leadership style is ideal for every situation. Fielder felt that the interrelationships between the group's leader and group members are the most important factors in determining the success of a group leader. Fielder also cited the task to be accomplished and the power associated with the leader's position as other key variables.

Blake and Mouton (1964) stated that the leadership style used by managers should combine "concern for people" and "concern for production." The grid they developed, which shows the various combinations of these concerns, has two axes that go from 0 to 9 with a total of 81 possible points. One axis of the grid represents "concern for people"; the other represents "concern for production." A leader can have a high or low position on one or both of these axes. Managers who show high concern for people and low concern for production place a high value on meeting employee needs, which leads to a relaxed work environment. Managers with high levels of concern for both people and production tend to be democratic consultive managers who work to maximize both the abilities and the output of their workers. Managers with low concern for people and high concern for production tend to utilize a traditional approach to management, as described in Chapter 2. Lastly, managers with both low concern for people and low concern for production tend to be permissive leaders who provide little structure or support for their staff.

Hersey and Blanchard (1977), expanding on the work of Fielder and of Blake and Mouton, stated that the maturity of the worker is an additional factor in determining the most appropriate leadership style for the manager. This maturity of the worker is not determined by chronological age or by the length of time the employee has been employed by the organization; rather, it represents the worker's familiarity with the task(s) to be accomplished. For example, novice nurses require greater structure than expert nurses. Hersey and Blanchard's theory focuses on the needs of the follower and the different expectations each follower has of an effective leader. These expectations are greatly influenced by the experiences of the follower in previous follower roles.

Additionally, Hersey and Blanchard (1977) stressed that each situation requires a different leadership style and that many variables determine the best leadership style for any given situation. Some of these variables include the type of follower, type of organization, job demands, time, resources, communication processes utilized, and individual and group goals. Given the number of variables that affect leadership success, a leader may be very successful with a specific leadership style in one situation and very unsuccessful the next time. For example, a nurse manager may find that firm discipline and highly structured work guidelines are very effective in helping a particular employee to achieve at a certain level. Another employee, however, might chafe against this rigidity and structure and might even become demotivated and less productive.

Other theorists have added to Hersey and Blanchard's work, saying that managers must alter their leadership styles as a means of actively promoting worker achievement. House and Mitchell (1974) developed the "path-goal" theory of leadership effectiveness, which states that leaders assist subordinates in attaining organizational objectives by removing the obstacles to goal attainment and by making personal rewards for employees contingent on attainment of those goals (Sullivan and Decker, 1988). In path-goal theory, leaders continuously alter their behavior or leadership styles in whatever manner is necessary to coach, guide, and provide incentives to subordinates. The roles leaders assume to accomplish these goals take one of four basic forms: supportive leadership, directive leadership, achievement-oriented leadership, and participative leadership (Sullivan and Decker, 1988).

Supportive leadership is behavior that is focused on meeting the affiliation needs of subordinates, i.e., strengthening the interpersonal relationship between managers and subordinates. Directive leadership focuses on the work to be accomplished. In this role, the behaviors exhibited by nurse managers are task centered, as they provide rules, procedures, and a plan for completion of the work. Achievement-oriented leadership is behavior that recognizes and encourages achievement by subordinates. In this role, managers assist subordinates in goal setting and reward high performance accordingly. The last role nurse managers assume in the path-goal theory of contingency leadership is participative. Participative leadership requires that managers seek out and utilize group feedback in making decisions.

Like other contingency theorists, House and Mitchell feel that the form of leader behavior most indicated for the leader will vary with situational factors such as the maturity of the subordinates, the environment, and the task to be accomplished. The work of all of these organizational theorists assists nursing managers in understanding and developing their own leadership styles and in selecting the most appropriate leadership for a group in a given situation.

PREPARING EFFECTIVE LEADERS AND MANAGERS

How do nursing managers learn to identify and interpret variables that alter their leadership styles? In other words, how do managers learn to manage? The traditional view of management development is that managers are born, not made, and that managers develop as a result of the survival of the fittest (Armstrong and Lorentzen, 1982).

More current views on management development stress that although management requires self-development and self-growth, the organization can take an active role in encouraging and guiding managers and providing them with opportunities for growth. Although many managers develop sensitivity and expertise through trial and error and past experiences, many other managers become discouraged and fail because of a lack of management theory and training. Their failure is not because of a lack of ability or potential to become effective managers. It is because they have not been taught how to be managers or to be supported in managerial roles. The *Pygmalion effect*, which refers to a self-fulfilling prophecy whereby individuals become what they expect to be, can be applied to nursing management. If novice nurse managers are coached, supported, and encouraged throughout the process of self-growth that is required to become an effective manager, they are more likely to gain the expertise and self-confidence essential for being successful in that role.

Management development should be a systematic process that is philosophically and economically supported by the organization at all levels. Primary goals of any management development program should be improving the performance of current managers, providing opportunities for managerial growth and development, and ensuring as much as possible that management succession within the organization is provided for (Armstrong and Lorentzen, 1982). The process, however, may vary widely from person to person. The National Commission on Nursing (1983) has recommended that nurse executives and nurse managers of patient care units be qualified by education and experience to promote, develop, and maintain an organizational climate conducive to quality nursing practice and effective management of the nursing resource. Many organizations limit management development to a series of appropriate courses at various points in a manager's career. Although these training courses may be extremely helpful, management development must also include personal growth obtained as a result of exposure to "real-life situations" that require decision-making. These experiences may be provided in a supportive and well-coached environment, or they may be provided vicariously through individual and group problem solving. Chapters 15, 16, and 17 addressed specific components that could be integrated into an individual's management development program. Generally, however, management development programs should consist of education and training, career planning, and succession planning activities that are derived from the outcome of the organization, manpower, and performance reviews (Armstrong and Lorentzen, 1982). Tool 18-2 is a check list to be used by an organization in assessing the adequacy of its management development program.

MANAGERIAL ROLES

Because management development programs must be tailored to meet the needs of each individual manager, it is necessary to assess exactly what roles will be assumed by managers in the implementation of their jobs. Mintzberg (1973) studied the management role extensively and identified ten working roles for every manager. These roles, which are frequently played simultaneously, can be grouped into three major categories: interpersonal, informational, and decisional.

The **interpersonal** roles, those of *figurehead, leader*, and *liaison*, are derived from managers' status and authority in the organization. In the figurehead role, top-level managers perform various symbolic or ceremonial duties, such as ribbon cutting or groundbreaking when a new wing opens in a hospital. Middle-level managers may function within the figurehead role by representing their units at meetings within the organization.

Tool 18-2   Management Development Check List

Philosophy

1. Does the stated or implied philosophy of the organization on management development make it clear that:
   a. Management development is primarily self-development, and the main role of the organization should be to provide conditions that favor growth in ability and potential.
   b. The training aspect of management development is mainly concerned with the modification of behavior through experience, which is best achieved if training is carried out in the normal course of a manager's work through coaching, projects, and guided self-analysis.
   c. Management development has three associated and equally important objectives:
      • to improve the performance of managers generally,
      • to identify managers with potential and to ensure that they receive the required development, training, and expertise to equip them for more senior posts,
      • to provide for management succession.
   d. While procedures and systems, such as management by objectives, management inventories and management succession charts, have a part to play in management development, they are less important than the concept of self-development under guidance for the whole management group?

Commitment

1. Is the top management of the organization fully committed to an understood philosophy and program of management development?
2. Do all levels of management understand the philosophy of management development in the organization, how they are affected by it, and the part they play in implementing it?

Manpower development programs

1. Is first priority given to coaching and developing managers on the job?
2. Have managers been given adequate training in performance review, counseling, and coaching techniques?
3. Is there a proper system for monitoring the effectiveness of on-the-job development?
4. Are appraisals and counseling based on objective reviews of achievement against previously agreed targets and standards?

5. If a management-by-objectives system is in use:
   a. Is there a reasonable degree of commitment to the program at all levels of management?
   b. Have managers been properly trained in the system?
   c. Are appropriate targets and standards being agreed on between managers and their subordinates?
   d. Are managers conducting effective review meetings in the sense that an objective and frank discussion of achievements takes place and areas for improvement and development are agreed upon?
   e. Is the procedure simple enough to operate, that is, not overloaded with paperwork?
6. Are management training activities planned in light of an analysis of management development needs, including management succession?
7. Is there a system for identifying and developing managers with potential and relating those available to present and future management requirements?

From Armstrong, M., and Lorentzen, J. F., *Handbook of Personnel Management Practice*, p. 163. Prentice-Hall, Englewood Cliffs, NJ, 1982.

In the leader role, managers utilize interpersonal skills with subordinates to create a milieu in the organization that allows for effective achievement of organizational goals (Kern et al., 1987). This role is probably the most well recognized of all management roles and is imperative in creating a positive and motivating work climate. The leader role for the top-level manager includes such functions as defining the philosophy, goals, policies and procedures of the organization and supervising middle-level managers. For middle-level managers, the leader role may include the implementation of the goals, philosophy, policies, and procedures at the unit level and the supervision of subordinates within that unit (Kern et al., 1987).

In the liaison role, managers use their interpersonal skills with people and agencies outside the organization. In this liaison role, which is most common in higher level positions, managers develop a network of contacts that can be used to obtain information or resources that may be useful in future negotiations (Kern et al., 1987). Much of this liaison role is carried out by personal contact with individuals from both within and outside the organization. In top-level management, this role frequently entails a liaison between professional and community groups and governmental and regulatory agencies. Middle managers in the liaison role may network with other professional groups in the organization or may serve as members of professional and community groups (Kern et al., 1987).

The **informational** roles, those of *monitor, disseminator*, and *spokesman*, entail the giving and receiving of information that has a direct impact on how the organization is perceived by its workers and by those outside the organization. The monitor role entails seeking and receiving internal and external information from many sources to obtain a thorough knowledge of the environment and the organization (Kern et al., 1987). Much of the information obtained in the monitor role is obtained informally through subordinate contact, written reports, and observations of the organizational environment. This information is invaluable to nursing managers in that it allows them to identify conditions that are ripe for conflict and intercede before conflict occurs. In the monitor role, top-level managers establish, manage, and monitor information and reporting systems within the organization. The middle-level manager implements these systems at the unit level, and receives reports, makes rounds, and provides quality assurance at the unit level (Kern et al., 1987).

In the disseminator role, the manager shares information gathered from inside and outside sources with subordinates. This sharing of information that was previously known only by the manager allows the manager to share his or her power base with subordinates (Kern et al., 1987). Top-level managers in the disseminator role design formal communication systems for the organization and share information with middle-level managers. Middle-level managers in this role may communicate organizational policy and directives to subordinates at the unit level. Frequently the channel for this communication is the department or unit meeting (Kern et al., 1987).

The role of spokesperson is the opposite of the role of disseminator. In the spokesperson role, the manager shares subordinate and organizational views with outsiders. The way that the manager's unit is viewed by others both within and outside the organization is due, at least in part, to how effective the manager is in the role of spokesperson. Top-level managers functioning in the spokesperson role speak for the organization at meetings and conferences inside and outside the organization. They may also represent the organization in meetings with visitors from other agencies. Middle-level managers may function in the spokesperson role by serving as unit representatives at department-level meetings and by acting as spokespersons to physicians, families, and patients regarding unit matters (Kern et al., 1987).

The third category of roles are the **decisional roles**, those of *entrepreneur, disturbance handler, allocator,* and *negotiator.* In the entrepreneur role, both top-level and middle-level managers serve as change agents, seeking out areas that need change and initiating a plan for that change. Most managers have several planned changes occurring simultaneously. The ability of the organization to adapt and to be current is directly related to the willingness and the ability of managers in the entrepreneur role.

In the disturbance handler role, managers are involved in solving conflict that occurs as part of the day-to-day operation within the organization. Top-level managers assist in handling disturbances that occur at the organizational level. Middle-level managers deal with disturbances occuring at the unit level. In this role, managers assist subordinates in conflict resolution to minimize impact on organizational productivity.

As resource allocators, top-level managers maintain control of organizational strategy through personnel planning, fiscal planning, and organizational design. In the resource allocator role, middle-level managers are responsible for personal time management and the determination of unit philosophy and goals. They are also responsible for designing the basic work design at the unit level. The resource allocator role also includes authorization of decisions, as well as responsibility for decisions made within the organization (Kern et al., 1987). A great deal of the success in the resource allocator role is dependent on the manager's ability to solve problems and the confidence that he or she has in that ability.

The final decisional role is that of negotiator. The negotiator deals with conflicts that occur with those outside the organization. An example of a negotiator role common to top-level managers is that of contract negotiations in collective bargaining or in political situations in which managerial expertise in smoothing and accommodation is required. The middle-level manager assumes the negotiator role in bargaining for resources from other units or from executive levels of management (Kern et al., 1987).

NURSING MANAGERS: ASSESSING THE ORGANIZATIONAL FIT

Earlier chapters in this book have stressed the importance of employees having value systems or goals that are congruent with those of the organization. This does not mean that nursing managers in the organization must be conformists, or that they must have a uniform way of thinking or a standardized approach to problem solving. It does mean, however, that managers' overall goals must not be in conflict with the organization and that the means by which managers plan to implement those goals are acceptable to both managers and their organizations.

In addition, the importance of careful employee placement to assure an "organizational fit" between employee and organizational expectations has been emphasized. The same careful planning that is utilized in subordinate placement is also necessary in the selection and placement of nursing managers. *Organizational fit* refers to the selection and placement of a manager into an organization so that both the manager and the organization are optimally productive and satisfied. Organizational fit does not refer to the potential ability of the individual to be a good manager. Many potentially good managers are set up for failure when they are placed in situations in which they are unqualified, incompetent, or understimulated.

Jennings (1988) suggested that nursing managers assess their organizational fit by asking the following questions:

1. *Am I incompetent and unqualified?* An individual who feels this way should not be placed in a management position without adequate training and education to gain the self-confidence and knowledge necessary to do the job well.

2. *Am I competent but unqualified?* It is possible to have the skills that are necessary to perform at the level of the position, but not the skills that are valued by the organization. Further education may help here, but only if it is congruent with organizational values.

3. *Am I competent, but personally unqualified?* Task competence alone is not enough. Managers must have good interpersonal and decision-making skills if they are to be unit leaders and maintain high morale and motivation at the unit level.

4. *Was I once competent?* Because health care is dynamic, skills quickly become obsolete, and many managers find themselves outdated and in need of further education and training. Managers who find themselves in this position need to reassess their career goals. If goals are unchanged the manager must seek this additional education or training. Otherwise, the manager may be better able to use currently existing expertise or talent in some other position.

5. *Am I qualified but not yet competent?* Novice managers are not expected to be experts. Just as novice nurses gain expertise and self-confidence with time and experience, so should managers.

6. *Have I reached the point where I can do it better than the rest?* This attitude may simply reflect the growth, expertise, and self-confidence one has achieved as a manager. It may, however, be perceived as threatening by the organization, as it may imply an early separation or parting from organizational goals and a spirit of cooperation.

7. *Have I reached the point where I am bored with my work?* Managers should feel challenged and stimulated if their work is to be motivating. Managers who feel bored with their work often become complacent. Managers who find themselves in this situation should alter the work environment in some way to make the work more meaningful or should seek new and more challenging positions.

It cannot be overemphasized that the quality of the organization is a direct reflection of the quality of the individuals that are employed in that organization. Perhaps no employees have greater impact on this quality than the managers within the organization. Organizations that actively seek to develop a management team with optimal leadership skills create a climate that fosters productivity, high morale, and retention.

KEY CONCEPTS CHAPTER 18

1. Although the terms *leadership* and *management* are used synonymously by many people, they are very different. Leadership is the art of getting work done through others

acting willingly. Management is the formal manipulation of people, the environment, money, time, and other resources to reach organizational goals.

2. Organizations need *both* good leaders and good managers.

3. Both leadership and management skills can be taught. The organization must actively develop and support an environment that emphasizes management development.

4. Organizational theorists have identified three primary and distinct patterns of leadership behavior, which are called leadership styles. These three styles are authoritarian, democratic, and laissez-faire.

5. The primary determinants of the most appropriate leadership style for a manager to use should be the situation itself, the abilities of the manager, and the abilities of the group members. This variation in leadership style according to situational variables is called *contingency leadership*.

6. The ten working roles every manager assumes can be grouped into three major categories: interpersonal, informational, and decisional. Often, these roles are assumed simultaneously.

7. The same careful planning that is utilized in employee placement is also necessary in the selection and placement of nursing managers. There must be a congruency in the expectations of the manager and the organization.

REFERENCES

Armstrong, M., and Lorentzen, J. F., *Handbook of Personnel Management Practice*, Prentice-Hall, Englewood Cliffs, NJ, 1982.

Beyers, M., and Phillips, C., *Nursing Management for Patient Care*, Second Edition, Little, Brown and Company, Boston, 1979.

Blake, R.R., and Mouton, J. S., *The Managerial Grid*, Gulf Publishing, Houston, 1964.

DiVincenti, M., *Administering Nursing Service*, Little, Brown and Company, Boston, 1972.

Fielder, F., *A Theory of Leadership Effectiveness*, McGraw-Hill, New York, 1967.

Hersey, P., and Blanchard, K., *Management of Organizational Behavior: Utilizing Human Resources*, Prentice-Hall, Englewood Cliffs, NJ, 1977.

House, R.J., and Mitchell, T. R., "Path-Goal Theory of Leadership," *Journal of Contemporary Business*, 3:81, 1974.

Jennings, E., as found in J. Newham-Javorek, "A Guide for Nurse Executives – Assessing Your Organizational Fit," *Nursing Management*, 19(5):94, 1988.

Kern, J.P., Riley, J.J., and Jones, L.N. (eds.), *Human Resources Management*, Marcel Dekker, New York, and ASQC Quality Press, Milwaukee, 1987.

Marquis, B., and Huston, C., *Management Decision Making for Nurses: 101 Case Studies*, J.B. Lippincott, Philadelphia, 1987.

Mintzberg, H., *The Nature of Managerial Work*, Harper and Row, New York, 1973.

National Commission on Nursing, *Summary Report and Recommendations*, American Hospital Association, Chicago, IL, 1983.

Stogdill, R., "Personal Factors Associated with Leadership: A Survey of the Literature," *Journal of Psychology*, 25:35–71, 1948.

Sullivan, E.J., and Decker, P.J. *Effective Management in Nursing*, Second Edition, Addison-Wesley, Menlo Park, CA, 1988.

Tannenbaum, R., and Schmidt, W., "How to Choose a Leadership Pattern," *Harvard Business Review*, 51:162–180, 1973.

ADDITIONAL READINGS

Argyris, C.T., *Increasing Leadership Effectiveness*, John Wiley and Sons, New York, 1976.

Burns, J. McG., *Leadership*, Harper and Row, New York, 1978.

Campbell, J.P., Dunnete, M. D., Lawler, E. E., and Weick, K. E., *Managerial Behavior, Performance, and Effectiveness*, McGraw-Hill, New York, 1970.

Kantor, R.H., *The Charge Masters*, Simon and Schuster, New York, 1983.

Vroom, V.H., and Deci, E.L. (eds.), *Management and Motivation*, Penguin, New York, 1982.

19
Providing a Motivating Climate

MOTIVATION IS the drive of individuals to satisfy their needs, or the willingness to put effort into achieving a goal or reward. It may also be defined as the drive to reduce tension caused by an unsatisfied need (Klatt et al., 1978). Because human beings constantly have needs and wants, the individual is always motivated to some extent. All human beings are motivated differently, however, because they have different needs and desires.

This difference in what motivates individuals can be explained in part by our large and small group cultures (Beach, 1980). For example, American culture values material goods and possessions much more than do many other cultures, and thus reward in America is frequently related to these values.

There are also organizational cultures and values. Motivators vary among organizations and even among units within organizations. For example, competition has been proven an effective motivator for company salesmen and college graduates but appears to do little to motivate blue collar factory workers (Beach, 1980). Competition may, however, be an effective motivator among blue collar workers when it is used in groups rather than between individuals (Strauss and Sayles, 1972).

Assessment of factors that promote employee motivation is not an easy task. Even in similar or nearly identical work environments, there is often great variation in individual and group motivation. A great deal of research has been undertaken by behavioral, psychological, and social scientists to develop theories and concepts of motivation. Economists and engineers have used financial incentive programs to improve performance and productivity, while human relations scientists stress intrinsic needs for recognition, self-esteem, and self-actualization (Lewis and Spicer, 1987).

Chapter 19 will examine motivational theories that have guided organizational efforts and resources in the last 80 years. The reader is encouraged to refer back to the human relations theorists discussed in Chapter 1. Special attention will be given to the concept of intrinsic versus extrinsic motivation and organizational versus self-motivation. In addition, the role of the supervisor in creating a motivating climate and the impact of motivation on human resource management will be examined. Tools for implementation include motivational check lists for management and self-evaluation.

THE HISTORY OF MOTIVATIONAL THEORY

Chapter 2 presented an introduction to traditional management philosophy, which emphasized paternalism, worker subordination, and bureaucracy as a means to predictable, but moderate, productivity. Much of this traditional management philosophy developed as a result of the work of Frederick Taylor and his "Scientific Management Method" in the early 1900s. Reducing work to its simplest elements by carefully controlled time and motion studies allowed for the greatest employee productivity. High productivity meant greater monetary incentives for workers. Workers were viewed as being motivated primarily by economic factors, and producing the most efficient worker was seen as beneficial to both the worker and management (Kirsch, 1988). This traditional management philosophy of what motivates humankind is still utilized today. Many factory jobs, assembly line production, and jobs that utilize production incentive pay are based on Taylor's principles.

The shift from traditional management philosophy to a greater focus on the human element and worker satisfaction as factors in productivity occurred with the human relations era, which began between 1930 and 1940. This era viewed the worker as a social being, requiring intrinsic as well as extrinsic rewards from work (Kirsch, 1988). This shifting focus in what motivates employees has had a tremendous impact on the value organizations place on workers today. Several of the prominent theorists of this era have already been discussed in Chapter 1.

B. F. Skinner was one of the theorists in the human relations era who contributed to our understanding of motivation, dissatisfaction, and productivity. Skinner's research on operant conditioning and behavior modification demonstrated that individuals can be conditioned to do or not to do certain behaviors based on a consistent reward or punishment system (Skinner, 1953). Behavior that is rewarded will be repeated, and behavior that is punished or that goes unrewarded will be extinguished. Skinner's work continues to be reflected today in how many managers view and utilize discipline in the work setting.

Another theorist who contributed immensely to our understanding of motivation was Frederick Herzberg. Herzberg (1959) believed that workers could be motivated by work itself and that people have an internal or personal need to meet organizational goals. He also felt that it was possible to separate personal motivators from job dissatisfiers (Marquis and Huston, 1987). This distinction between hygiene/maintenance factors and motivation factors was called *motivation-hygiene theory*, or *two-factor theory*. This chapter will deal primarily with motivator factors. Chapter 20 will focus primarily on creating an organizational climate that reduces job dissatisfiers and increases hygiene or maintenance factors.

Table 19-1 lists motivator and hygiene factors as identified by Herzberg. Herzberg maintained that motivators (also called *job satisfiers*) are present in the work itself and encourage people to want to work and to do that work well. Hygiene and maintenance factors keep workers from being dissatisfied or demotivated but do not act as real motivators. It is important to remember that the opposite of dissatisfaction may not be satisfaction. When hygiene factors are met, there is a lack of dissatisfaction, rather than the existence of satisfaction. Likewise, the absence of motivators does not necessarily cause dissatisfaction.

For example, salary is a hygiene factor. It does not motivate in itself, although when used in conjunction with other motivators,

Table 19-1. Herzberg's Motivator and Hygiene Factors

Motivators	*Hygiene Factors*
Achievement	Salary
Recognition	Supervision
Work itself	Job security
Responsibility	Positive working conditions
Advancement	Personal life
Possibility for growth	Interpersonal relations/peers
	Company policy
	Status

such as recognition or advancement, it can be a powerful motivator. If salary is, however, deficient, it can result in employee dissatisfaction. Some individuals argue that money can truly be a motivator and that this is demonstrated by individuals who work insufferable hours at jobs they do not enjoy. Most theorists would argue that money (salary) in this case may be taking the place of some deep-felt need the individual is not fully conscious of (Beach, 1980).

It should also be noted that some individuals in Herzberg's studies (1959) did report job satisfaction solely from hygiene or maintenance factors. Herzberg asserts that such individuals show only a temporary satisfaction when hygiene factors are improved, show little interest in the kind and quality of their work, experience little satisfaction from accomplishments, and tend to show chronic dissatisfaction with other hygiene factors such as salary, status, and job security.

As a result of Herzberg's work, managers recognize that although hygiene or maintenance factors provide an essential base for the organization to build upon, the motivating climate must actively include the worker. The worker must be given greater responsibilities, challenges, and recognition for work well done (Marquis and Huston, 1987). Table 19-2 identifies techniques managers may utilize in meeting each of the motivator factors identified by Herzberg.

Another motivational theorist in the humanistic era was Victor Vroom. Vroom (1964) developed an "expectancy model"

Table 19-2. Implementing Herzberg's Motivator Factors

Motivator	Technique
Achievement	1. Nothing succeeds like achievement itself, so provide assignments that the employee can achieve. 2. Increase the employee's accountability for his or her work.
Recognition	1. Assess each individual employee to ascertain the employee's values and reward accordingly, whenever possible, i.e., • Verbal praise, to worker alone and in front of others • Employee of the Month • Written letters of commendation • Certificates of achievement • Change in title or status
Work itself	1. Identify individual worker's strengths and talents and assign work accordingly. 2. Whenever possible, vary the work to be performed and avoid routine, repetitive, and boring assignments. 3. Assign work that requires the full attention of the employee.
Responsibility	1. Challenge employees on a regular basis. Stretch them, but not beyond what they are capable of achieving and not all the time. 2. Assign employees to departmental and organizational committees. 3. Increase worker autonomy.
Advancement	1. Promote or transfer employees upward in the organization. 2. Add new roles or responsibilities.
Possibility for growth	1. Agree to be a mentor to a novice nurse manager. 2. Provide the opportunities for additional education and new learning experiences.

that examined motivation in terms of the individual's valence or preferences, based on social values. In contrast to operant conditioning, which focuses on observable behaviors, the expectancy model says that people's expectations about their environment or a certain event will influence their behavior (Sullivan and Decker, 1988).

Individuals, therefore, will look at all actions as having a cause and an effect. The effect may be immediate or it may be delayed, but there is a reward inherent in the behavior that will motivate individuals to undertake the risks of action. In the expectancy model, people make conscious decisions in anticipation of a reward, whereas in operant conditioning they react in a stimulus/response mode. Managers using the expectancy theory must know their workers personally so as to gain an understanding of the employees' individual values, reward system, strengths, and willingness to take risks (Marquis and Huston, 1987).

McClelland (1961) also contributed to motivational theory in examining the motives that lead individuals to take action. McClelland's studies identified three basic needs that motivate all people: achievement, affiliation, and power. Achievement-oriented individuals actively focus their lives on improving what is. They transform ideas into action, judiciously and wisely, taking risks when necessary.

In contrast, affiliation-oriented individuals focus their energies on families and friends. Their overt productivity is less, as they view their contribution to society in a different light from achievement-oriented individuals. Research has shown that women, and especially nurses, frequently have high affiliation needs, and this is a major reason many more young women than men enter nursing (Simms et al., 1985).

Power-oriented individuals are motivated by the power that can be gained as a result of a specific action. They want to command attention, get recognition, and control others. McClelland theorized that managers in organizations can identify the achievement, affiliation, or power needs of their employees and develop motivational strategies that meet those needs. Tool 19-1 is a self-evaluation tool that can be used to assess individual achievement, affiliation, and power needs.

Gellerman (1963), another humanistic motivational theorist, identified three methods to positively motivate people. The first of these is "stretching." This is the assignment of tasks to individuals that generally are more difficult than what they are used to doing. Stretching, however, must be used sparingly and infrequently (Beyers and Phillips, 1979). A second method is "management by objectives," which was discussed in Chapter 14. The third method is "participation," which consists of actively drawing employees into decisions affecting their work.

Tool 19-1   Assessing Achievement, Affiliation, and Power Needs:
A Self-Evaluation Tool

List ten goals you hope to accomplish in the next 25 years.

1. _____

2. _____

3. _____

4. _____

5. _____

6. _____

7. _____

8. _____

9. _____

10. _____

Look at the ten goals you have identified. Identify which goals are more closely related to achievement needs by placing an (*A*) beside them. Do the same for affiliation (*AF*) and power (*P*). Remember that most individuals are motivated at least in part by all three needs and that no one motivational need is better than the others. It is important, however, that each individual be self-aware enough to recognize and understand which basic needs have the greatest motivation in his or her life.

Gellerman felt strongly that motivation problems are usually due to the way the organization manages and not to an unwillingness of the staff to work hard (DiVincenti, 1972). Gellerman stated that most managers in organizations "overmanage"; that is, they make employee's jobs too narrow and fail to give employees any decision-making power.

The work of motivational theorists such as Taylor, Skinner, Herzberg, McClelland, and Gellerman has added greatly to our understanding of what motivates individuals, both in and out of the work setting. Their research, however, has also revealed that motivation is extremely complex and that there is tremendous variation in which factors and settings motivate different individuals. It therefore is important for managers to understand what aspects of motivation the organization can affect as well as how.

INTRINSIC VERSUS EXTRINSIC MOTIVATION

Intrinsic motivation can be defined as the motivation that comes from within the individual. It is an internal reward and occurs as a direct result of the completed work. Intrinsic or internalized motivation is satisfaction that is gained internally from accomplishing work at a high level.

The intrinsic motivation individuals have to achieve and accomplish is directly related to level of aspiration. Parental and peer influence play a major role in shaping values about what individuals want to do and be. Parents who set high, but attainable, expectations for their children and who provide continuous encouragement in a nonauthoritarian environment tend to impart a strong achievement drive in their children (Beach, 1980).

Even an individual with a strong achievement drive must internalize two other beliefs before he or she will be intrinsically motivated to behave in a certain way. First, the individual must believe that improved performance will lead to outcomes that are congruent with his or her value system. Second, the individual must believe that increased effort will lead to improved performance and therefore that the required energy expenditure will be worth the cost (Milkovich and Glueck, 1985).

Lawler (1969) also identified characteristics required for jobs to be intrinsically motivating:

1. *Feedback* — Individuals must receive meaningful feedback regarding their performance. Ideally, feedback should be given following a self-evaluation by the individual.

2. *Use of abilities* — Individuals must perceive that effective performance of the job will require abilities they value.

3. *Self-control* — Individuals must feel a high degree of self-control over their own goals and the means by which they implement them.

Extrinsic motivation is motivation that is enhanced by the job environment or by external rewards. This reward occurs after the work has been completed. Although all individuals are intrinsically motivated to some degree, it is unrealistic for the organization to assume that all workers have an adequate level of intrinsic motivation to meet organizational goals. Thus, it is important for the organization to provide a climate that extrinsically motivates its workers, as well as provides a climate that meets intrinsic motivational needs.

CREATING A MOTIVATING CLIMATE

Because the organization has such an impact on the factors that extrinsically motivate employees, it is important to examine organizational climates or attitudes that have a direct influence on worker morale and motivation. For example, frequently organizations overtly or covertly reinforce the image that each and every employee is expendable and that a great deal of individual recognition is in some way detrimental to both the individual and that individual's productivity within the organization. Just the opposite is true. Individuals who have a strong self-concept and perceive themselves to be winners are willing to take risks and increase their productivity to achieve additional recognition. Peters and Waterman (1982) stress that organizations must be designed to make individual employees feel like winners. The focus must be on degrees of winning rather than on degrees of losing.

Another erroneous attitude held by some organizations is at the opposite extreme. This is the belief that if a small reward results in desired behavior, then a larger reward will result in even more of the desired behavior. Thus they feel an employee's motivation should increase proportionately with the amount of the incentive or reward. In a study of navy recruits, Korman and associates (1981) found little support of this concept; to the contrary, more incentives were actually less motivating, as they engendered a feeling of distrust or being bought. Increasing incentives may be perceived as a violation of individual norms or of guilt (Bowin, 1987). Thus, there appears to be a perceived threshold beyond which increases in incentives result in no additional motivation. Organizations must be cognizant of the need to offer incentives at a level at which they are valued by employees. Thus, organizations must have some understanding of the collective values held by their employees and must use a reward system that is consonant with the employees' value system.

In addition to the climate created by the organization's beliefs and attitudes, the supervisor or unit manager also has a tremendous impact on motivation at the unit level (Milkovich and Glueck, 1985). Longest (1974) affirmed that interpersonal relations between employees and their supervisors are one of the most critical factors affecting job satisfaction. Because motivation comes from within the individual, nurse managers can not directly motivate their employees. They can, however, play an integral part in motivating employees by providing a climate that encourages growth and productivity. This requires that they recognize each employee as a unique individual who is motivated by different things and in different ways. Each employee must be rewarded in a manner that is consistent with what he or she values.

One of the most powerful motivators the manager can use to create a motivating climate, and one that is frequently overlooked or underutilized, is positive reinforcement. Peters and Waterman (1982) identified the following simple schemes and approaches necessary for an effective reward-feedback system that utilizes positive reinforcement.

1. Positive reinforcement must be *specific*, or relevant, to a particular performance. The manager should give praise to an employee for a specific task accomplished or goal met, and this praise should not be general in nature. For example, "Your nursing care is good," has less meaning and reward than, "The communication skills you showed today as an advocate for Mr. Jones were excellent. I feel you made a tremendous difference in his life."

2. The positive reinforcement must have *immediacy*. The positive reinforcement must occur as soon after the event as possible.

3. The reward-feedback system must be *achievable*. All performance goals must be achievable, and both large and small achievements should be recognized or rewarded in some way.

4. Rewards should be *unpredictable* and *intermittent*. If rewards are given routinely, they tend to lose their value.

Although there is value in not allowing rewards to be taken for granted, we disagree with Peters and Waterman, our feeling being that there must be some consistency in when and how rewards are given.

Rewards that lack consistency may themselves become a source of competition and lowered morale. The attitude prevails that, "There are a limited number of awards and an award received by anyone else limits my chances of getting one; thus I cannot support recognition for my peers." Likewise, rewarding the behavior of one individual and not that of another who has accomplished a similar task at a similar level promotes jealousy and can demotivate.

Since rewards are given in response to a genuine accomplishment on the part of the individual, it is essential that they be individual in nature if they are to be effective as a motivational strategy. For example, many managers erroneously consider annual merit pay increases as rewards that motivate employees. Most employees, however, recognize annual merit pay increases as a universal "given." Thus, this reward has little meaning and little power to motivate.

Nurse managers should think excellence and achievable goals, and reward performance in a way that is valued by their staff. These are the cardinal elements for a successful motivation-reward system for the nursing organization (Kirsch, 1988). Tool 19-2 identifies 12 golden rules that should be followed in using praise and reward to create a motivating climate.

Managers can also create a motivating climate by being positive and enthusiastic role models in the clinical setting. Studies by Jenkins and Henderson (1984) demonstrated that supervisors' or managers' personal motivations are the most important factor affecting their staffs' commitments to duties and morale. Positive outlooks, enthusiasm, productivity, and accomplishment are contagious. Radzik (1985) stated that employees frequently gauge their job security and their employer's satisfaction with their job performance by the expression they see on their manager's face. Unhappy managers frequently project their unhappiness on their subordinates and contribute greatly to low unit morale. Tool 19-3 can be used to measure morale or cohesiveness at the unit level.

Managers must be positive and encouraging in their interactions with their subordinates. Losoncy (1977) identified the following essential characteristics of the "encouraging person" or "encouraging manager":

Tool 19-2   Rewards and Praise: 12 Golden Rules

1. The employee's behavior that you reward is very likely to be the behavior they will repeat.

2. When rewarding, your first concern is to reinforce good performance.

3. Managers confuse employees when they reward not only performance, but also nonperformance factors such as loyalty, compliance, and friendship.

4. Good performers may become demotivated by the manager's rewarding on a nonperformance basis.

5. If you want full value from rewards for good performance, make sure that all employees know exactly what you reward.

6. If you try to treat everyone equally in giving rewards, you may create demotivation in better performers.

7. Praise is one of the most effective rewards you have.

8. Praise is effective only when it is genuine and deserved.

9. The more specific the praise is, the more effective it will be.

10. Do not praise personality traits. Praise the behavior that reflects the personality trait.

11. Criticism should always be done in private. Praise should be in public when appropriate.

12. When everything is rewarded, nothing is.

Adapted from Quick, T. L., "Review of Getting and Maintaining the Behavior You Want," *The Manager's Motivation Deskbook*, John Wiley and Sons, New York, 1985, pp. 404–405.

---

1. The encouraging person *sees only individuals in the world.* When faced with groups of people, he or she views each individual as unique—with interests, problems, and goals that must be acknowledged.

2. The encouraging person is a *safe, totally accepting person.* He or she believes that the discouraged individual hasn't consistently experienced safe relationships and hence has developed a mask.

Tool 19-3   Assessing Unit Morale/Cohesiveness

Directions: Use the following tool to assess the morale/cohesiveness of your unit. Next to each of the 15 characteristics, write the number that most closely reflects your assessment. Use the following key to guide your choice of numbers:

0 = Not at all
1 = Infrequently
2 = Frequently
3 = Almost all the time

Characteristics	*Examples*
＿＿ 1. Members value unit goals.	• Members accept long- and short-term unit goals. • Members accept leader's priorities. • Members participate in formulating unit goals. • Members perceive unit and its work as meaningful. • Members are willing to work hard to achieve goals.
＿＿ 2. Individual goals mesh with unit goals.	• Members feel they benefit personally from unit membership. • Unit membership brings individuals closer to long-term career goals.
＿＿ 3. Unit works to attain difficult as well as easy goals.	• Difficulties are defined as challenges or opportunities. • Difficult jobs are fairly assigned to all members. • Leader recognizes and rewards successful completion of difficult tasks.
＿＿ 4. Relationships are friendly and enjoyable.	• Members socialize at breaks and mealtime. • Subgroups interact easily and amicably. • Members enjoy being together.
＿＿ 5. Relationships are trusting and open.	• Communication is direct, honest, and respectful. • Members discuss controversial issues without fear of reprisal. • Confidentiality is honored. • Members resolve conflicts constructively.

____ 6. Relationships are loyal and supportive.	• Members defend unit to outside critics. • Members avoid criticizing unit or its members in front of nonmembers. • Members handle conflict internally. • Members receive support when speaking up in a meeting. • Help is offered when members need it. • Risk-taking is encouraged and rewarded. • Members praise and recognize one another's accomplishments.
____ 7. Participation is stable, reliable, and consistent.	• Turnover is low. • Call-outs are infrequent. • Use of floats or temporary help is minimal. • Members arrive on time and complete work on time. • Members follow through on commitments.
____ 8. Participation is flexible.	• Members readily accept assigned tasks or roles. • Members help those who need help. • Members willingly fill in for those absent. • Members can fulfill a variety of roles. • Members are willing to adapt to change.
____ 9. Participation is goal directed.	• Members understand and fulfill their responsibilities. • Leader guides unit toward goal achievement. • Leader assists ineffective or resistant members to alter unacceptable behavior.
____ 10. Participation is interdependent.	• Leadership is democratic. • Members cooperate in achieving goals. • "We, us" is used to describe the unit, not "us vs. them," or "I." • Contributions of all members are valued and respected. • Members do not compete against each other.
____ 11. Participation is guided by group norms.	• Job descriptions specify expected behavior. • Rules are applied fairly and consistently. • Rules facilitate rather than hinder. • Policies and procedures are clear and relevant. • Violations of norms are censured.
____ 12. Participation is productive.	• Productivity levels are achieved. • Members manage time effectively. • Groups function within budget. • Conflict does not consume or drain unit energy.

_____ 13.	Participation yields high-quality output.	• Professional standards are met. • Quality assurance audits yield positive results. • Patients/clients offer positive feedback. • Members work to their best abilities.
_____ 14.	Participation improves the security and self-esteem of members.	• Members develop technical job skills. • Individuality is respected and valued. • Members interact respectfully. • Rewards of membership are both tangible and intangible.
_____ 15.	Participation is satisfying.	• Members are proud to be unit members. • Members praise unit to outsiders. • Work of the unit challenges members to grow. • Members feel competent to do job and fulfill roles.

_____ **TOTAL SCORE:** Record the number that correlates with your total on the graph below for a picture of the morale/cohesiveness of your unit.

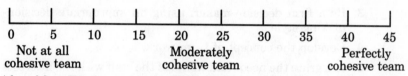

Adapted from Hamilton, J. M., and Kiefer, M. E., *Survival Skills for the New Nurse*, p. 142. J. B. Lippincott, Philadelphia, 1986.

---

3. The encouraging person is *skilled at looking for uniqueness or differences* in individuals. This is almost a second-nature skill that the helper develops along the way. Once the individual's uniqueness is noticed, he or she begins to develop a sense of self-worth and the courage to take risks and change.

4. The encouraging person not only has *faith in human nature,* but has *faith in the discouraged individual.*

5. The encouraging person is *sincerely enthusiastic about the growth of the discouraged individual* and *communicates* this enthusiasm to others.

6. The encouraging person is *ultrasensitive to the self-defeated person's goals, values, and purposes,* believing that each behavior is significant and consequential. The encourager helps this person learn to see himself or herself in a more powerful light.

7. The encouraging person realizes that *knowledge of the discouraged individual's past proud moments — his or her "claim to fame" —* is important to a new, more positive identity. Encouraged to feel worthwhile, the formerly defeated individual will now take risks, formulate goals, and evaluate self-growth.

8. The encouraging person is sensitive to *overdependency* in the relationship and *helps the discouraged person develop self-encouragement.* As a result, this person begins to develop new relationships in which the same encouragement process is used to help others. This person then becomes an encourager.

In addition to positive reinforcement, role-modeling, and encouragement, the following actions should assist nurse managers in creating a motivating climate (Marquis and Huston, 1987):

1. Have clear expectations for workers, and communicate these expectations clearly and effectively.

2. Be fair and consistent in dealing with all employees.

3. Be a firm decision-maker, using an appropriate decision-making style.

4. Develop the concept of team work.

5. Integrate the needs and wants of the staff with the interests and purpose of the organization.

6. Know the uniqueness of each employee and let the employees know that you understand their unique qualities.

7. Remove the traditional blocks between employees and the work to be done.

8. Provide experiences that intermittently challenge or "stretch" employees and allow opportunity for growth.

9. When appropriate, request participation and input from all subordinates in decision-making.

10. Whenever possible, give recognition and credit to subordinates.

11. Be certain that employees understand the reason behind decisions and actions.

12. Reward desirable behavior. Be consistent in how you handle undesirable behavior.

13. Let employees exercise individual judgment as much as possible.

14. Create a trustful and helping relationship with employees.

15. Let employees exercise as much control as possible over their work environment.

Tool 19-4 provides a self-evaluation tool assessing career motivation.

THE IMPACT OF MOTIVATION ON HUMAN RESOURCE MANAGEMENT

Creating a motivating climate in order to increase productivity and retention is an integral component of optimum human resource management. Research by Longest (1974) reported serious problems among registered nurses in terms of lack of motivation and subsequent turnover. The cost of turnover as a significant factor in the labor-intensive budgets of most hospitals was discussed in Chapter 1. If goals of human resource management are to increase retention and productivity, it is imperative that the organization identify what factors motivate its employees and that it works to create an environment that meets employee needs. By taking a humanistic approach, the nurse manager can create an environment in which the development of human potential can be maximized (Simms et al., 1985). Motivated employees are satisfied employees, and satisfied employees have higher retention and productivity.

KEY CONCEPTS CHAPTER 19

1. Because human beings constantly have needs and wants, the individual is always motivated to some extent. All human beings are motivated differently, however, because they have different needs and desires.

2. Skinner's research on operant conditioning and behavior modification demonstrated that individuals can be conditioned to do or not to do certain behaviors based on a consistent reward or punishment system.

3. McClelland's studies identified that all people are motivated by three basic needs: achievement, affiliation, and power.

4. Gellerman stated that most managers in organizations over-manage; that is, they make the jobs of employees too narrow and fail to give employees any decision-making power.

Tool 19-4   Assessing Motivation: Tool for Self-Analysis

Diagram the motivational levels you have felt at different points in your career. Think about the periods during which you felt the highest and lowest motivation. What factors can you identify that made the greatest difference in your motivational levels? Which of these factors were intrinsic? Which were extrinsic?

High
M
O
T
I
V
A
T
I
O
N
Low

Novice Nurse	2 years experience	5 years experience	10 years experience	20 years experience	30 years + experience

---

5. Herzberg maintained that motivators (also called *job satis-fiers*) are present in the work itself and encourage people to want to work and to do that work well. Hygiene or maintenance factors keep workers from being dissatisfied or demotivated, but do not act as real motivators for workers.

6. *Intrinsic* motivation can be defined as the motivation that comes from within the individual. *Extrinsic* motivation is motivation that is enhanced by the job environment or by external rewards.

7. Peters and Waterman (1982) stress that organizations must be designed to make the individual employee feel like a winner. The focus must be on degrees of winning rather than on degrees of losing.

8. There appears to be a perceived threshold beyond which increasing the incentive results in no additional motivation.

9. Because motivation comes from within the individual, nurse managers cannot directly motivate their employees. They can, however, play an integral part in motivating employees by providing a climate that encourages growth and productivity.

10. One of the most powerful motivators that nurse managers can use, and one that is frequently overlooked or under-utilized, is positive reinforcement.

11. The supervisor or manager's personal motivation is an important factor affecting the staff's commitment to duties and morale.

REFERENCES

Beach, D., *Personnel: The Management of People at Work*, Fourth Edition, MacMillan, New York, 1980.

Beyers, M., and Phillips, C., *Nursing Management for Patient Care*, Second Edition, Little, Brown and Company, Boston, 1979.

Bowin, R.B., *Human Resource Problem Solving*, Prentice-Hall, Engelwood Cliffs, NJ, 1987.

DiVincenti, M., *Administering Nursing Service*, Little, Brown and Company, Boston, 1972.

Gellerman, S.W., *Motivation and Productivity*, American Management Association, New York, 1963.

Herzberg, F., *The Motivation to Work*, John Wiley and Sons, New York, 1959.

Jenkins, R.L., and Henderson, R.L., "Motivating the Staff: What Nurses Expect from their Supervisors," *Nursing Management*, 15(2):13–14, 1984.

Kirsch, J., *The Middle Manager and the Nursing Organization: Human Resources, Fiscal Resources*, Appleton & Lange, Norwalk, CT, 1988.

Klatt, L.A., Murdick, R.G., and Schuster, F.E., *Human Resources Management: A Behavioral Systems Approach*, Richard D. Irwin, Homewood, IL, 1978.

Korman, A.K., Glickman, A.S., and Frey, R.L., "More Is Not Better: Two Failures of Incentive Theory," *Journal of Applied Psychology*, 66:255–259, 1981.

Lawler, E.E., "Job Design and Employee Motivation," *Personnel Psychology*, 22:426–435, 1969.

Lewis, E.M., and Spicer, J.G., *Human Resource Management Handbook; Contemporary Strategies for Nursing Managers*, Aspen Publishers, Rockville, MD, 1987.

Longest, B.B., "Job Satisfaction for Registered Nurses in the Hospital Setting," *JONA*, 4(3): 46, 1974.

Losoncy, L.E., *Turning People On: How To Be an Encouraging Person*, Prentice-Hall, Englewood Cliffs, NJ, 1977.

Marquis, B., and Huston, C., *Management Decision Making for Nurses: 101 Case Studies*, J.B. Lippincott, Philadelphia, 1987.

Milkovich, G.T., and Glueck, W.F., *Personnel, Human Resource Management: A Diagnostic Approach*, Business Publications, Plano, TX, 1985.

Peters, T., and Waterman, R.H., *In Search of Excellence*, Harper and Row, New York, 1982.

Radzik, A., "What Managers Want to Know," *Nations Business*, 73(8):37, 1985.

Simms, L. M., Price, S.A., and Ervin, N.E., *The Professional Practice of Nursing Administration*, John Wiley and Sons, New York, 1985.

Skinner, B.F., *Science and Human Behavior*, Free Press, New York, 1953.

Strauss, G., and Sayles, L.R., *Personnel: The Human Problems of Management*, Third Edition, Prentice-Hall, Englewood Cliffs, NJ, 1972.

Sullivan, E.J., and Decker, P.J., *Effective Management in Nursing*, Second Edition, Addison-Wesley, Menlo Park, CA, 1988.

Vroom, V.H., *Work and Motivation*, John Wiley and Sons, New York, 1964.

ADDITIONAL READINGS

Bristol, C.M., *The Magic of Believing*, Cornerstone Library, Simon and Schuster, New York, 1979.

Case, B.B., "Motivating Your Staff Toward Excellent Performance," *Nursing Management*, 14(12):45–48, 1983.

Levinson, H., *Psychological Man*, The Levinson Institute, Cambridge, MA, 1976.

Likert, R., *The Human Organization*, McGraw-Hill, New York, 1967.

McCormack, M.H., *What They Don't Teach You at Harvard Business School*, Bantam Books, New York, 1984.

Nadler, D., Hackman, J.R., and Lawler, E.E., *Managing Organizational Behavior*, Little, Brown and Company, Boston, 1979.

Nelson, G.M., and Schaefer, M.J., "An Integrated Approach to Developing Administrators and Organizations," *JONA*, 10(2): 37–42, 1980.

Peters, T., and Austin, N., *A Passion for Excellence*, Random House, New York, 1985.

Stubbs, I.R., and Parker, E.R., "Motivating for Management 'Effectiveness'," *Legal Economics* 5(5):38–40, 1979.

Wysenki, N.J., "Motivating Your Staff to Do Their Best," *Nursing Life*, 6(1):52–53, 1986.

20
Quality of Work Life – Reducing the Dissatisfiers

AN EFFECTIVE reward system meets both motivation and hygiene needs, and the emphasis given by the manager should vary with the situation and employee involved. Although hygiene factors in themselves do not motivate the worker, they are necessary to create an environment that encourages the worker to move on to higher level needs. They also keep the employee from being dissatisfied and may be very useful in recruiting an adequate employee pool.

Chapter 19 discussed the components of the motivating climate and how the organization and its supervisors can work to create a climate that meets the higher level needs or motivators as identified in Herzberg's two-factor theory. Chapter 20 will examine several of Herzberg's hygiene factors and job dissatisfiers and will discuss organizational and managerial strategies that can be implemented to improve the quality of work life in the organization. Special emphasis will be given to salary, benefits, guaranteed job security, provision of child care, positive working conditions, and employee assistance programs. Tools for implementation include a fringe benefit assessment tool.

SALARY

Management's primary objective in developing an appropriate wage payment system is to see that maximum productivity and quality are obtained at minimum cost (Armstrong and Lorentzen, 1982). The assumption behind most wage payment systems is that salary is a key motivating factor. This is *not* a valid assumption, but it *is* reasonable to assume that pay is an important factor in obtaining and recruiting workers, and that an inadequate salary can be a major cause of dissatisfaction for workers. It is also important to remember that salary is important to many people because it is frequently tied to motivators such as recognition and achievement.

Employee dissatisfaction with salaries occurs for several common reasons: inadequate number of steps in the salary schedule, inadequate pay differentials between job classifications or pay steps, inconsistency in application of salary administration, and general inadequacy of paid salary.

A typical graded salary schedule consists of a sequence of salary ranges or bands, each of which has a defined minimum and maximum (Armstrong and Lorentzen, 1982). It is assumed that all the jobs allocated into a range are broadly of the same value, although actual salaries earned by individuals will depend on their performance and length of service. Current practice is to aim for 7 to 10 pay steps covering all nursing personnel and to have salary range maximums generally about 20% above the average salary being paid for that job in the organization (Armstrong and Lorentzen, 1982).

It is important to have adequate pay differentials between each grade so that a significantly increased reward results from an upgrading, and to avoid the arguments about regradings that result if the increases between grades are too small (Armstrong and Lorentzen, 1982). It is also important to recognize that employees who have reached the top step of the salary progression must be rewarded in additional ways if their continuing productivity is desired.

There are basically three methods of determining pay progression throughout a range: (1) length of service, (2) performance, and (3) a combination of performance and merit (Beach, 1980). Most motivational theorists believe that salaries or wages should reflect performance and not length of service. Individuals should be advanced through the salary schedule as they improve their performances or through promotion. If salary increases are given solely on the basis of years of service and do not reflect the quality or the productivity of the employee, the rewarding or motivating capability of the salary decreases greatly. American workers in general need to understand that in order for employers to increase salaries, workers must improve their performance at a level that will produce economic return to justify the increased remuneration (Laliberty and Christopher, 1984). If employees want greater remuneration, they must do more, not just demand more.

Historically, management has believed that the most important element in the employees' demand package is salary. Thus, when worker dissatisfaction has been high, management often has opted to increase wages as the primary solution. Research, however, has demonstrated that when the basic wage is adequate to meet normal expected standard-of-living requirements, wages actually take a low priority (Laliberty and Christopher, 1984).

Then, are nursing salaries today adequate to meet expected standards of living requirements, and are inadequate salaries a primary cause of dissatisfaction for nurses? Historically, low nursing salaries have been a primary dissatisfier for nurses. Chapter 19, however, identified research showing that salaries, although still a very important factor to most nurses, have become less important in the last few years as a primary dissatisfier or as a reason given for turnover in nursing. This has occurred in great part due to the approximate doubling of nursing salaries within the last ten years.

As a result of the nursing shortage of the 1970s, nursing salaries have increased tremendously, and today nursing is considered one of the highest paid of traditional female occupations. This is especially true for the novice nurse, whose starting salary looks very good in comparison with other professional occupations. However, because of the current salary structure in nursing, nurses very quickly reach peak salary, giving little financial incentive to the experienced nurse. The salary of the professional nurse with 20 years of experience trails far behind that of individuals in other professions who had a comparable starting salary.

Although nursing salaries have increased greatly in the last 15 years, nursing salaries are anticipated to increase only 4% to

6% in 1988. This moderate increase reflects the health care industry's continued cost consciousness and the projected low inflation rate for 1988 (Young, 1987). However, nurses in anticipated high-demand areas such as oncology, management, open-heart surgery, and neonatal intensive care may receive even greater increases. Table 20-1 identifies projected average salaries for nurses in selected positions for 1988. Many of these salaries are at least competitive with comparable professional positions, and salary may cease to be a dissatisfier for many nurses in the future.

In evaluating the fairness and equity of a salary schedule, the nurse must examine more than the basic hourly range. There are many other income factors that must be considered, including pay for overtime and differentials. Table 20-2 identifies components of the salary schedule.

BENEFITS

Although recruitment success is often based, at least in part, on salary offered, retention is frequently based on fringe benefits (Laliberty and Christopher, 1984). Fringe benefits — compensation other than wages or salaries — today constitute about one third of the compensation of the typical U.S. employee (Sullivan and Decker, 1988), and this figure is increasing. In 1929, benefits cost the employer 3% of total wages and salaries. In 1949, the cost had increased to 16%, and by the 1970s, it had increased to between 30% and 50% (Glueck, 1978). In examining the total representative cost of fringe benefits in the organization, the

Table 20-1. 1988 Salary Forecast for Nurses

Position	Projected Median Salary
Chief nursing administrator	$53,600
Asst. or assoc. nursing administrator	$44,250
Intensive care (ICU/CCU) supervisor	$39,100
Head nurse	$38,600
Clinical nurse specialist	$37,750
Staff nurse	$28,450

From Young, R., " '88 U.S. Nursing Profession Salary Outlook," Roth Young Personnel Service Inc., as found in *Nursing Life*, 7(6):10, 1987.

Table 20-2. Components of the Salary Schedule: Income Factors

---

1. *Hourly rate* — The hourly rate is typically based on type and amount of prior work experience and on educational preparation.
2. *Weekday, evening, and night shift differential* — These shift differentials usually represent a set percentage over the base rate, i.e., 15% for evenings and 25% for nights.
3. *Weekend differential* — Weekend differentials also represent a set percentage over the basic rate for work on either Saturday or Sunday.
4. *Holiday differential* — Typically, holiday differential is 1½ times normal hourly pay (but may be double pay) for scheduled holiday work.
5. *Charge nurse differential* — This differential is generally 5%–10% over the basic hourly rate.
6. *On-call differential* — This differential is generally funded in two ways. One rate is for those hours spent at home while on call, and the other rate is for those hours at work for which one has been called in.
7. *Education or specialty area certification differential* (i.e., MICN, CCU, etc.) — Typically this is a small differential (less than 5%), but may be substantial, depending on the difficulty in hiring adequate numbers of adequately trained nurses in that specialty.
8. *Overtime pay* — Overtime pay may be calculated using a 40-hour work week or an 80-hour 2-week pay period. It is important to know which pay period is used by the organization to determine overtime. Overtime pay is typically 1½ times the normal pay rate for a set number of hours and then is advanced to double pay.
9. *Profit sharing* — These plans are available in for-profit institutions and allow the employee to purchase stock in the corporation that owns the institution or to have money placed in an investment fund for retirement. Employees receive a share, fixed in advance, of the profits.

---

manager should examine four aspects of benefit cost and compare the results with other organizations within the industry (Foegen, 1974):

1. Total cost of benefits annually for all employees

2. Cost per employee per year ÷ number of employee hours worked

3. Percentage of payroll ÷ annual payroll

4. Cost per employee per hour ÷ employee hours worked

Because benefits have traditionally been paid only to full-time workers, many organizations, in an attempt to reduce benefit costs, have attempted to change the base worker population by increasing the number of part-time workers or increasing overtime. This shift from the more stable full-time worker to part-time employment has tremendous implications regarding organizational stability and the ability to meet organizational goals. In the last 30 years, the organizational cost of providing fringe benefits has increased twice as fast as salaries and wages (Glueck, 1978; Strauss and Sayles, 1972). These increases in the cost of fringe benefits can be attributed to the rising cost of social security, pensions, vacations, and insurance, as well as a general increase in the number of fringe benefits that have been made available to employees in the last 20 years (Schuster, 1985).

The term *fringe* is really a misnomer. Fringes are no longer "extras," and a vast majority of Americans rely on them as their first line of defense against illness, unemployment, and old age, as well as their source of vacations and holidays (Schuster, 1985). These fringe benefits provide security to the employee, and their absence may be a prime dissatisfier. Likewise, because fringe benefits are not allocated in response to performance levels, most employees feel fringes are a basic entitlement and a right (Milkovich and Glueck, 1985).

Many proactive organizations have attempted to include benefit planning in their long-term strategic planning. In 1976, 150 experts predicted the following trends in benefits (Paul, 1976):

1. Increased coverage of health insurance plans
   a. Hospitalization for 120 days
   b. 100% surgical expense coverage
   c. Major medical coverage with 10% employee co-payment on total cost of coverage
2. Newer coverage in allied health fields
   a. Dental coverage, probably added primarily as an extension to a Blue Cross type of coverage
   b. Drug insurance: coverage of major prescription drug costs by employer-paid insurance
   c. Vision care: payment of eye examination and provision of glasses/contact lenses as needed
   d. Preventive care: coverage for regular physical examinations
3. Group auto insurance: provision of liability and collision coverage by employer-paid group auto insurance.

Many of these 1976 predictions are now a reality. Predictions for the 1990s focus on the emergence of prepaid legal services, group auto insurance, employee counseling/assistance programs, and child care centers as priority benefits (Glueck, 1978). Child care and employee assistance programs will be discussed later in this chapter.

The provision of employer-paid benefits represents a tremendous cost to most organizations. Research has shown it to be an effective tool for retention, but few empirical studies exist to show the effects of benefits on productivity. Despite this, organizations have responded to unions, competition, and industry trends by expending tremendous sums of money on benefits (Glueck, 1978). Benefits programs must be better planned and coordinated. Important decisions regarding benefits unfortunately are often made autocratically by top-level managers without thorough examination of what goals will be met by the benefit increase for either the worker or the organization. Input from middle- and first-level managers should be used to provide insight into the potential value of the benefit to increased productivity or retention at the unit level.

In addition, the employee work pool should be examined and an assessment made regarding which benefits are valued the most in a particular organization. For example, at present, more educated, older, higher status employees generally prefer greater benefits to pay increases, as fringe benefits provide a form of tax-free income; in contrast, the majority of employees still prefer pay raises (Glueck, 1978). In addition, medical insurance in corporate America is a preferred benefit and shorter work hours are not, and stock plans are preferred and early retirement is not (Glueck, 1978). The wise organization will seek to eliminate benefits that are not valued highly by employees or to provide less costly substitutes.

In addition to better planning and communication in the management hierarchy, there must be better communication about the benefits package to employees. Research studies have shown that most employees have limited understanding of the details of their benefits and the cost to the organization in providing and administering such benefits (Glueck, 1978). Tool 20-1 identifies some of the more common fringe benefits available to employees as well as questions that should be asked in assessing the quality of the benefit package.

All individuals affected by personnel planning should be encouraged to be involved in the planning process. When employees share in benefits planning, they show greater interest in, and appreciation for, the benefits that are provided by the organization.

For benefits to have a positive effect on employee satisfaction, Glueck (1978) states that the employees must know about their

Tool 20-1   Assessing the Benefits Package

1. *Worker's compensation* – provides compensation for injuries, disabilities, or death occurring as a result of the employment situation. Generally, workmen's compensation is designed to take care of short-term disabilities.

   Assessment questions: Are medical expenses paid as well as lost salary or wages? Are wages reimbursed in full or part for work time missed?

2. *Health insurance* – basic coverage generally provides for some or all of the costs for hospitalization (room and board and other hospital service charges), surgery, and medical care.

   Assessment questions: Is the cost of the health insurance covered fully or partially by the organization? Is there an additional charge for family members? Is this a major medical policy? What copayment is required by the policy owner? Is the organization self-insured? Does the employee have a choice of health care providers? Are prescription drugs covered under the plan? Are there special provisions for mental health or maternity care? If multiple health plans are offered, are there limited enrollment periods for employees who elect to change to a different plan? If you leave your job, can your insurance plan be converted to an individual plan?

3. *Group life insurance* – one of the oldest and most widely available employee benefits. Coverage is provided to all employees without physical examinations, with premiums based upon the characteristics of the group as a whole.

   Assessment questions: What is the face value of the policy? Is the policy whole life or term insurance? Does the face value of the policy increase as salary increases? Are there limitations to coverage on the policy? Is there a copayment required by the employee? Does life insurance coverage continue after retirement from the organization?

4. *Dental and vision insurance* – these insurance coverages may expand upon the health insurance policy provided by the employer or may be separate and distinct forms of insurance coverage.

   Assessment questions: Is the cost of the dental insurance covered fully or partially by the organization? Is there an additional charge for family members? What copayment is required by the policy owner?

5. *Retirement plan* – this benefit, which is typically based on years of service and salary at time of retirement, provides an ongoing source of income to the employee after retirement.

   Assessment questions: Is there a fixed retirement age? How long must employees work before they become vested or able to collect benefits? Does the contribution of the employer match or exceed that of the employee? Can retirement funds be withdrawn early, and if so, what is the penalty for doing so? Are there tax advantages to the retirement plan sponsored by the organization? Does the retirement plan include an inflation factor?

6. *Disability insurance* — this coverage provides for disabled employees who have a long-term or permanent disability that is not covered by worker's compensation.

   Assessment questions: Is the cost of this policy covered fully or partially by the organization? How long must the employee be disabled before benefits can be collected? What percentage of salary compensation is provided in the policy? Is coverage tied to salary level? Is pregnancy considered a disability?

7. *Professional liability insurance premium* — this coverage for professional liability or malpractice typically covers work that would be performed according to established standards of care within the organization.

   Assessment questions: What are the limits of coverage? Are the limitations of coverage adequate for the types of damages awarded for nurses functioning in a specialty area? Does the organization provide an individual policy for employees or are they covered under the organizational umbrella? Is there any personal liability coverage associated with the policy?

8. *Parking and transportation fees* — this benefit may include financial remuneration for parking and transportation or refer to methods of access provided by the organization.

   Assessment questions: Is a company car provided? How many miles will I be required to travel each year? Can the business car be used for personal reasons? If I use my personal car, will I be reimbursed and at what rate? Is there adequate access to parking? Are parking facilities adequate and safe?

---

benefits, prefer the organization's benefits to those offered by other organizations, and perceive the organization's benefits as satisfying more of their needs than competing organizations' benefits. Glueck goes on to say that, for benefits to affect employee performance, employees must see them as a strongly preferred end and perceive that by performing better, they can increase their benefits.

CHILD CARE IN THE WORK PLACE

Employee needs in American businesses today have changed as a result of the influx of women into the work place. Although nursing has always been primarily a female profession, women for the first time hold the majority of professional jobs in the United States today (Moskowitz and Townsend, 1986). Women now make up 52% of the college population and 25% to 52% of the enrollment in schools of architecture, medicine, economics, law, accounting, and pharmacy. Likewise, the number of working mothers has doubled since 1970, and over half of women with children under 1 year of age now have jobs outside the home (Moskowitz and Townsend, 1986).

Proactive organizations recognize that the working woman and mother is a major part of the work force and that they must recognize the unique needs of this group of employees if they desire increased retention and productivity. Working mothers list "inadequate child care" as the most important problem they face (Ornati and Buckham, 1983). Nurses have additional difficulties in finding child care because of work hours that differ from the norm, including evenings, nights, and weekends.

The provision of child care in the work place continues to gain popularity and results in increased recruitment, retention, and productivity for the organization. Milkovich and Gomez (1976) studied one of the largest day care centers in the United States and found that employees who used the day care center had much lower rates of absenteeism and turnover. A 1983 research study showed that employees who used employer-sponsored child care worked harder, had less absenteeism, and were more productive because they wanted to keep their jobs. Child care was also cited as the most effective recruitment tool, resulted in significant improvement in retention, and was a positive public relations tool (Burud et al., 1983).

Moskowitz and Townsend (1986) studied companies across the United States and identified the 30 best companies for working mothers. All of these companies stress the motivational factors identified by Herzberg as well as superior benefits, and most of these companies have made inroads into the provision of child care for their employees. In 1970, only 6% of employers surveyed by the Bureau of National Affairs provided child care centers for the children of employees (Bureau of National Affairs, 1974). Clearly, this is not adequate to meet the need. As of March 1988, fewer than 200 U.S. hospitals provided on-site child care centers (Piller 1988). Information about these facilities and the resultant increases in productivity and retention associated with work-site child care can be obtained from:

> Coalition for Employer Supported Child Care
> Creative Partnerships
> Child Care Information Service
> Pasadena, CA 91103
> (213) 796-4341

JOB SECURITY

Job security is a fundamental human need that for many people is more important than either salary or advancement. Organizations that are committed to job security "make every effort to provide continuous employment or income for at least some segment of its workforce, and put into place at least some activities or programs to support this commitment" (Luxenberg, 1983). Many of the forces driving employees toward unionism, serious conflicts in superior-subordinate relationships, and fear of change are linked to humankind's grasp for security (Strauss and Sayles, 1972). Unions provide a guarantee to employees, through an established grievance process, that they will not be disciplined or terminated unjustly and without due process. All nonunion organizations should also provide a grievance procedure to increase worker security so that employees need not fear being terminated unjustly as a result of arbitrary managerial action.

POSITIVE WORKING CONDITIONS

Positive working conditions are a hygiene factor that may be reflected superficially in the esthetics of the work environment. What is the organization's age and location? Are the nursing units attractive, bright, and spacious? Are there adequate climate controls? Do the noise levels provide an environment that is soothing and conducive to high productivity? Is lighting adequate? Are employees attired neatly? Do middle-level nursing managers have their own offices? Is there adequate ancillary or secretarial help? Although positive working conditions do not motivate workers, they do increase retention of candidates, and their absence can lead to dissatisfaction.

Another factor that contributes to the esthetics of the organizational environment is the use of uniforms or some required standard of professional dress. Although the argument is frequently heard that "uniforms do not a nurse make," they do contribute to a professional-appearing environment. When the organization agrees to financially support the use of uniforms in the work place, they impart a message to employees that the desired image of the organization and its employees is one of professionalism.

Another working condition that is very important to some employees is time off. Many organizations now have incentive programs that offer additional paid time off as a type of reward system. For the individual who has a family or who has adequate fiscal resources, time off may be a powerful tool for retention. Organizations that recognize and see that all individuals have time away from their work to rest, regroup, and set new goals have more productive employees. Traditionally, the United States has had one of the lowest hours of time off per hours worked ratio of any industrialized country in the world. Because the American culture is very achievement oriented, frequently the value of time away from work as a means of increasing or maintaining high productivity is overlooked.

SOCIAL AND RECREATIONAL PROGRAMS

Another positive working condition that has gained popularity in recent years is the provision of social and recreational programs for employees. Social programs may include functions such as teas, dinners, and receptions to honor employee accomplishments and longevity of employment. Other social events may include annual Christmas parties and summer barbecues or picnics. These social programs allow the workers and their families to form social relationships both inside and outside the organizational environment.

In addition to social needs, the humanistic management view recognizes that humans have recreational needs. More than

50,000 American businesses had developed some form of recreation program for their employees by the early 1970s (Famularo, 1986). These programs are frequently used to link employee affiliation and achievement needs, thus generating a feeling of belonging, improving morale, and increasing employer loyalty. These programs also may keep employees physically fit, and strengthen employees' perceived obligation to their employers ("Operation Outdoors," 1974). Employees find it easier to identify with a company that cares about their off-the-job human needs and to form meaningful relationships with fellow employees who work together cooperatively both within and outside the organization.

In many institutions, the recreation program is formalized into a fitness program either on or off site. Although traditionally reserved for management only in corporate America, fitness programs are now common for all employees, as they have been in Japan for many years. The primary reason is simple economics — an unhealthy worker costs more to keep on the job. Sedentary employees have 30% more hospital days than those who get adequate exercise. Fit, happy employees produce more, are less likely to be absent, and are less likely to be injured (Bergstrom, 1988).

In implementing a recreational or social program, the organization must follow several principles (Famularo, 1986). First, the program should provide the greatest opportunity for the greatest amount of participation by the greatest number of employees. Second, the recreation must be more than "play"; it must include a wide variety of activities to accommodate the wide variety of interests in a group of individuals. Third, the program must be flexible so that it can grow and change as new needs and activities arise. The organization should also be cognizant that recreational and social programs are most successful when the interested employees play an active part in organizing and administering the activities (Beach, 1980).

The inclusion of recreational and social programs as a means of increasing the quality of the work environment is gaining recognition, although studies of the preferences of employees indicated that recreational services are the least preferred of all benefits and services offered by organizations (Glueck, 1978). Managers must carefully evaluate their worker needs and values in evaluating the potential costs and benefits of such a program in their organizations.

EMPLOYEE ASSISTANCE PROGRAMS

As a result of worker shortages and an increased movement toward humanistic management, organizations have begun examining ways to help rather than terminate discouraged or impaired employees. Employee assistance programs are in-house programs that provide both inside and outside counseling for employee problems.

Although a primary purpose of employee assistance programs has traditionally been to help employees with addiction problems (drug and alcohol), the types of employee problems and needs dealt with are varied. Table 20-3 identifies the areas of personal and work assistance requested in 1974 of Employee Advisory Resource, a Control Data employee assistance program (Reed, 1983). The employee assistance program can also be invaluable in helping employees who have family members or significant others who are impaired in some way.

Employee assistance programs have traditionally been focused on helping employees deal with problems in their personal lives that could be affecting their work lives. Currently, there is an increasing trend to utilize these programs to proactively assist employees in their growth and development. Programs are offered on health and fitness, parenting, stress management, aging, and so on. This new focus is proactive rather than reactive and should prevent some employee problems from ever occurring.

The quality of the work life in the organization is affected by many factors. Managers must assess motivational and hygiene factors that are present or should be present at the unit and organizational level. Each factor should be examined in terms of its direct and indirect implementation costs for the organization. The organization should attempt to emphasize those factors that result in the greatest increase in productivity and satisfaction for both the organization and its employees. Any factors that result in a dissatisfying work environment should be eliminated or modified in such a way that the changed work environment results in both increased productivity and retention.

KEY CONCEPTS CHAPTER 20

1. Although salary is not a true motivator, it is an important factor in obtaining and recruiting workers, and can be a major cause of dissatisfaction for the worker.

Table 20-3. Problems Reported to an Employee Assistance Program

Personal Problems	*Percentage of Calls*
1. Financial (bankruptcy, poor financial management, inflation)	26%
2. Legal (family conflict and tenant-landlord conflict)	21%
3. Chemical (10% alcohol, 3% drugs)	13%
4. Mental health (primarily depression)	9%
5. Familial (parent-child and parent-relative conflict)	8%
6. Marital difficulties	8%
7. Personal (identity, self-esteem, relationships, and sex)	5%
8. Physical health	5%
9. Miscellaneous	6%

Work Problems	*Percentage of Calls*
1. Compensation and benefits	22%
2. Performance appraisals and disciplinary actions	19%
3. Transfers and promotions	7%
4. Requests for familiarization of specific policies and procedures	14%
5. Interpersonal relations with coworkers and management	10%
6. Career counseling	8%
7. Miscellaneous (includes complaints about working conditions, discrimination, and others)	20%

2. Generally, salaries or wages should reflect performance and not time of service.

3. Current practice is to aim for 7 to 10 pay steps covering all nursing personnel and to have salary range maximums generally about 20% above the average salary being paid for that job in the organization.

4. Fringe benefits—compensation other than wages or salaries—today constitute about one third of the compensation of the typical U.S. employee, and this figure is expected to continue to increase.

5. At present, there is little evidence that fringe benefits motivate performance or increase productivity. Benefits do, however, have a significant impact on worker retention.

6. Proactive organizations recognize that working women and mothers are a major part of the work force and that their

need for adequate child care must be met if the goal of increased retention and productivity is to be met.

7. The inclusion of recreational and social programs as a means of linking employee achievement and affiliation needs is gaining recognition, although studies of the preferences of employees indicated that recreational services are the least preferred of all benefits and services offered by organizations.

8. As a result of worker shortages and an increased movement toward humanistic management, organizations have begun developing employee assistance programs as a means of helping discouraged or impaired employees, rather than terminating them.

REFERENCES

Armstrong, M., and Lorentzen, J.F., *Handbook of Personnel Management Practice*, Prentice-Hall, Englewood Cliffs, NJ, 1982.

Beach, D.S., *Personnel: The Management of People at Work*, Fourth Edition, Macmillan, New York, 1980.

Bergstrom, W.S., "Fitness Programs Move to Plant Floors," *Sacramento Bee*, June 12, 1988, p. E2.

Bureau of National Affairs, *Employee Health and Welfare Benefits*, Personnel Policies Forum Survey 107, Washington, DC, 1974.

Burud, S.L., et al., *Child Care: The New Business Tool*, National Employment Supported Child Care Project, Pasadena, CA, 1983.

Famularo, J.J. (ed.), *Handbook of Human Resources Administration*, Second Edition, McGraw-Hill, New York, 1986.

Foegen, J.H., "The Fringe Benefit Spiral," *Human Resource Management*, 13(3):23–26, 1974.

Glueck, W.F., *Personnel: A Diagnostic Approach*, Revised Edition, Business Publications, Dallas, TX, 1978.

Laliberty, R., and Christopher, W.I., *Enhancing Productivity in Health Care Facilities*, National Health Publishing, Owing Mills, MD, 1984.

Luxenberg, S., "Lifetime Employment, U.S. Style," *New York Times*, April 17, 1983, p. 12F.

Milkovich, G.T., and Glueck, W.F., *Personnel, Human Resource Management: A Diagnostic Approach*, Business Publications, Plano, TX, 1985.

Milkovich, G., and Gomez, L., "Day Care and Selected Employee Work Behaviors," *Academy of Management Journal*, 19(1): 111–115, 1976.

Moskowitz, M., and Townsend, C., "The 30 Best Companies for Working Mothers," *Working Mother*, 9(8):25–28, 1986.

"Operations Outdoors," *Time*, December, 16, 1974.

Ornati, O., and Buckham, C., "Day Care: Still Waiting Its Turn as a Standard Benefit," *Management Review*, 72:57–62, 1983.

Paul, R., *Employee Benefits Factbook*, Martin Segal Company, New York, 1976.

Piller, B., "Proposing a Child Care Center for Your Hospital," *Nursing Management*, 19(3):114–115, 1988.

Reed, D.J., "One Approach to Employee Assistance," *Personnel Journal*, 62:648–652, 1983.

Schuster, F.E., *Human Resource Management: Concepts, Cases and Readings*, Reston Publishing, Reston, VA, 1985.

Strauss, G., and Sayles, L.R., *Personnel: The Human Problems of Management*, Third Edition, Prentice-Hall, Englewood Cliffs, NJ, 1972.

Sullivan, E.J., and Decker, P.J., *Effective Management in Nursing*, Second Edition, Addison-Wesley, Menlo Park, CA, 1988.

Young, R. "88 Nursing Profession Salary Outlook," *Nursing Life* 7(6):10, 1987.

ADDITIONAL READINGS

Bright, W.E., "How One Company Manages Its Human Resources," *Harvard Business Review*, 54:81–93, 1976.

Kamerman, S.B., "Child Care Services: A National Picture," *Monthly Labor Review*, 106:35–39, 1983.

Klatt, L.A., Murdick, R.G., and Schuster, F.E., *Human Resources Management: A Behavioral Systems Approach*, Richard D. Irwin, Homewood, IL, 1978.

Nauright, L.P., "Toward a Comprehensive Personnel System: The Reward System – Part V," *Nursing Management*, 18(9):58–64, 1987.

Potter, D.O. (ed.), "Salary and Benefits – Options You Can Bargain For," Entry 61 in *Practices*. Nursing 85 Books, Nursing Reference Library, Springhouse Corporation, 1985, p. 392–398.

· UNIT EIGHT
Management of Personnel Problems

IF AN organization is to reach maximum efficiency and productivity, there must be a highly coordinated effort by all the individuals who work in that organization. Even small numbers of employees not performing at the expected level can affect unit and organizational functioning. An analogy to this might be a rowing team. If even one member of the rowing team is asynchronous, the scull is unable to achieve maximum velocity or accuracy in direction.

The role of managers is that of helmsman or coordinator. Their initial role is to identify employees who are having difficulty achieving organizational goals or working at expected levels of achievement. Their subsequent responsibilities are ascertaining that these employees understand the expectations of the organization, implementing a disciplinary program examining why an employee is not achieving at satisfactory levels, intervening appropriately and evaluating the effects of remediation.

Frequent causes of performance problems are lack of self-direction, resistance to authority, and lack of motivation on the part of the employee and poorly written and communicated rules on the part of the organization. The manager should help the employee develop a remediation plan that addresses these factors. If the employee is not meeting acceptable performance standards because of chemical or psychological impairment, the manager must assume a different role. The manager's responsibility then is no longer to administer discipline, but to confront the employee and refer the individual for needed professional help. The managerial role in counseling should not be confused with that of a therapeutic counselor (i.e., the management role is not that of a counselor). Although the manager should consider the causes of the employee's performance problems in selecting the most appropriate remediation plan, the manager's primary responsibility is to ensure that the employee performs at acceptable standards.

The main purpose of the plan for remediation should be employee growth. With counseling and guidance, most employees are capable of achieving at an acceptable level. When this does not occur despite a progressive disciplinary plan, it may be necessary for the employee to be terminated. Although managers have a commitment to help employees achieve, they also have a commitment to the organization to remove employees whose repeated inability to follow rules or meet expected standards negatively affect organizational functioning.

Constructive discipline can be a growth-producing experience for the employee. When, however, the employee perceives that discipline has been administered arbitrarily or that rules have been applied unjustly, it becomes destructive and results in high levels of conflict. Unresolved employee conflict may be just as deleterious to organizational functioning and productivity as the original disciplinary problem was, perhaps even more so. Because of this, most organizations have in place a grievance procedure that allows employees to resolve these conflicts through an impartial review. This process, which should be available to employees in both union and nonunion organizations, increases the likelihood of constructive conflict resolution.

21

Discipline as a Means of Producing Growth

UNIT 7 in this book focused on the organizational environment necessary for employee satisfaction and high productivity. Employee satisfaction and organizational productivity are greatest when employees are successful in meeting organizational goals. The coordination and cooperation necessary to meet organizational goals require that managers control the individual urges of subordinates that are counterproductive to these goals. The manager does this by enforcing established rules, policies, and procedures. Subordinates do this by self-control.

When employees are unsuccessful in meeting organizational goals, the manager must attempt to identify reasons for this failure and counsel the employees accordingly. If employees fail because they are unable to follow rules or established policies and procedures, or if they are unable to perform their duties adequately despite assistance and encouragement, the manager has an obligation to discipline them. However, there are some problem employees, such as impaired employees, who should be handled differently. These employees require special assistance and counseling, not progressive discipline. Guidance of impaired employees will be discussed in Chapter 23.

Chapter 21 will focus on discipline as a necessary and positive tool in promoting subordinate growth. The normal progression of steps taken in disciplinary action will be delineated. Suggested components of disciplinary and termination conferences will be reviewed, and strategies for the manager to use in administering discipline fairly and effectively will be discussed. Tools for implementation include a guide for progressive discipline and a formal reprimand documentation form.

CONSTRUCTIVE VERSUS DESTRUCTIVE DISCIPLINE

Traditionally, management has viewed discipline as a necessary means for controlling an "unmotivated and self-centered work force." Because of this traditional philosophy about humans and the organization, managers utilized threats and fear as the primary means of controlling behavior. Written warnings and threats of termination were rampant, and employees were always alert to impending penalty or termination. This "big stick" approach to management focused on eliminating all behavior that could be considered in conflict with organizational goals, without regard for employee growth. Although this approach is successful on a short-term basis, it is demotivating and reduces productivity in the long term. This occurs because individuals will achieve only at the level they feel is necessary to avoid punishment. This approach is also destructive and demoralizing, as discipline is often arbitrarily administered and is unfair either in the application of rules or in the resulting punishment (Marquis and Huston, 1987). "In examining the history of crime, punishment has never been shown to be an effective deterrent. The individual who breaks rules does not plan that far head. They are not thinking of the consequences of their actions, only their immediate needs" (Beach, 1980).

Constructive discipline is a means of helping employees grow, not a punitive measure. Webster includes punishment in the definition of *discipline* but also defines the word as meaning "to instruct, educate, train, regulate or govern" (Webster, 1979). In fact, the origin of the word *discipline* comes from the Latin *disciplina*, which means teaching or learning (Lewis and Spicer, 1987). In constructive discipline, punishment may be applied for improper behavior, but this is carried out in a supportive, corrective manner. Employees are reassured that the punishment given is because of their actions and not because of who they are as people.

The primary emphasis in constructive discipline is assisting employees to behave in a manner that allows them to be self-directive in meeting organizational goals. Before employees can focus their energies on meeting organizational goals, they must feel a sense of security in the work place. This security can develop only when employees know and understand organizational rules and penalties, and when rules are applied in a fair and consistent manner. In an environment that promotes constructive discipline, employees generally are self-disciplined to conform with established rules and regulations, and the primary role of the manager becomes that of coordinator and helper rather than enforcer.

SELF-DISCIPLINE

Ideally, all employees have adequate self-control and are self-directed in their pursuit of organizational goals. Unfortunately, this is not always the case. There are, however, four basic factors managers can influence in creating an environment that promotes the development of self-discipline in their employees (Health Care Education Associates, 1987). The first of these factors is employee awareness and understanding of the rules and regulations that govern behavior. Rules and regulations must be clearly written and communicated to subordinates. Managers must discuss these rules and policies with subordinates, explain the rationale for their existence, and encourage questions. It is impossible for employees to have self-control if they do not understand what are acceptable boundaries for their behavior. Likewise, individuals can not be self-directed if they do not understand what is expected of them.

The second factor is an atmosphere of mutual trust. Managers must believe that employees are capable of, and actively seeking, self-discipline. Likewise, employees must perceive their managers as honest and trustworthy. Employees lack the security to discipline themselves if they do not trust their managers' motives.

The third factor is the judicious use of formal authority. If formal discipline is quickly and widely used, subordinates do not have the opportunity to discipline themselves.

The last important factor in self-discipline is employee identification with the goals of the organization. When employees accept the goals and objectives of an organization, they are more likely to accept the standards of conduct deemed acceptable by that organization.

FAIR AND EFFECTIVE RULES

There are several rules that should be followed if employees are to perceive the manager's purpose for discipline as growth producing and not punitive. This does not imply that subordinates enjoy being disciplined or that discipline should be a regular means of promoting employee growth. However, correctly implemented discipline should not result in permanent alienation and demoralization of a subordinate.

McGregor (1967) developed a set of rules for enforcing discipline so as to make discipline as fair and growth producing as possible. These rules were called "hot stove rules" because they can be applied to someone touching a hot stove. The following rules explain this theory:

1. All individuals must be *forewarned* that if they touch the hot stove (i.e., break a rule), they will be burned (punished or disciplined). They must know the rule beforehand and be aware of the punishment.

2. If the individual touches the stove (i.e., breaks a rule), there will be *immediate* consequences (getting burned). All discipline should be administered immediately after rules are broken.

3. If the individual touches the stove again, he or she will again be burned. Therefore, there is *consistency*. Each time the rule is broken, there are immediate and consistent consequences.

4. If any other individual touches the hot stove, he or she will also get burned. Discipline must be *impartial*; everyone breaking the rule must be treated in the same manner.

Unfortunately, most rule breaking is not enforced according to McGregor's rules. For example, many individuals exceed the speed limit when driving. Generally, individuals are aware of speed limit regulations, and signs are posted along roads to remind individuals of the rules. Thus, there is forewarning. There is not, however, immediacy, consistency, or impartiality. Many individuals exceed the speed limit for long periods of time before they are stopped and disciplined, or they may never be disciplined at all. Likewise, an individual may be stopped and disciplined one day and not the next. Lastly, the punishment is inconsistent in that some individuals are punished for their rule breaking and others are not. Even the penalty different individuals pay may not be the same.

Continuing with this example, imagine that some day an automobile will be developed that requires the driver to place a built-in electronic sensor on the end of a finger before the automobile will operate. The purpose of this sensor would be to deliver a low-charge, but painful electric shock to the driver every time the car exceeds the posted speed limit. The driver would be forewarned regarding the consequences of breaking the speed limit rule. If the driver immediately received an electric shock each time the rule was broken, and if all automobiles included this feature, speeding would be virtually eliminated.

If a rule or regulation is worth having, it should be enforced (Marquis and Huston, 1987). When rule breaking is allowed to go unpunished, groups generally adjust to and replicate the low-level performance of the rule breaker (Strauss and Sayles, 1972). Likewise, the average worker's natural inclination to obey rules can be dissipated by lax or inept enforcement policies, and employees develop contempt for managers who allow rules to be disregarded (Beyers and Phillips, 1979). The enforcement of rules using McGregor's guide for rule fairness keeps morale from breaking down and allows structure within the organization.

There should, however, be as few rules and regulations as possible in the organization, and all rules, regulations, and policies should be reviewed on a regular basis to see if they should be deleted or modified in some way. If managers find themselves spending all their time enforcing one particular rule, it would be wise to re-examine the rule and to consider whether there is something wrong with the rule or how it is communicated (Marquis and Huston, 1987).

DISCIPLINE AS A PROGRESSIVE PROCESS

Occasionally, employees continue to behave undesirably, either breaking rules or not performing their job duties adequately. Further action should be taken in these situations. Managers have the authority and the responsibility to use progressively stronger forms of discipline when employees continue to fail to meet expected standards of achievement. Most progressive discipline systems utilize the following steps:

1. Generally, the first step of the disciplinary process is the *informal reprimand* or *verbal admonishment*. This reprimand includes an informal meeting between the employee and the manager to discuss the broken rule, policy, or performance deficiency. Suggestions are given to the employee on how behavior might be altered to keep the rule from being broken again. Often an informal reprimand is all that is needed for behavior modification.

2. The second step is a *formal reprimand* or *written admonishment*. If rule-breaking behavior recurs after a verbal admonishment, the manager again meets with the employee and issues a written warning about the behaviors that must be corrected. This written warning is very specific about what rules or policies have been violated as well as what the consequences will be if behavior is not altered to meet the expectations of the organization. The written admonishment should also include any reference to prior informal reprimands, an employee explanation of the incident(s) in question, a plan of action to achieve expected change or improvement, and an employee opinion of that plan (Health Care Education Associates, 1987). Tool 21-1 is a form that could be used for a written reprimand. Both the employee and the manager should sign the written warning. One copy of the written admonishment is then given to the employee, and another copy is retained in the employee's personnel file.

3. The third step in progressive discipline is usually a *suspension from work without pay*. If the employee continues the undesired behavior despite verbal and written warnings, the manager should remove the employee from the job for a brief period of time, generally a few days to several weeks.

4. The last step in progressive discipline is *involuntary termination* or *dismissal*. Termination should always be the last resort in dealing with poor performance. However, if the

Tool 21-1   Sample Written Admonishment Form

Employee name_____
Position _____ Date of hire_____
Person completing report_____
Position _____ Date report competed_____

Date of incident(s) _____ Time_____

Description of incident:

_____
_____
_____
_____
_____
_____

Prior attempt to counsel employee regarding this behavior (cite date and results of disciplinary conferences):

_____
_____
_____
_____
_____
_____

Disciplinary contract (plan for correction) and timelines:

_____
_____
_____
_____
_____
_____

Consequences of future repetition:

_____
_____
_____
_____

Employee comments (additional documentation or rebuttal may be attached):

_____

_____

_____

_____

_____

_____   _____

Signature of Individual   Employee Signature
Making the Report

_____   _____

   Date   Date

Date and time of follow-up appointment to review disciplinary contract:

_____

_____

manager has given repeated warnings, and the employee continues to break rules or violate policy, the employee should be terminated. Although this is difficult and traumatic for the employee, the manager, and the unit, the cost in terms of managerial and employee time and unit morale for keeping such an employee in the organization is enormous.

It is important to remember that the disciplinary steps are followed progressively only for repeated infractions of the same rule. For example, even though an employee has received a prior formal reprimand for an unexcused absence, discipline for a first-time offense of tardiness should begin at the first step of the process. It is also important to remember that although discipline is generally administered progressively, some rule breaking is so serious that the employee may be suspended or dismissed with the first infraction. Tool 21-2 presents a guide for managers of progressive discipline for specific offenses.

In progressive discipline it is also important, in all but the most serious infractions, that the "slate" be wiped clean after a

Tool 21-2   Guide to Progressive Discipline

Offense	First Infraction	Second Infraction	Third Infraction	Fourth Infraction
Gross mistreatment of a patient	Dismissal			
Discourtesy to a patient	Verbal admonishment	Written admonishment	Suspension	Dismissal
Insubordination	Written admonishment	Suspension	Dismissal	
Intoxication while on duty (this offense is difficult to prove)	Verbal admonishment	Written admonishment	Dismissal	
Use of intoxicants while on duty	Dismissal			
Neglect of duty	Verbal admonishment	Written admonishment	Suspension	Dismissal
Theft or willful damage of property	Written admonishment or dismissal	Dismissal		
Falsehood	Verbal admonishment	Written admonishment	Dismissal	
Unauthorized absence	Verbal admonishment	Written admonishment	Dismissal	
Abuse of leave	Verbal admonishment	Written admonishment	Suspension	Dismissal
Deliberate violation of instruction	Verbal admonishment	Written admonishment	Suspension	Dismissal
Violation of safety rules	Verbal admonishment	Written admonishment	Dismissal	
Fighting	Verbal admonishment	Written admonishment	Suspension	Dismissal
Inability to maintain work standards	Verbal admonishment	Written admonishment	Suspension	Dismissal
Excessive unexcused tardiness*	Verbal admonishment	Written admonishment	Dismissal	

*The first, second, and third infractions do not mean the first, second, and third time an employee is late, but the first, second, and third time that unexcused tardiness becomes excessive as determined by the manager.

From Marquis, B., and Huston, C. J., *Management Decision Making for Nurses: 101 Case Studies*, p. 339. J. B. Lippincott, Philadelphia, 1987.

predesignated period, generally 1 to 2 years (Beach, 1980). There is little justification for holding infractions against employees in perpetuity if the employees have since modified their behavior.

DISCIPLINARY STRATEGIES FOR THE NURSE MANAGER

It is vital that nurse managers recognize the power they hold in evaluating and correcting employees' behavior. Because individuals' jobs are very important to them (often a part of their self-esteem as well as livelihood), taking away an individual's job is a very serious action that should not be undertaken lightly (Marquis and Huston, 1987). There are several strategies managers can implement to assure that discipline is fair and growth producing.

The first thing the manager must do is thoroughly investigate the situation that has prompted the employee discipline. Has this employee been involved in a situation like this before? Was he or she disciplined for it? What was his or her reaction to the corrective action? How serious or potentially serious is the current problem or infraction? Who else was involved in the situation? Does this employee have a history of other types of disciplinary problems? What is the quality of this employee's performance in the work setting? Have other employees in the organization also experienced the problem? How were they disciplined? Could there be a problem with the rule or policy? Were there any special circumstances that could have contributed to the problem in this situation? What disciplinary action is suggested by the organizational manual for this type of offense? Will this type of disciplinary action keep the infraction from recurring? The wise manager will ask himself or herself all of these questions so that a wise and fair decision can be reached about an appropriate course of action.

Another thing wise managers will do is always consult with either their superiors or the personnel department before dismissing employees. Most organizations have very clear policies about which actions constitute grounds for dismissal as well as how dismissals should be handled. In an effort to protect themselves from charges of willful or discriminatory termination, nurse managers should carefully document the behavior(s) that occurred, as well as any attempts to counsel the employee. They must also be careful not to discuss with other employees the reasons for terminating one employee or to make negative comments regarding past employees that might discourage other employees or reduce their trust in their superiors (Health Care Education Associates, 1987).

THE DISCIPLINARY CONFERENCE

After having thoroughly investigated employee offenses, managers must confront employees with their findings. This occurs in the form of a disciplinary conference. Health Care Education Associates (1987) have identified the following steps in the disciplinary conference:

1. *State the problem clearly and specifically, and refer to previous discussions of the rule violation.* It is important for the manager not to be hesitant or apologetic. Novice nurse managers often feel uncomfortable with the disciplinary process and may provide unclear or mixed messages to employees regarding the nature or seriousness of a disciplinary problem. Managers must assume the authority given to them by their role. A major responsibility in this role is evaluating employee performance and suggesting appropriate action for improved or acceptable performance. Disciplinary problems, if unrecognized or ignored, generally do not go away; they get worse.

2. *Get input from the employee regarding why there has been no improvement.* It is always important to give the employee an opportunity to explain any limiting or extraneous factors of which you may not be aware. Allowing employees to provide feedback in the disciplinary process assures them recognition as human beings and reassures them that the manager's ultimate goal is to be fair and promote employee growth.

3. *Explain the disciplinary action you are going to take and why you are going to take it.* Although the manager must be open to new information that might be gathered in Step 2, he or she should already have made some preliminary assessments regarding the disciplinary action that is appropriate for the offense. This discipline should be communicated to the employee. The employee who has been counseled at previous disciplinary conferences should not be surprised at the punishment to be given.

4. *Describe the behavioral change that is expected, and list the steps needed to achieve this change. Explain the consequences of failure to change.* Again, it is important here that the manager not be apologetic or hesitant. This will create confusion in the employee's mind about the manager's seriousness about carrying out the threat. Employees who have repeatedly broken rules lack self-control and need firm direction. It must be made very clear to the employee that follow-up in a timely manner will occur.

5. *Get agreement and acceptance of the plan. Let the employee know that you are interested in him or her as a person, and give your support.* Because discipline is being given to promote employee growth, rather than just to punish, the manager must be a humanist. Although the expected standards must be very clear, the manager should impart a sense of genuine concern for the employee and desire to help the employee grow. This approach helps the employee recognize that the discipline is directed at the offensive behavior and not at the individual. The manager must be careful, however, not to relinquish the management role in an effort to nurture and become a counselor for the employee. The manager's role is to provide a supportive environment and structure so that the employee can make the necessary changes.

In addition to understanding what should be covered in the disciplinary conference, managers must be sensitive to the environment in which discipline is given. All discipline, even informal admonishments, should be done in private. Although managers should administer feedback to employees about the rule breaking or inappropriate behavior as soon as possible after it has occurred, it is never acceptable to do this in front of patients or peers. If more than an informal admonishment is required, managers should inform employees of the unacceptable action and then schedule formal disciplinary conferences for further discussion and follow-up later.

All formal disciplinary conferences should be scheduled in advance at a time agreeable to both the employee and the manager, each of whom will want time to reflect on what has happened. Allowing a lag time should reduce the emotionalism of the situation. It also promotes employee self-discipline, since it gives the employee time to develop his or her own plan for keeping the behavior from recurring.

In addition to privacy and advance scheduling, the length of the disciplinary conference is important. It should not be so long that it degenerates into a debate, nor so short that the employee and manager cannot state their positions. The facts of the situation should be stated, and each party should provide input. If the employee seems overly emotional or if there are great discrepancies between the perception of the manager and that of the employee, an additional conference should be scheduled. Employees often need time to absorb what they have been told and to develop a plan that is not defensive.

THE TERMINATION CONFERENCE

Occasionally, the disciplinary conference must be a termination conference. Although many of the principles are the same, the termination conference differs from a disciplinary conference in that planning for future improvement is eliminated. The following steps should be followed in the termination conference (Health Care Education Associates, 1987):

1. *Calmly state the facts of the situation, and explain the reasons for termination.* It is important that the manager not appear angry or defensive. Although the manager may express regret that the outcome is termination, he or she must not dwell on this or give the employee reason to think that the decision is not final. The manager should be prepared to give examples of the behavior(s) in question.

2. *Explain the termination process.* State the date of termination, as well as the employee's and organization's role in the process.

3. *Ask for employee input and respond calmly and openly.* Listen to the employee, but do not allow yourself to be drawn emotionally into his or her anger or sorrow. Always stay focused on the facts of the case.

4. *End the meeting on a positive note.* It is important that the manager express confidence in the employee and offer wishes for success in the future. The manager should also inform the employee what, if any, references will be supplied to prospective employers in the future. Lastly, it is usually best to allow the employee who has been terminated to leave the organization immediately. If the employee continues to work on the unit after termination has been discussed, it can be demoralizing for all the employees who work on that unit (Health Care Education Associates, 1987).

DISCIPLINING THE UNIONIZED EMPLOYEE

It is hoped that all managers will be fair and consistent in disciplining employees regardless of whether a union is present. However, the presence of a union does usually entail more procedural, legalistic safeguards in the administration of discipline as well as a well-defined grievance process for employees who feel they have been disciplined unfairly. The grievance process will be discussed in detail in Chapter 22.

For example, managers of nonunionized employees have greater latitude in selecting what disciplinary measure is appropriate for a specific infraction. This gives managers greater flexibility and latitude but may result in inconsistency of discipline between employees. In contrast, unionized employees generally must be disciplined according to specific, pre-established steps and penalties within an established time frame (Yaney, 1986). For example, the union contract may be very clear that unexcused absence from work must be disciplined first by a written reprimand, then by a 3-day suspension from work, and then by termination. This type of discipline structure is generally fairer to the employee, but it allows the manager little flexibility in evaluating extenuating circumstances.

Another aspect of discipline that may differ between unionized and nonunionized employees is the need for management to follow "due process" in disciplining union employees. Due process means that management must provide union employees with a written statement outlining disciplinary charges, the resulting penalty, and reasons for the penalty. Employees then have the right to defend themselves against such charges and to settle any disagreement through formal grievance hearings (Beach, 1980).

Another difference between unionized and nonunionized employee discipline lies in the burden of proof. In disciplinary situations with union employees, the burden of proof for the wrongdoing and the need for subsequent discipline falls on management. This means that managers disciplining union employees must keep detailed records regarding misconduct and attempts to counsel employees. Among nonunionized employees, the burden of proof typically falls on the employee.

The contract language used by unions regarding discipline may be very specific, or it may be very general. Most contracts recognize the right of management to discipline, suspend, or dismiss employees for "just cause." *Just cause* means that the manager must be able to prove three things: (1) this employee did commit this offense or breach of rule, (2) the offense does, in fact, merit some corrective action or penalty, and (3) the proposed penalty is appropriate to the offense (Metzger and Pointer, 1972). Contracts also generally recognize the right of employees to submit grievances when they feel these actions have been taken unfairly or are somehow discriminatory. Managers must be responsible for knowing all union contract provisions regarding discipline that may affect how discipline is administered on their units.

Good managerial practice greatly reduces the need for discipline. Even with good management, however, some employees need external direction and discipline to accomplish organizational goals. Discipline allows the violating employee, as well as all the employees on the unit, to clearly understand the expectations of the organization as well as the penalty for failure to meet those expectations. When constructive discipline is fair and consistent, it provides the structure necessary for increased unit morale and productivity.

KEY CONCEPTS CHAPTER 21

1. Discipline is a necessary and positive tool in promoting subordinate growth.

2. In the history of crime, punishment alone has never been shown to be an effective deterrent.

3. The optimal goal in constructive discipline is assisting employees to behave in a manner that allows them to be self-directive in meeting organizational goals.

4. To assure fairness, rules should include the components of forewarning, immediacy, consistency, and impartiality.

5. If a rule or regulation is worth having, it should be enforced. When rule breaking is allowed to go unpunished, groups generally adjust to and replicate the low-level performance of the rule breaker, and the average worker's natural inclination to obey rules is dissipated.

6. There should, however, be as few rules and regulations as possible in the organization, and all rules, regulations, and policies should be reviewed on a regular basis to see if they should be deleted or modified in some way.

7. Except for the most serious infractions, discipline should be administered in progressive steps, starting with verbal admonishment and going to written admonishment, suspension, and finally termination.

8. The disciplinary conference provides the opportunity for the manager to clearly delineate to the employee what behavior(s) is unacceptable to the organization and for the two to work together in making a plan to alter that behavior.

9. The presence of a union generally entails more procedural, legalistic safeguards in the administration of discipline, as well as a well-defined grievance process for employees who feel they have been disciplined unfairly.

REFERENCES

Beach, D. S., *Personnel: The Management of People at Work*, Fourth Edition, Macmillan, New York, 1980.

Beyers, M., and Phillips, C., *Nursing Management for Patient Care*, Second Edition, Little, Brown and Company, Boston, 1979.

Health Care Education Associates, *Models of Excellence for Nurse Managers*, C. V. Mosby Company, St. Louis, 1987.

Lewis, E.M., and Spicer, J.G., *Human Resource Management Handbook: Contemporary Strategies for Nursing Managers*, Aspen Publications, Rockville, MD, 1987.

McGregor, D., *The Professional Manager*, McGraw-Hill, New York, 1967.

Marquis, B., and Huston, C.J., *Management Decision Making for Nurses: 101 Case Studies*, J. B. Lippincott, Philadelphia, 1987.

Metzger, N., and Pointer, D., *Labor Management Relations in the Health Service Industry*. The Science and Health Publications, New York, 1972.

Strauss, G., and Sayles, L.R., *Personnel: The Human Problems of Management*, Third Edition, Prentice-Hall, Englewood Cliffs, NJ, 1972.

Webster, D., *Webster's Unabridged Dictionary*, Second Edition, Simon and Schuster, New York, 1979.

Yaney, J.P., "Union and Nonunion Employees," in Famularo, J. J., *Handbook of Human Resources Administration*, Second Edition, McGraw-Hill, New York, 1986, p. 54.

ADDITIONAL READINGS

Beletz, E.E., "Discipline: Establishing Just Cause for Correction," *Nursing Management*, 17(8):63–67, 1986.

Donnelly, G., "The Insubordination Game: Graceful Strategies for Maintaining Control," *RN*, 43(4):56–69, 1980.

Glende, N.H., "Constructive Criticism: Building Blocks to Improved Performance," *Nursing Life*, 7(2):46–48, 1987.

Holle, M.L., "What to do When Your Staff Won't Follow Your Lead," *Nursing Life*, 6(6):48–50, 1986.

Jernigan, D., "Keeping the Gears Meshing: 5 Steps for Managing the Problem Employee," *Nursing Life* 6(2):50–54, 1986.

Lee, I.M., "Angry Nurse," *Nursing Life*, 5(4):26, 1985.

Mager, R., and Pipe, P., *Analyzing Performance Problems*, Fearon Publishers, Palo Alto, CA, 1970.

Marriner-Tomey, A., *Guide to Nursing Management*, Third Edition, C.V. Mosby, St. Louis, 1988.

Steinmetz, L., *Managing the Marginal and Unsatisfactory Performer*, Addison-Wesley, Reading, MA, 1969.

22

Grievances and Arbitration

CHAPTER 21 discussed discipline as a means of producing employee growth. This growth can occur only when employees perceive that the constructive feedback and discipline they have received is fair and just. When employees' perceptions of fair and just discipline differ from those of managers, most nonunion and virtually all unionized organizations have an established procedure that must be followed to resolve the discrepancy. This grievance procedure, as it is called, is a procedure to follow when one feels that a wrong has been committed (Marquis and Huston, 1987). The grievance procedure is not limited to resolving discipline discrepancies and can be used by employees any time they feel they have been treated unfairly by management. Yarbrough (1987) states that grievance procedures are appropriate when an employee perceives that management actions are (1) not in compliance with the union contract, (2) unfair and without just cause in the administration of discipline, and (3) in violation of past practice. Although most grievances are filed against management, management can also file grievances, also referred to as *disciplinary actions*, against employees (Potter, 1984).

Most grievances or conflicts between employees and management can be resolved informally through communication, negotiation, compromise, and collaboration. Generally, though, even this informal process has well-defined steps that should be followed in seeking resolution. If the employee and management are unable to resolve their differences informally, the formal grievance process begins. The steps to the formal grievance process are outlined clearly in all union contracts or administration policy and procedure manuals. If the differences can not be settled through a formal grievance process, the matter is finally resolved in a process known as *arbitration*.

Although grievance procedures require a great deal of time and energy of both the employee and the manager, they serve several valuable and needed purposes. Grievances can settle smaller problems earlier, thus preventing larger problems, such as strikes, from occurring later. They can also serve as a source of data to focus attention on ambiguous contract language for negotiation at a later date (Milkovich and Glueck, 1985). Perhaps, though, the most important outcome of a grievance is the legitimate opportunity it provides for employees to resolve conflicts with their superiors. Employees who are not given an outlet for resolving work conflicts can become demoralized, angry, and dissatisfied. This affects unit functioning and productivity. Even if the outcome of the grievance is not in the favor of the individual filing the grievance (grievant), he or she will have had the opportunity to present the case to an objective third party, and the chances of constructive conflict resolution will thereby have been greatly increased. In addition, managers tend to be fairer and more consistent when they know that employees have a method of redress for arbitrary managerial action.

This chapter will discuss the informal versus formal grievance process and the process of arbitration. The determination of what is grievable as well as the most common grievances in the work place will be presented. Differences between grievance procedures in organizations with and without unions will be discussed. In addition, the rights and responsibilities of both the employee and the employer in resolving grievances or conflicts will be presented. Tools for implementation will include American Nurses' Association (ANA) guidelines for labor contract grievance issues and a listing of 24 rules that increase the likelihood of a positive grievance outcome.

THE CLEARLY WRITTEN LABOR CONTRACT

The labor contract is a lengthy document that deals with employee rights relating to wages, hours, fringe benefits, promotions, layoffs, discipline and transfers (Strauss and Sayles, 1972). Many grievances or differences between managers and employees are directly attributable to poorly written, incomplete, or unclear labor contracts. As in all policies and procedures, if contracts are written unclearly, there is great room for varying interpretation and conflict. Because unions hold the belief that grievances are valid only if there has been a violation of the labor contract, organizations with unions generally have comprehensive, clearly written contracts outlining employee rights. It is impossible, however, to write a contract that is so complete and conclusive that it covers every possible situation or extenuating circumstance. In addition, because written contracts, as well as all written communication, do not allow for verbal clarification, conflict may occur due to differing interpretations by different individuals. Frequently the differing interpretations are between management and the union.

When there is a conflict in interpreting work conditions or discipline standards in the labor contract, it becomes necessary to utilize the grievance process, spelled out in the labor contract. This grievance process should be clear and explicit regarding the steps that should be taken in resolving the complaint. Tool 22-1 outlines the ANA guidelines for the grievance process in a labor contract. Although the contract language or process may seem lengthy or cumbersome, it is imperative that both the employee and the employer follow the procedure exactly as outlined. Failure to do so often results in either a dismissal of the grievance or an automatic victory for the opposite side.

THE INFORMAL GRIEVANCE PROCESS

To begin the grievance process, both parties must meet informally to attempt to resolve their differences. In an employee grievance against management, the employee generally must

---

Tool 22-1 American Nurses' Association Guidelines for the Individual Nurse Contract: The Grievance Procedure

---

Suggested contract language

It is the intention of the parties that an employee grievance that arises out of alleged violation, misinterpretation, or misapplication of this agreement shall be resolved in accordance with provisions set forth within.

Definition of a grievance: The term *grievance* as used in this agreement shall mean a complaint filed by the employee alleging a violation, misinterpretation, or misapplication, of a specific provision of this agreement occurring after its effective date. A grievance shall, whenever possible, be discussed and settled informally between the employee and his or her immediate supervisor. The employee may, if so desired, be assisted by a representative of his or her nurses' association.

Formal steps

1. If the matter is not satisfactorily settled on an informal basis, the employee may institute a formal grievance by setting forth in writing the nature of the complaint, the specific term or provision of the agreement allegedly violated, and the remedy sought.

   The grievance shall be presented to the appropriate employer representative in writing within 14 days after the occurrence of the alleged violation.

   After the presentation of the grievance, the employee and the Nurses' Association representative shall be offered the opportunity to meet with the appropriate employer representative in an attempt to settle the grievance. The decision of the employer representative shall be in writing and shall be transmitted to the employee within 14 days after receipt of the written grievance unless extended by mutual consent.

2. Arbitration: If the matter is not satisfactorily settled at Step 1 and the employee decides to proceed with arbitration, the employee shall serve written notice on the employer of the desire to arbitrate within 5 days of receipt of the written decision of the employer under Step 1.

   Selection of an arbitrator shall be by agreement, if possible or, if the parties cannot so agree within 5 days, from a list of arbitrators obtained by request from the Federal Mediation and Conciliation Service or American Arbitration Association, with the parties alternately striking names until only one name remains.

The award of the arbitrator shall be accepted as final and binding. There shall be no appeal from the arbitrator's decision by either party if such decision is within the scope of the arbitrator's authority as described by the following:

a. The arbitrator shall not have the power to add, subtract from, disregard, alter, or modify any of the terms of this agreement.

b. His or her power shall be limited to deciding whether the employer has violated any terms of this agreement. It is understood that any matter that is not specifically set forth in this agreement shall not be subject to arbitration.

c. In any case of discipline or discharge where the arbitrator finds that such discipline or discharge was improper, the arbitrator may set aside, reduce, or modify the action taken by the employer. If the penalty is set aside, reduced, or otherwise changed, the arbitrator may award back pay to compensate the employee wholly or partially for any wages or other benefits lost because of the penalty.

The fees and expenses of the arbitrator shall be shared equally by the employer and the employee.

These guidelines were produced in joint effort by the American Nurses' Association Economic and General Welfare Department and the Council of Nurse Practitioners in the Nursing of Children (Economic and General Welfare Department, American Nurses Association).

---

meet directly with the manager with whom there is a conflict and verbally identify the conflict that has occurred. If the manager and the employee cannot reach agreement on the issue(s) at hand, the employee has the right of appeal to the next higher level of management. This process may be repeated again and again until the employee has appealed to the highest management level in the organization. The employee and management are encouraged to have a representative or advocate present at all levels of the informal process.

For example, an employee who feels discriminated against in patient care assignments should initially present his or her concerns to the first-level manager who made out the patient care assignments. If the employee cannot resolve the conflict at this level the case should then be presented to the supervisor or appropriate middle-level manager. If the conflict cannot be re-solved again, the employee should continue up the organizational chart and meet with the chief nursing executive or the personnel department manager, as specified in the organization's policy or grievance contract. Although higher level managers should be more objective and detached in their outlook, it is impossible for them to be totally impartial. They are managers involved in a management-versus-employee conflict, and a well-established principle of democratic government says that the executive and judicial bodies within government should be separate (Beach, 1980). Thus, the employee must have another means of redress to an impartial third party; this occurs in the form of the formal grievance process.

THE FORMAL GRIEVANCE PROCESS

Although the key elements and number of steps in a formal grievance process may vary considerably among institutions, there are generally several common elements. These include reasonable time limits for filing the grievance and making a decision, procedures to appeal a grievance to a higher union-management level if the grievance is not resolved, assignment of priority to crucial grievances (such as worker suspensions or dismissals), and an opportunity for both sides to investigate the complaint (Potter, 1984).

After the employee has exhausted all means of informal resolution, the grievant begins the formal process by putting the complaint or grievance in writing. This written notification of grievance should include the name of the grievant, the alleged adversity, dates of occurrence and discovery by the grievant, and the specific remedy sought. This must occur within a pre-specified time period, generally within 2 to 4 weeks after the incident has occurred and after informal resolution has been unsuccessful. The individual against whom the grievance is filed (the respondent) must respond in writing to the grievant, outlining why the contested action was taken against the employee and that an informal means of resolution cannot be reached.

After this occurs, unionized organizations begin a series of formal union management meetings. The alleged wrongdoing is first reported by the employee to the shop steward or a union representative. This union management representative assists the individual in determining whether the offense is even grievable (a contract issue).

If the contract specifies that the alleged misconduct of management is grievable, the union representative actively assists the employee in seeking formal resolution. Meetings are scheduled among the grievant, the respondent, and the shop steward. The respondent will also have a representative present. More than 75% of grievances are settled at this first step (U.S. Department of Labor, 1984). If conflict resolution does not occur at this meeting, another meeting is scheduled, generally between a chief steward and a middle- or top-level manager. An additional 20% of grievances are resolved at this level (U.S. Department of Labor, 1984). If this meeting is again unsuccessful, regional or district union representatives meet with top corporate managers. Unsatisfactory resolution at this level usually results in an appeal for an arbitration hearing.

In contrast, nonunionized organizations generally progress directly from the informal process to a formal in-house grievance hearing. The date selected for this hearing must be agreed to by both parties; it should allow enough time for both parties to prepare their cases but should also encourage prompt resolution. An in-house grievance panel or committee is charged with reviewing the case. This panel, similar to a jury, is charged with determining the grievance outcome. Generally, this panel is composed of three to five members, with one person being designated as the facilitator or chair. This facilitator chairs the hearing and makes rulings on procedural matters and the relevance of evidence. It is recommended that the facilitator have some legal background or training whenever possible. The following persons cannot serve on the grievance panel:

- Friends of either party
- Persons involved with the grievance in any way
- Any person who is serving as an advocate for employees or management

This panel is charged with making a final decision in favor of either the grievant or the respondent, or reaching a compromise resolution. Following a presentation of evidence by both parties, the panel votes by secret ballot, and the vote is recorded by the facilitator. The facilitator informs both the grievant and the respondent of the panel's final decision in writing.

ARBITRATION: THE FINAL DECISION

In contrast to nonunion organizations, 94% of all union collective bargaining agreements provide for arbitration as the final step in the grievance process (Beach, 1980). However, it is not automatic, and one party must call for arbitration in writing if the grievance has not been resolved. In arbitration, an objective third party, called an *arbitrator*, reviews evidence submitted by both management and the employee and makes a final ruling or decision in the case. The arbitrator, who usually is a professor or lawyer, functions in a role similar to that of a judge. He or she can interpret, apply, or determine compliance with the provisions of union or management contracts but cannot add to, subtract, or alter the provisions of the contract.

Union and management can select an arbitrator in one of two basic ways, usually spelled out in the labor contract (Beach, 1980). One is the permanent arbitrator or umpire system; the other is the ad hoc system. The permanent arbitrator system allows organizations to contract with an arbitrator who works full time as a salaried arbitrator, generally for a large corporation or the government. Permanent arbitrators are experts at what they do and usually are able to bring rapid closure to a grievance. The more commonly used ad hoc system allows for the selection of an arbitrator on a case-by-case basis. This is more time consuming but does allow an arbitrator to be selected who has special expertise in the area of the particular grievance. The American Arbitration Association and the Federal Mediation and Conciliation Service are primary sources for professional arbitrators (Marriner-Tomey, 1988).

The means by which the arbitrator settles the conflict is in the form of a quasi-judicial process known as an *arbitration hearing*. Although many aspects of an arbitration hearing resemble a hearing in a court of law, it is less formal. Both the arbitrator and the opposing sides are present at the hearing and may ask questions or call witnesses to clarify evidence that has been presented; however, the side calling for arbitration has the responsibility of burden of proof. The arbitration hearing consists of (1) statement of issue, (2) presentation of facts, and (3) closing arguments.

Both the grievant and the respondent are encouraged to have a representative assist in preparing and presenting evidence at the grievance hearing. A unionized employee generally has a shop steward or union representative do this. A manager may have a managerial colleague or the immediate supervisor function in this role. Although the use of representatives may complicate the process somewhat, as additional parties are involved, they are very helpful in keeping the grievance hearing more objective and less emotional. Because the grievant and the respondent are going to be emotionally charged, the representatives are often able to calm their respective parties and identify new perspectives or compromise resolutions that may be appropriate (Huston, 1986).

The actual grievance hearing is generally a closed hearing and is limited to the grievant, the respondent, their representatives, witnesses (while they are giving evidence), the grievance panel, and the facilitator. The content of the proceedings and the outcome are not generally made public by participants in the hearing.

During the hearing, both the grievant and the respondent may make an opening statement. Then evidence is presented by both sides. This may include calling witnesses. Witnesses must leave the hearing after presenting their testimony and should not discuss the content of their testimony or the hearing with other witnesses who may be waiting to present evidence. Both parties will end the hearing with closing statements.

The arbitrator is then charged with making a decision in favor of either the grievant or the respondent. Only the evidence presented at the hearing can be used in considering the outcome of the case. A written decision is generally rendered several weeks, or even several months, after the hearing. If, however, both sides request an immediate response, the arbitrator can issue an oral decision and withhold a written explanation of the decision unless requested by both sides (Potter, 1984). In contrast to a court of law in the United States, where a judge's decision can be appealed, the arbitrator's decision is binding and usually is used to set a precedent for future administration or practice (Yarbrough, 1987).

DETERMINING WHAT IS GRIEVABLE

Potter (1984) makes a distinction between "grievances" and "gripes." Grievances are substantive complaints that usually involve definitive contract violations. Although this is a fairly narrow definition of a *grievance*, it is the one generally accepted by both management and unions. Gripes are personal problems or interpersonal problems that are not related to an established contract or standard. Generally, the shop steward or union representative will advise an employee if a complaint is a grievance or a gripe.

Grievances should meet the following criteria to be considered valid:

1. Grievants must show that they have been adversely affected by whatever action was taken against them.

2. Grievants must be able to demonstrate that an official action was taken that was either unreasonable or not generally or specifically authorized in the labor contract.

3. If the action follows a written or implied policy, grievants must demonstrate that the policy is either unreasonable or not generally or specifically authorized.

4. Grievants must show that the remedy sought will not effectively result in special favoritism for them or prejudice against others.

If the employee can demonstrate these criteria, the issue should be followed through in a formal grievance process.

On the other hand, gripes should be settled informally through conflict resolution and should not be a part of the formal grievance process. An example of a gripe might be a nurse who perpetually defies authority and has recurrent interpersonal conflicts with her supervisor. This nurse might file a grievance to harass the supervisor, although there may not have been any contract or policy violation. Likewise, a manager can misuse authority in an effort to tyrannically rule and thus file inappropriate grievances against employees who question his or her method of management.

COMMON GRIEVANCES

Grievances can reflect an almost infinite number of problems, but several occur consistently. Potter (1984) identified the most common grievances or disciplinary actions filed by management against employees as the following:

1. Allowing personal problems to interfere with work performance
2. Failing to perform assigned duties
3. Poor work habits, such as tardiness or absenteeism
4. Antagonistic attitude toward management in labor relations when serving in union positions

The U.S. Department of Labor (1984) found that the most common incidents resulting in employees filing grievances against managers were employee discipline, seniority decisions at promotion or layoff time, work assignment, management rights, and compensation and benefits. Potter (1984) reinforced these findings, stating that employee grievances frequently occur because managers:

1. Dispense discipline inconsistently
2. Show favoritism
3. Treat employees unfairly
4. Discriminate against some employees in hiring, promotions, shift assignments, disciplinary actions, and merit salary increases

Table 22-1 lists five types of grievances filed by employees against management (Potter, 1984).

THE IMPACT OF UNIONIZATION ON THE GRIEVANCE PROCESS

One of the most common differences between unionized and nonunionized organizations is the formality of the process used to resolve management/employee conflict. Most union organizations utilize a grievance process as the formal tool for conflict resolution, whereas nonunion organizations tend to resolve these conflicts more informally. Typically, the unionized organization has specific and detailed contracts that outline when an employee may file a grievance, what is considered a grievable offense, and the steps the employee must follow in filing a grievance.

In a nonunionized organization, there may be no formal grievance procedure, or the procedure may be more informal. First-level managers in decentralized management are expected to resolve disturbances of conflicts at the unit level. Often this

---

Table 22-1. Five Types of Grievances Filed by Employees Against Management

---

Contract Violations

The employment contract between the employer and the employee is binding. When this contract is violated, the employee has a valid grievance. An example of a contract violation would be discipline without just cause or that did not follow progressive discipline guidelines that had been established.

Federal and State Law Violations

Any action by the employer that violates federal or state law is grievable, even if this action is not in direct violation of the contract. An example would be the employee who is discriminated against in promotions on the basis of race, sex, or religion.

Past Practice Violations

A past-practice—any practice that has been accepted by both parties over an extended period of time and that is suddenly discontinued by the employer without notification—is grievable. For example, if the employer has consistently rewarded employees who have worked within the organization for 25 years with a monetary bonus, they can not withdraw this bonus on the day before you will have completed 25 years of service, particularly if you were promised this bonus at the time of hire.

Health and Safety Violations

Grievances in this category involve working conditions that an employer is responsible for, regardless of whether they are covered in the contract. An example would be excessive radiation exposure of an employee because of inadequate or defective protective devices in the x-ray department.

Employer Policy Violations

If an employer violates its own rules, this is considered a justifiable grievance. The employer can, however, change the rules unilaterally. An example would be if the manager is overdue in scheduling the employee's annual performance appraisal and thus the employee did not receive a merit pay increase, despite clearly written policy about how often performance appraisals must be completed.

---

results in greater flexibility in resolving conflicts between managers and employees; however, it may result in some inconsistency in the treatment of employees, and it gives management an advantage over employees because of the inherent authority structure.

Generally, nonunion organizations have fewer grievances filed than their union counterparts. This does not mean that nonunion employees are any more content than union employees. Because the nonunionized employees lack a formalized support system such as a union, they lack power and may not be as well informed about their rights as unionized employees, and thus they may not seek and receive appropriate redress. Even if employees file and win grievances in a nonunion organization, the personal cost to them in doing so may be high because of future retaliation by management. With few exceptions, the absence of a union gives managers greater unchecked authority and this presents a potential danger, as most managerial orders and decisions must go unchallenged.

In contrast, the presence of a union in an organization is generally an impetus to better personnel policies and clearer definitions of employee rights. If union employees feel they have been dealt with unfairly, they know that it is fully legitimate to submit complaints and grievances to management, and they immediately enter into a formal and systematic process of doing so. The union representative's contract expertise and moral support are invaluable to employees during grievances, although they can also be a deterrent to conflict resolution. Although a grievant may withdraw the grievance or accept an informal solution at any time in the formal process, there is some concern that the involvement of a third person who may be antimanagement may hamper informal resolution of conflicts. This occurs because some union officials strongly encourage the expression of grievances as a means of "keeping management in line," not only for a particular case, but as a reminder in the future. As a result, a grievant may be reluctant to withdraw a complaint or settle for a compromise if the union representative has put time and energy in the case or if the union representative is encouraging the employee to seek full recourse in the process.

RIGHTS AND RESPONSIBILITIES OF THE EMPLOYEE AND EMPLOYER

Although the employee and employer have some separate and distinct rights and responsibilities in grievance situations, it is more common for such rights and responsibilities to overlap. It is easy to be drawn into the emotionalism of a grievance that focuses on "one's perceived contractual rights," but it is imperative that both the employer and the employee remember that both individuals in a grievance have rights and that these rights have concomitant responsibilities. For example, given that both parties have the right to be heard, there is an equal responsibility for both parties to listen without interrupting. The employee has the right to a positive work environment and accordingly has the responsibility to communicate needs and discontents to the supervisor. The employer has the right to expect a certain level of productivity from the employee and accordingly has the responsibility to provide a work environment that makes this possible. The employer has the right to expect employees to follow rules and has the responsibility to see that these rules are clearly communicated and fairly enforced.

Smooth labor relations require both the employee and the employer to honor existing labor contracts and to show good will in resolving differences when grievances arise. This means that both parties must be open to discussion, negotiation, and compromise (Potter, 1984) and that an attempt should be made to solve the grievance at the earliest possible point in the process. The ultimate goal of the grievance should not be to win, but to seek a resolution that results in maximal worker and unit productivity and satisfaction. Tool 22-2 identifies 24 rules that should be followed by both parties in the grievance process to increase the likelihood of a positive outcome.

In many cases, the manager can eliminate or reduce the risk of being involved in a grievance by fostering a work environment that emphasizes clear communication and fair, constructive discipline. To create such an environment, the manager must agree to be responsible for:

1. Using clearly defined objective criteria as the basis for performance evaluations.

2. Using fair, consistent, and impartial discipline that follows established policy or contract guidelines for its administration.

3. Maintaining complete and objective records regarding employee disciplinary problems, including dates of infractions, type of infractions, and any attempts to counsel.

4. Being attentive to employee needs and discontent. Unexpressed dissatisfaction is just as important as verbalized dissatisfaction.

5. Being well informed regarding the contents of the labor contract. Ignorance of the contract is not a legitimate excuse for its violation.

Tool 22-2   Twenty-Four Rules That Increase the Likelihood of a Positive Grievance Outcome

Beletz (1977) identified the following suggestions, for both parties in a grievance, that increase the likelihood of a positive outcome:

1. The final objective of the grievance should not be conquest; the parties should treat each other with courtesy and respect. It is important to remember that the grievant and the respondent will probably have to work together again after the grievance is settled.

2. Do not threaten or bluff. The other party will probably recognize this strategy for what it is.

3. Don't withhold information that could help resolve the grievance.

4. Do not, whatever your position, exhibit internal disagreements or disputes. Both the bargaining unit and management must present a unified front when faced with each other.

5. Although time must be allowed for all the facts to be gathered, work to expedite the grievance outcome whenever possible. Delaying the outcome only increases the emotionalism associated with the grievance.

6. Own up to your own mistakes and don't waste time and energy trying to blame the other side for your mistakes.

7. Be as objective as possible.

8. Be proactive. Anticipate responses from the opposing side in planning your strategy.

9. Utilize all appropriate resources, especially human resources, that may be able to help you.

10. Never refuse to meet with the grievant or the representative. The right to representation is under the auspices of the collective-bargaining contract.

11. Remember that the bargaining unit representative is not immune from reprimand or discipline. When not actively involved as the grievant's advocate, the bargaining unit representative must meet organizational requirements just as any other employee must.

12. If a grievance meeting degenerates and becomes overly emotional or destructive, the meeting should be adjourned and rescheduled for a later date or time.

13. Even if management denies the validity of a grievance, the employee may pursue the grievance and seek redress at the next step in the procedure.

14. What is "fair" is what has been determined by the labor contract. Individual interpretation of what is fair has no relevance.

15. Always be open to compromise.

16. Know the strengths and weaknesses of the issue for both sides.

17. Always plan ahead in identifying grievance solutions that may accommodate future changes and needs.

18. There is no one standard way to settle grievances or solve problems. Case-by-case flexibility is required.

19. Be honest with yourself and your representative about what your bottom line is for compromise.

20. Observe the time limits in the contract or be prepared to lose the grievance.

21. Some grievances have a chain reaction. Be prepared for the worst possible outcome.

22. Knowledge is very important in adjusting a grievance, and interpretation of facts is colored by the values and temperament of the individuals involved.

23. Do not be overconfident. Just because you won one grievance does not mean that you will win the next.

24. Gather enough information to adequately respond to the grievance. Call appropriate witnesses. See if a precedent has been set for this type of grievance in the past.

---

6. Maintaining an open and positive attitude toward labor relations as a means of reducing conflict in the work place and thus increasing employee satisfaction and productivity.

Employees also can eliminate or reduce their risk of being involved in a grievance by:

1. Being well informed regarding the labor contract, policies and procedures, and rules in the organization in which they work.

2. Openly communicating with their immediate supervisors about work conditions or managerial actions that are perceived as unfair or discriminatory in some way.

If both the employee and the employer recognize their rights and responsibilities, the incidence of grievances in the work place should decrease. In those situations in which mutual problem solving, negotiation, and compromise are ineffective at resolving conflicts, the grievance process can provide a positive and growth-producing resolution to conflicts.

KEY CONCEPTS CHAPTER 22

1. A grievance procedure is broadly defined as a statement of wrongdoing or a procedure to follow when one feels that a wrong has been committed. Unions look at this definition more narrowly and utilize the grievance procedure only when there has been some violation of some aspect of a labor contract.

2. Most grievances or conflicts between employees and management can be resolved informally through communication, negotiation, compromise, and collaboration.

3. If the employee and management are unable to resolve their differences informally, a formal grievance process begins that includes in-house grievance hearings in nonunion organizations and union-management meetings and arbitration in unionized organizations.

4. Approximately three quarters of grievances are resolved either informally or early in formal union-management meetings. Only 5% of grievances must be resolved in arbitration.

5. In arbitration, an objective third party, called an *arbitrator*, reviews evidence submitted by both management and the employee and makes a final ruling or decision in the case. This decision is considered binding in a court of law.

6. The grievance process is often absent or informal in non-unionized organizations. This results in greater flexibility in resolving conflicts between managers and employees, but may result in some inconsistency in the treatment of employees and gives management an advantage over employees because of the inherent authority structure.

7. The presence of a union in an organization is generally an impetus to better personnel policies and clearer definitions of employee rights. It also reduces the possibility of arbitrary treatment by managers.

REFERENCES

American Nurses Association, *Guidelines for the Individual Nurse Contract*, American Nurses Association, Kansas City, MO, 1974.

Beach, D.S., *Personnel: The Management of People at Work*, Fourth Edition, Macmillan, New York, 1980.

Beletz, E., "Some Pointers for Grievance Handlers," *Supervisor Nurse*, 8:56, 1977.

Huston, C.J., "Preparing for Student Grievances," *Nursing Outlook* 34(6):304, 1986.

Marquis, B., and Huston, C., *Management Decision Making for Nurses: 101 Case Studies*, J. B. Lippincott, Philadelphia, 1987.

Marriner-Tomey, A., *Guide to Nursing Management*, Third Edition, C.V. Mosby, St. Louis, 1988.

Milkovich, G.T., and Glueck, W.F., *Personnel: Human Resource Management/A Diagnostic Approach*, Fourth Edition, Business Publications, Plano, TX, 1985.

Potter, D.O. (ed.), *Practices*, Nurses Reference Library, Nursing 85 Books, Springhouse Corporation, Springhouse, PA, 1984.

Strauss, G., and Sayles, L.R., *Personnel: The Human Problems of Management*, Third Edition, Prentice-Hall, Englewood Cliffs, NJ, 1972.

U.S. Department of Labor, Federal Mediation and Conciliation Service, Thirty Sixth Annual Report, Fiscal Year 1983, U.S. Government Printing Office, Washington, DC, 1984.

Yarbrough, M.G., "Successful Contract Management," in Lewis, E.M., and Spicer, J.G., *Human Resource Management Handbook*, Aspen Publications, Rockville, MD, 1987, p. 295–311.

ADDITIONAL READINGS

Elkouri, F., and Elkouri, E.A., *How Arbitration Works*, Third Edition, Bureau of National Affairs, Washington, D.C., 1973, Chapter 12.

The Guide to Basic Law and Procedures under the National Labor Relations Act, U.S. Government Printing Office, Washington, D.C., 1978.

Klaus, R.C., "The Ins and Outs of Collective Bargaining," *JONA*, 10(9):18–21, 1980.

Levenstein, A., "The Art and Science of Supervision: Caught in a Bind," *Supervisor Nurse*, 11:63–64, 1980.

Stessin, L. and Smedkesman, L., *The Encyclopedia of Collective Bargaining Contract Clauses*, Business Research Publications, New York, 1980.

Trotta, M.S., *Handling Grievance: A Guide for Management and Labor*, Bureau of National Affairs, Washington D.C., 1976.

23
The Impaired Employee

O'CONNOR (1985) estimates that at least 12% of the entire work force has serious personal problems, with over half of these problems being related to alcohol or drug use. These personal problems impair affected employees' performances to such a degree that they are unable to follow established rules or to meet organizational goals. Impairment may be manifested in an individual's judgment, behavior, memory, interpersonal relationships, technical skills, and even hygiene and appearance (Landry, 1987).

Chapter 21 discussed the need for progressive discipline in dealing with employees who are unable to follow established rules or procedures or to meet organizational goals. However, progressive discipline is inappropriate for impaired employees, as it cannot result in employee growth. These employees are impaired as a result of a disease and need professional counseling to stop their self-destructive behavior and to again become productive. Thus, it is essential that managers learn to identify and distinguish between an employee who needs progressive discipline and an impaired employee so that the employee can be managed in the most appropriate manner.

Assisting the impaired employee to again become an effective and productive member of the work force should not be viewed as an altruistic or benevolent action on the part of the employer. The cost of absenteeism, work-related accidents, lowered productivity, and turnover associated with impaired employees is immense. In addition, the impaired employee places the organization at greater liability for patient care errors in judgment. The impaired employee also reduces group morale and efficiency of unit-wide functioning. "As drug dependency behaviors manifest in the employee, complex emotional barriers develop between the manager, the impaired employee and other staff members" (Robinson and Spicer, 1987).

Therefore, effective human resource management demands that the organization take an active role in helping impaired employees. Planning strategies that counsel and assist these employees in an effort to return them as productive members of the work force are not only humanistic, but cost effective and necessary.

Although employees can have many types of impairments, Chapter 23 will focus on chemical impairments. *Chemical impairment* refers to impairment due to drug and/or alcohol addiction. The scope of the problem of chemical addiction among nurses will be discussed. Behaviors common to chemically impaired nurses will be identified to aid managers in identifying these employees. In addition, the manager's role in confronting and assisting impaired employees will be presented. Also, steps in the recovery process and the re-entry of recovering impaired nurses into the work force will be discussed. Tools for implementation include a 20-question check list for identifying employees who are at high risk for alcohol impairment, a four-question adaptation of the CAGE questionnaire to assess actual or potential chemical dependency, and an interview guide for evaluating the readiness of recovering chemically impaired employees to return to the work force.

CHEMICAL IMPAIRMENT – SCOPE OF THE PROBLEM

Chemical dependency in the health professions was first documented in studies by Modlin and Montes (1964) in the late 1940s, although there is little doubt that chemical dependency has been around as long as alcohol and drugs have been. Substance abuse accounts for almost 70% of cases of nurses having their licenses withdrawn or revoked (Curtin, 1987). Robbins (1987) and Bissell (1979) estimate that there are 40,000 to 75,000 chemically impaired nurses in the workforce. Landry (1987) estimates that 8% to 10% of all registered nurses and licensed practical nurses in the United States have either a drug or alcohol dependency. This translates to approximately 135,000 to 170,000 impaired nurses. The American Nurses' Association (ANA) estimates the number of chemically impaired nurses to be as high as 200,000 (Morse et al., 1984). These statistics suggest that at least 1 in 20 nurses in the hospital setting are working under the influence of some sort of mood-altering drug (Robinson and Spicer, 1987).

The rate of narcotic addiction of nurses is estimated to approximate that of physicians which is estimated to be 30 to 100 times that of the general population (Curtin, 1987; Fox, 1957; and Murray, 1974). The nursing profession as a whole has a 50% higher risk of becoming chemically addicted than do other professions (Robinson and Spicer, 1987).

This heightened risk occurs in part because nursing is primarily a female occupation, and current literature clearly documents that women have a greater susceptibility to drug abuse than do men. This may occur because women use more prescription mood-altering drugs, such as tranquilizers, than men do (Naegle, 1988; Robinson and Spicer, 1987). Women are also more apt than men to see their physicians for medical and emotional problems, and as a result they have over twice as many prescriptions filled as do men (Robinson and Spicer, 1987). Studies have also shown that most chemically addicted nurses first began abusing drugs with legally prescribed drugs that they legitimately obtained for physical, emotional, personal, or job-related problems (Poplar, 1969).

Demerol and alcohol are the most commonly abused chemicals. Ninety-four percent of the members of the San Francisco Support Group for Chemically Dependent Nurses reported Demerol as their primary drug of use (Buxton and Jessup, 1983). Other frequently abused chemicals include the benzodiazepines, such as Valium, and other narcotic drugs, such as morphine and pentazocine (Talwin) (Landry, 1987). Employees may use barbiturates instead of alcohol in the work place so as to feel a similar effect without having alcohol detectable on their breath. Likewise, addicted nurses may use amphetamines in combination with central nervous system depressants to facilitate their performance and mediate the depressed effect (Landry, 1987).

Clearly, the incidence of chemical impairment in health professionals is substantial. On a personal level, the tragedy is that individuals suffer from an illness that may go undetected and untreated for many years. On a professional level, the entire health care system is affected by impaired employees. Patient care is jeopardized by nurses with impaired skills and judgment, and teamwork and continuity are compromised as team members attempt to pick up the slack of their impaired colleagues (Jefferson and Ensor, 1982). The personal and professional cost of chemical impairment demands, then, that nursing managers recognize chemically impaired employees as early as possible and intervene.

RECOGNIZING THE CHEMICALLY IMPAIRED EMPLOYEE

Although most nurses have finely tuned assessment skills for identifying patient problems, they generally lack sensitivity in identifying behaviors and actions that could signify chemical impairment of a nursing employee or colleague. The profile of the impaired nurse may vary greatly, but several behavior patterns and behavior changes have been frequently noted. These behavior changes can be grouped into three primary areas: personality/behavior changes, job performance changes, and time and attendance changes (Landry, 1987). Tables 23-1, 23-2, and 23-3 show characteristics of each of these categories, respectively.

As the employee progresses into a deeper stage of chemical dependency, it should become easier for the manager to recognize these behaviors. Typically, in the earliest stages of chemical dependency, the individual uses the addictive substance primarily for pleasure, and although the alcohol or drug use is excessive, it is primarily recreational and social. Thus, substance use does not generally occur during work hours, although some effects of its use, such as absenteeism, judgment errors, and changes in interpersonal relationships, may be apparent (Robinson and Spicer, 1987).

Table 23-1.   Common Personality/Behavior Changes of the Chemically Impaired Employee

---

Increased irritability with patients and colleagues, often followed by extreme calm

Social isolation: eats alone, avoids unit social functions

Extreme and rapid mood swings

Euphoric recall of events or elaborate excuses for behaviors

Unusually strong interest in narcotics or the narcotic cabinet

Sudden dramatic change in personal grooming

Any dramatic change from normal affect

Forgetfulness ranging from simple short-term memory loss to blackouts

Change in physical appearance that may include weight loss, flushed face, red or bleary eyes, unsteady gait, slurred speech, tremors, restlessness, diaphoresis, cigarette burns and bruises, jaundice, and ascites

Extreme defensiveness regarding medication errors

Table 23-2.   Common Job Performance Changes of the Chemically Impaired Employee

---

Difficulty meeting schedules and deadlines

Illogical or sloppy charting

High-frequency medication errors or errors in judgment affecting patient care

Frequent volunteering to be medication nurse

High number of assigned patients who complain that their pain medication is ineffective in relieving their pain

Work performance consistently marginal; minimum acceptable amount of work done

Judgment errors

Sleeping or dozing on duty

Complaints from other staff members about the quality and quantity of employee's work

---

As the employee moves deeper into chemical dependency, tolerance to the chemical has occurred and the individual must use the substance in greater quantities and more frequently to achieve the same effect. At this point, the individual has made a conscious decision to use chemicals as part of his or her lifestyle, although there frequently is a high use of defense mechanisms such as justification, denial, and bargaining about the drug use

**Table 23-3.   Common Time and Attendance Changes of the Chemically
Impaired Employee**

Increasing absences from work without adequate explanation or notification; most
frequent absences are on a Monday or Friday

Long lunch hours

Excessive use of sick leave or requests for sick leave after days off

Frequent calling in to request compensatory time at the beginning of shifts

Arriving at work late or staying late for no apparent reason

Consistent lateness

Long lunch hours

Frequent "disappearances" from the unit without explanation

(Hutchinson, 1987). Often, the employee in this stage begins to
use the chemical substance both at work and during unsched-
uled work hours. Work performance generally declines in the
areas of attendance, judgment, quality, and interpersonal relationships, and an appreciable decline in unit morale, as the
result of an unreliable and unproductive worker, begins to be
apparent (Robinson and Spicer, 1987).

In the final stages of chemical dependency, the employee
must continually use the chemical substance, even though it is
no longer associated with pleasure or gratification of any sort.
The employee is physically and psychologically addicted. There
is total disregard for self and others. Because the need for the
addictive substance is so great, the employee's personal and
professional life is focused around the need for the drug. The
employee in this stage is totally unpredictable and undependable
in the work area. Assignments are incomplete or not done at all.
Charting may be sloppy or illegible, and judgment errors are
frequent. Because the employee in this stage must use the
substance frequently, there are often signs of use during work
hours. Narcotic vials are unaccounted for. The employee may be
absent from the unit for brief periods of time with no plausible
excuse. Mood swings are excessive, and the employee often looks
physically ill. It is hoped that, as managers gain greater expertise in identifying chemically impaired employees, they will be
able to remove such employees from the work setting prior to
this final stage. Figure 23-1 summarizes behavior phases, crisis

points, and visible signs of the chemically dependent employee.

It is also important that the manager examine which clinical area the suspected impaired nurse has been working in. Buxton and Jessup (1983) found that 55% of addicted female nurses and 75% of addicted male nurses first self-administered a psychoactive drug while working in critical care areas such as an intensive care unit, critical care unit, and emergency room. Whether these nurses took these drugs as a result of their inability to cope with the higher stress levels associated with these clinical areas or whether these nurses sought work in these areas because of the greater availability of psychoactive drugs is unclear.

Another factor that contributes to managerial difficulty in identifying impaired employees is that most managers have some preconceived ideas about what chemically impaired nurses look or act like. Frequently, these preconceptions include unkempt, marginally bright employees with a history of poor work performance and little self-motivation. In reality, in a study of 100 alcoholic nurses, Bissell (1979) found that most:

- were in the top third of their class,
- held advanced degrees,
- held demanding and responsible jobs,
- were highly respected for excellent work, which continued long after they began to drink heavily, and
- were ambitious and achievement oriented.

These characteristics generally do not fit the stereotyped image managers have of chemically impaired individuals, much less chemically impaired nurses. Surveys of health professionals indicate that most nurses view substance abuse as a treatable disease unless the abuser is a colleague. When the abuser is a colleague, nurses tend to hold the belief that such behavior results from a moral defect (Curtin, 1987). It becomes clear that nursing managers need extensive education about chemical abuse. Sixty-one percent of employers in a recent study said that they have not provided staff education programs on substance abuse (Naegle, 1988). It is also clear that nursing managers must examine their values, biases, and beliefs about chemical abuse before they can recognize impaired employees and implement an appropriate strategy to help impaired nurses overcome this disease.

(Text continued on p. 426)

BEHAVIOR	EFFICIENCY	CRISIS POINTS DURING DETERIORATION	VISIBLE SIGNS
EARLY PHASE Drinks to relieve tension			Late (after lunch) Leaves job early Absent from office
Alcohol tolerance increases			Fellow workers complain Overreacts to real or imagined criticism Complains of not feeling well Lies
Blackouts (memory blanks)	90%		Misses deadlines Mistakes through inattention or poor judgment Decreased efficiency
Lies about drinking habits		CRITICISM FROM BOSS	
MIDDLE PHASE Surreptitious drinks	75%	FAMILY PROBLEMS LOSS OF JOB ADVANCEMENT	Frequent days off for vague ailments or implausible reasons
Guilt about drinking		FINANCIAL PROBLEMS, e.g. WAGE GARNISHMENT	Statements become undependable Begins to avoid associates Borrows money from co-workers Exaggerates work accomplishments Hospitalized more than average Repeated minor injuries on and off the job Unreasonable resentment
Tremors during hangovers Loss of interest		WARNING FROM BOSS	General deterioration Spasmodic work pace Attention wanders; lack of concentration

SUPERVISOR'S EVALUATION

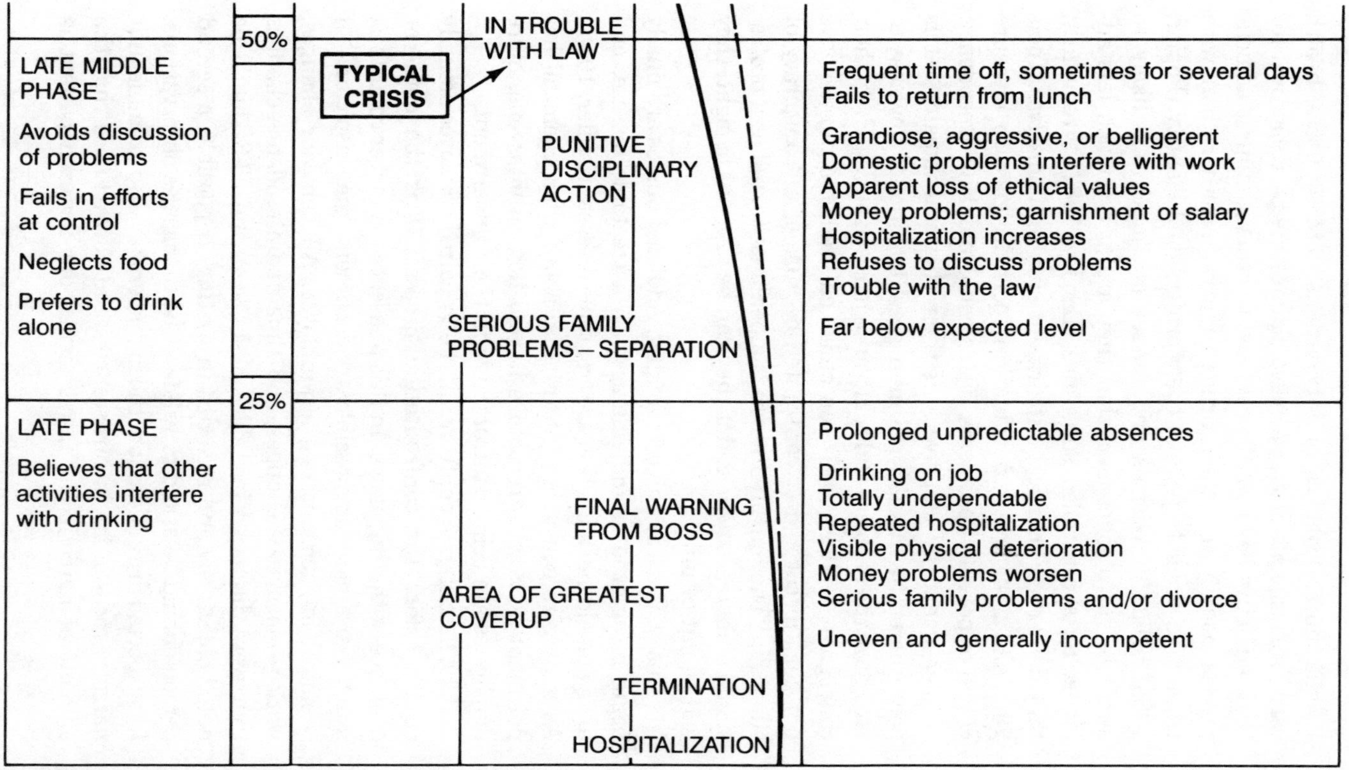

LATE MIDDLE PHASE	50%			IN TROUBLE WITH LAW	Frequent time off, sometimes for several days Fails to return from lunch
Avoids discussion of problems					Grandiose, aggressive, or belligerent Domestic problems interfere with work Apparent loss of ethical values Money problems; garnishment of salary Hospitalization increases Refuses to discuss problems Trouble with the law
Fails in efforts at control			TYPICAL CRISIS	PUNITIVE DISCIPLINARY ACTION	
Neglects food					
Prefers to drink alone				SERIOUS FAMILY PROBLEMS—SEPARATION	Far below expected level
LATE PHASE	25%			FINAL WARNING FROM BOSS	Prolonged unpredictable absences
Believes that other activities interfere with drinking			AREA OF GREATEST COVERUP		Drinking on job Totally undependable Repeated hospitalization Visible physical deterioration Money problems worsen Serious family problems and/or divorce
				TERMINATION	
				HOSPITALIZATION	Uneven and generally incompetent

FIGURE 23-1. *How a chemically dependent employee behaves*
From Charter Medical Corporation, Addictive Disease Division, 11050 Crabtree Road, Roswell, Georgia 30075.

425

CONFRONTING THE CHEMICALLY IMPAIRED EMPLOYEE

Unlike most alcoholics or intravenous narcotic users, health care professionals do not achieve clandestine peer approval for their addictive behavior. In contrast to other nonnurse addicts, nurses usually use their drugs in private rather than with friends, in order to protect their professional identity (Poplar, 1969). Thus, physicians and nurses are much less likely to admit, even to colleagues, that they are using, much less addicted to, a controlled substance (Landry, 1987). Frequently, they deny their chemical impairment even to themselves. Tools 23-1 and 23-2 are self-evaluation tools designed to measure actual or potential problems with alcohol and drug dependency.

The denial by employees of their chemical impairment is perpetuated by nurses' and managers' traditional slowness to recognize the problem and reluctance to reach out and help their colleagues. Leffler (1986) contends that addicted nurses have not been discovered or confronted because of a "conspiracy of silence": "The impaired nurse is a personal as well as a professional embarrassment and if they can be kept out of sight, they will be out of mind."

This attitude is slowly changing. Addicted nurses are finally being recognized as individuals with a treatable disease, and drug and alcohol addiction are treatable diseases (Leffler, 1986). As managers gain more information about what chemical impairment is, how to recognize it, and how to intervene, more employees are being confronted with their impairment.

The first step to confronting the impaired employee actually occurs before the confrontation process. It is the data- or evidence-gathering phase. In this phase, the manager collects as much hard data as possible to document the suspicions of chemical impairment in the employee. All behavior changes, work performance changes, and time and attendance changes that were discussed in Tables 23-1, 23-2, and 23-3 should be noted objectively and recorded in writing. If possible, a second person should be asked to validate the manager's observations. In suspected drug addiction, the manager may also examine unit narcotic records for inconsistencies and check to see that the amount of narcotic the nurse signed out for each patient is

---

**Tool 23-1   Twenty-Question Check List — Identifying Employees at
High Risk for Alcohol Impairment**

Are you an alcoholic? To answer this question, ask yourself the
following questions and answer them as *honestly* as you can.

1. Do you lose time from work due to drinking?

2. Is drinking making your home life unhappy?

3. Do you drink because you are shy with other people?

4. Is drinking affecting your reputation?

5. Have you ever felt remorse after drinking?

6. Have you gotten into financial difficulties as a result of drinking?

7. Do you turn to lower companions and an inferior environment when
   drinking?

8. Does your drinking make you careless of your family's welfare?

9. Has your ambition decreased since drinking?

10. Do you crave a drink at a definite time daily?

11. Do you want a drink the next morning?

12. Does drinking cause you to have difficulty in sleeping?

13. Has your efficiency decreased since drinking?

14. Is drinking jeopardizing your job or business?

15. Do you drink to escape from worries or trouble?

16. Do you drink alone?

17. Have you ever had a complete loss of memory as a result of drinking?

18. Has your physician ever treated you for drinking?

19. Do you drink to build up your self-confidence?

20. Have you ever been to a hospital or institution on account of drinking?

If you have answered YES to any one of the questions, there is a
definite warning that you *may* be an alcoholic. If you have answered
YES to any two, the chances are that you *are* and alcoholic. If you have
answered YES to three or more, you *are definitely* an alcoholic.

From Seliger, R. V., and Sanford, V., *A Guide on Alcoholism for Social Workers.*
Alcoholism Publications, Baltimore, 1945.

Tool 23-2   Predicting Actual or Potential Problems with Chemical Dependency Using the CAGE Questionnaire

---

The following four questions have been adapted from the **CAGE** questionnaire (Ewing, 1984). Although there is no formal scoring mechanism, individuals who answer yes to any of the following questions are at risk for chemical impairment.

1. Do you now or have you ever felt that you should **C**ut down on your alcohol, drug, or medication use?

2. Have you ever felt angry or **A**nnoyed by other people's criticism of your alcohol, drug, or medication use?

3. Do you now or have you ever had **G**uilty feelings about using alcohol, drugs, or medications?

4. Do you take a morning **E**ye opener of drugs or medicine?

Adapted from Ewing, J. A., "Detecting Alcoholism — The CAGE Questionnaire," *JAMA* 252:1905, 1984. Copyright 1984, American Medical Association.

---

congruent with the amount that was ordered for that patient (Doyle, 1986).

It is more difficult to prove alcohol impairment, as it is easier for an employee to hide alcoholism than drug addiction (Doyle, 1986). Because few nurses drink while on duty, the manager will have to observe the employee for more subtle clues, such as the smell of alcohol on the employee's breath. If the organization's policy allows for it, the manager may wish to require an employee suspected of alcohol impairment to have a serum alcohol analysis while on duty. If the employee refuses to cooperate, the organization's policy for documenting and reporting this incident should be followed (Doyle, 1986).

If at any time the manager suspects that an employee is chemically influenced and thus presents a potential hazard to patient safety, the employee must be immediately pulled off the unit and privately confronted with the manager's perceptions. The employee should be decisively and unemotionally told that he or she will not be allowed to return to the work area because of the manager's perception that he or she is chemically impaired. The manager should make arrangements for the employee to be taken home, so that the employee does not drive while impaired. A formal meeting to discuss this incident should be scheduled within the next 24 hours (Jefferson and Ensor, 1982).

This type of direct confrontation between the manager and the employee is the second phase in dealing with the employee suspected of chemical impairment. Many employees admit their problem when directly confronted, although the use of defense mechanisms (including denial) are common in impaired employees, who may not, in fact, have admitted the problem even to themselves. Denial and anger should be expected in the confrontation, and the manager must assume responsibility for controlling the situation (Robinson and Spicer, 1987). If an employee denies having a problem, documented evidence demonstrating a decline in work performance should be shared with him or her. The manager must be careful to keep the confrontation focused on the performance deficits of the employee and not allow the discussion to be directed to the cause of the underlying problem or addiction. These are issues and concerns that the manager is unable to address. The manager must also be careful not to preach, moralize, scold, or blame.

Confrontation should always occur before the problem escalates beyond approach. In some situations the manager may have only limited direct evidence but still feel that the employee should be confronted because of rapidly declining employee performance or unit morale. There is, however, a greater risk that confrontation at this point may not help the employee. If direct confrontation is unsuccessful, it may have been too early, the employee may not have been desperate enough, or the employee may still be in the denial stage. In these situations, job performance will probably continue to be marginal to unsatisfactory, and progressive discipline may be necessary. If the employee continues to deny chemical impairment and work performance continues to be unsatisfactory despite repeated constructive confrontation, it may be necessary to terminate the employee (Robinson and Spicer, 1987).

The last phase of the confrontation process is outlining the organization's plan or expectations for helping the employee overcome the chemical impairment. This plan is similar to the disciplinary contract discussed in Chapter 21 in that it is usually written and outlines clearly what rehabilitative measures should be undertaken by the employee as well as the consequences if the employee does not seek the remedial action. Although the employee is generally referred informally by the manager to outside sources to help in dealing with the impairment, the employee is given the responsibility for correcting his or her work deficiencies. Timelines are included in the plan, and the manager and employee must agree on and sign a copy of the contract.

THE ROLE OF THE MANAGER IN ASSISTING THE IMPAIRED EMPLOYEE

Because of the general nature of nursing, many managers find themselves wanting to nurture impaired employees, much as they would any other individual who is sick. In addition, the employee who already has a greatly diminished sense of self-esteem and a perceived loss of self-control may ask the manager to be an active participant in helping in the recovery process. This is one of the most difficult aspects of working with the impaired employee. The manager must be very careful *not* to assume the role of counselor or treatment provider. There are other individuals with greater expertise and objectivity that can and should assume this role.

The manager must also be careful not to feel the need to diagnose the cause of the chemical addiction or to justify its existence. Protecting patients must be the top priority for the manager, and this takes precedence over any tendency to protect or excuse subordinates. The manager's role is to clearly identify performance expectations for the employee and to confront the employee when those expectations are not met. This is not to say that the manager should not recognize the problem as a disease and not a disciplinary problem or that the manager should be unwilling to refer the employee for needed help; however, the manager's primary responsibility is to see that the employee becomes functional again and can meet organizational expectations prior to returning to the unit.

In addition, the manager can play a vital role in creating an environment that decreases the chances of chemical impairment in the work setting. This may be done by controlling or reducing work-related stressors, whenever possible, and by providing mechanisms for stress management for employees. The manager should also control drug accessibility by implementing, enforcing, and monitoring policies and procedures related to medication distribution. Lastly, the manager should provide opportunities for the staff to learn about substance abuse, its recognition, and available resources (Robinson and Spicer, 1987).

THE RECOVERY PROCESS

Although there is disagreement on the name or number of steps in the recovery process, most authors concur that there are phases or progressive observable behaviors that suggest recovery from chemical impairment (Veatch, 1987). The first of these phases is called the *premotivation phase*. In this phase, the impaired employee continues to utilize denial about the significance or severity of the chemical impairment but does reduce or suspend chemical use to appease family, peers, or management. The employee in this phase hopes to continue or re-establish the substance abuse in the future.

The second phase of recovery is the *breakthrough phase*. As denial subsides, the impaired employee begins to see that the chemical addiction is having a negative impact on his or her life and begins to want to change. Frequently, individuals in this phase are buoyant with hope and commitment but lack maturity about the struggles that will face them in doing so. This phase generally lasts about 3 months.

The third phase of recovery is *early recovery*. During this phase, the individual examines his or her values and coping skills and works to develop more effective coping skills. Frequently this is done by alignment with support groups who will reinforce a chemical-free lifestyle. In this stage, individuals realize how sick they were in the active stage of their disease and are fraught with feelings of humiliation and shame (Jaffe, 1982).

The last phase of recovering is called *extended recovery*. In this phase individuals have gained self-awareness regarding why they became chemically addicted and have developed coping skills that will help them deal more effectively with stressors. As a result of this self-awareness, self-esteem and self-respect have increased. When this happens, individuals are able to make a conscious decision regarding whether they wish to and should return to the work place.

REENTRY OF THE CHEMICALLY IMPAIRED EMPLOYEE INTO THE WORK PLACE

Because impaired nurses recover at varying rates, it is difficult to predict how long this process will take. Many experts feel that impaired employees must devote at least one year to their recovery without the stresses of drug availability, overtime, and shift rotation.

With active treatment programs, employees return to the work place as productive employees in 85% to 90% of the cases (Robbins, 1987). Their success in reentering the work force is dependent on factors such as the extent of the recovery process and individual circumstances. Again, although the manager must show a genuine personal interest in the employee's rehabilitation, the manager's primary role is to be sure that the employee understands that the organization has the right to insist on unimpaired performance in the work place. Buxton and colleagues (1985) and Curtin (1987) suggest the following reentry guidelines for the recovering nurse:

- The employee must be told that no psychoactive drug use will be tolerated.

- The employee should be assigned to the day shift for the first year.

- The employee should be paired or "buddied" with a successful recovering nurse whenever possible.

- The employee should give approval for random urine screening twice weekly, with toxicology and/or alcohol screens.

- The employee should agree to participate in weekly nurses' group meetings with the option of open communication with facilitators.

- The employee must give evidence of continuing involvement with support groups such as AA (Alcoholics Anonymous) or NA (Narcotics Anonymous). The employee should be encouraged to attend meetings four times per week.

- The employee should be urged to participate in a recommended aftercare program.

- The employee should be encouraged to seek individual psychotherapy (optional).

- The employee should be encouraged to take Antabuse or Naltrene on the recommendation of a physician (optional).

These guidelines should be a part of the employee's return-to-work contract, although mandatory drug testing invokes questions about privacy rights and generally should not be implemented without advice from human resource personnel or legal counsel (Robinson and Spicer, 1987).

One of the tools most frequently used in evaluating whether the recovering impaired nurse is ready to return to the work force is the interview. It is important that the nurse manager be cognizant of what types of questions are appropriate to ask in such an interview. Tool 23-3 presents key questions that can be used to evaluate the nurse's level of recovery and to reestablish the nurse's credibility with both the employer and the profession.

Nurse managers have the responsibility to be proactive in identifying and confronting impaired employees. Prompt and appropriate intervention by nurse managers is essential for positive outcomes. With an estimated 10% to 20% of the already critically shorthanded nursing work force chemically impaired, organizations must actively assist these employees, in any way they can, to return as productive members of the work force.

KEY CONCEPTS CHAPTER 23

1. Because chemical impairment is a disease, progressive discipline is inappropriate for impaired employees, as it can not result in employee growth.

2. Planning strategies that counsel and assist impaired employees in an effort to return them as productive members of the work force are not only humanistic but also cost effective.

3. Current estimates are that there are 40,000 to 75,000 chemically impaired nurses in the work force. Eight percent to 10% of all registered nurses and licensed practical nurses in the United States have either a drug or alcohol dependency.

4. The rate of narcotic addiction among nurses is estimated to be 30 to 100 times that of the general population.

5. The profile of the impaired nurse may vary greatly, but typically behavior changes are seen in three areas: personality/behavior changes, job performance changes, and time and attendance changes.

(Text continued on p. 436)

Tool 23-3   Interview Guide for Evaluating the
Recovering Impaired Nurse

Interview questions

1. *Is there anything I need to know that will affect or impair your functioning on the job?*
   Analysis: Recovering nurses are concerned about obtaining a job, but really have no choice. They must acknowledge their illness to begin to reestablish credibility (Buxton and Jessup, 1982).

2. *Is there anything you want to tell me about your recovery?*
   Analysis: Nurses who are able to give some basic information are at least at the point where they can admit they have a chemical impairment that is destructive to their current and future lives.

3. *Is there any way I can validate what you have told me?*
   Analysis: It is reassuring to both the recovering nurse and to the interviewer to have data confirmed. Again, it allows the recovering nurse to continue to rebuild her credibility.

4. *What were the stresses in your previous job?*
   Analysis: Nurses who are self-aware regarding the stressors in their lives and how they cope with them are probably more advanced in their recovery than individuals who have not examined these issues.

5. *What do you expect the job stressors to be here? (Or: Is there anything about this job that might cause you difficulty?)*
   Analysis: Nurses who provide concrete answers to these questions have obviously examined the specific challenges to them in returning to the work force and thus are more prepared to meet these challenges. For example, recognizing possible stressors, such as having access to a narcotic supply or peer concern regarding their reliability, are valid concerns and demonstrate a nurse who is beginning to problem solve these stressors.

6. *Where do you get your support?*
   Analysis: Nurses who have a formalized peer support system have a greater likelihood of overcoming their chemical dependence. Often the relationships formed in these support systems assist the employee in forming their new drug-free identity (Buxton and Jessup, 1982).

7. *What other activities are you involved in?*
   Analysis: Nurses who are involved with family, friends, community activities, recreation, music, hobbies, sports, or church activities are generally more advanced in their recovery.

8. *If you are hired, we both need to feel comfortable. What orientation time frames do you need to assume different responsibilities?*
Analysis: Generally, recovering impaired nurses require a more prolonged orientation. This prolonged orientation allows nurses to face the stresses of the work place on a more gradual basis and to be resocialized in their roles. The manager should also ascertain that the employees are willing to cooperate in random urine or blood drug screens, at the hospital's cost, to assure safe patient care.

General analysis   (to be evaluated by interviewer after the interview)

1. *What was the nurse's attitude toward addiction?*
Analysis: It is imperative that the nurse accept his or her illness. The nurse should have been able to answer the questions directly and openly. It is also important that the nurse assume responsibility for how he or she has dealt with prior stressors.

2. *Did the nurse sound genuine?*
Analysis: The interviewer should trust his or her intuitive nature. If the nurse gave all the "right answers" but did not sound genuine, the employee's need to acquire a job may be greater than the readiness to do so.

3. *Did the nurse appear fearful and anxious?*
Analysis: Fearfulness and anxiety would be expected reactions in a situation where a recovering impaired nurse is unsure of the attitude or biases of the interviewer.

4. *Did the nurse appear highly vested in staying in the profession?*
Analysis: The nurse's commitment to the profession is one indicator of his or her values and fortitude in dealing with difficult situations.

5. *Did the nurse present with a sense of humility and a quality of serenity?*
Analysis: When nurses become self-aware about what they have done to themselves and their patients, they often have a profound sense of humility and serenity about their former addiction.

Adapted from Veatch, D., "When Is the Recovering Impaired Nurse Ready to Work? A Job Interview Guide," *JONA*, 17(2):14–16, 1987.

6. Nurses and managers traditionally have been slow to recognize and reluctant to reach out and help their colleagues who are impaired.

7. It is easier for an employee to hide alcoholism than drug addiction.

8. Confrontation of an employee suspected of chemical impairment should always occur before the problem escalates beyond approach or before patient safety is jeopardized.

9. The manager should *not* assume the role of counselor or treatment provider or feel the need to diagnose the cause of the chemical addiction. The manager's role is to clearly identify performance expectations for the employee and to confront the employee when those expectations are not met.

10. There are phases or progressive observable behaviors that the manager should be able to observe in evaluating whether the recovering impaired employee is ready to return to the work setting. Many experts feel that impaired employees must devote at least 1 year to their recovery without the stresses of drug availability, overtime, and shift rotation.

REFERENCES

Bissell L., "Alcoholism and the Health Professional," Paper presented at the Summer School on Alcohol Studies, Rutgers University, June 27, 1979.

Buxton, M., and Jessup, M., "The Development of Peer Support Group in California: Recovery Is Possible," unpublished, 1982.

Buxton, M., and Jessup, M., Unpublished Survey in the San Francisco Support Group for Chemically Dependent Nurses, 1983.

Buxton, M., Jessup, M., and Landry, M., "Treatment of the Chemically Dependent Health Professional," in Milkman, H., and Shaffer, H. (eds.), *The Addictions: Multi-disciplinary Perspectives and Treatments*, Lexington Books, D.C. Heath and Company, Lexington, MA, 1985.

Curtin, L., "Throw Away Nurses: Editorial Opinion," *Nursing Management* 18(7):7–8, 1987.

Doyle, S., "How Managers Can Help," in Leffler, D., "Addicted Nurses: How You Can Lend Them a Helping Hand," *Nursing Life*, 6(3):41–43, 1986.

Fox, J.D., "Narcotic Addiction Among Physicians," *Journal of the Michigan Medical Society*, 56:214–217, 1957.

Hutchinson, S.A., "Chemically Dependent Nurses: Implications for Nurse Executives," *JONA*, 17(9):23–29, 1987.

Jaffe, S., "Help for the Helper: First-Hand Views of Recovery," *AJN*, 82(4):578–579, 1982.

Jefferson, L.V., and Ensor, B.E., "Help for the Helper: Confronting a Chemically Impaired Colleague," *AJN*, 82(4):574-577, 1982.

Landry, M., "The Impaired Nurse," *California Nursing Review*, 9(6): 14–18, 1987.

Leffler, D., "Addicted Nurses: How You Can Lend Them a Helping Hand," *Nursing Life*, 6(3):41–43, 1986.

Modlin, H.C., and Montes, A., "Narcotics Addiction in Physicians," *The American Journal of Psychiatry*, 121:358–363, 1964.

Morse, R.M., Martin, M.A., Swenson, W. M., and Niven, R.G., "Prognosis of Physicians Treated for Alcoholism and Drug Dependence," *Journal of the American Medical Association*, 251(6):743-746, 1984.

Murray, R.M., "Psychiatric Illnesses in Doctors," *Lancet*, 1: 1211–1213, 1974.

Naegle, M.A., "Drug and Alcohol Abuse in Nursing: An Occupational Hazard?" *Nursing Life*, 8(1):42–54, 1988.

O'Connor, P., "Managing Impaired Nurses," *Nursing Administration Quarterly*, 9(2):1–6, 1985.

Poplar, J.F., "Characteristics of Nurse Addicts," *AJN*, 16(1): 117–119, 1969.

Robbins, C.E., "A Monitored Treatment Program for Impaired Health Care Professionals," *JONA*, 17(2):17–21, 1987.

Robinson, M., and Spicer, J.G., "Impaired Employee – Confrontation Process," in Lewis, E.M., and Spicer, J.G., *Human Resource Management Handbook*, Aspen Publications, Rockville, MD, 1987, pp. 217–227.

Veatch, D., "When is the Recovering Impaired Nurse Ready to Work?: A Job Interview Guide," *JONA*, 17(2):14–16, 1987.

ADDITIONAL READINGS

American Nurses' Association, *Addictions and Psychological Dysfunctions in Nursing: The Profession's Response to the Problem*, Kansas City, MO, 1985.

Bilski, A., "Substance Abuse in Nursing: How to Recognize It, What to Do," *Imprint*, 32(2):42–47, 1985.

Creighton, H., "Legal Implications of the Impaired Nurse – Part II," *Nursing Management*, 19(2):20–21, 1988.

Naegle, M.A., "Impaired Nursing Practice: Ethical and Legal Issues," *Imprint*, 32(2):48–56, 1985.

Neill, M.M., "Impaired Employee – Administrative Strategy," in Lewis, E.M., and Spicer, J.G., *Human Resource Management Handbook*, Aspen Publications, Rockville, MD, 1987, pp. 229–246.

Shaffer, S., "Attitudes and Perceptions Held by Impaired Nurses," *Nursing Management*, 19(4):46–50, 1988.

Tobin, B., "What Our Readers Said About Entrapping a Colleague," *Nursing Life*, 5(3):54–55, 1985.

▪ UNIT NINE
Ethical Considerations of Human Resource Management

HUMAN RESOURCE management is in essence the manipulation of human resources to meet both organizational and individual goals. Human resource management is easiest when physical, fiscal, and human resources are abundant. Unfortunately, in an age of cost containment and health care worker shortages, managers are forced to make many decisions regarding how limited resources can be used most appropriately. Any time there are limited or inadequate resources, the decisions made about how to utilize those resources involves an ethical component.

Ethics is defined by the *World Book Dictionary* (1979) as "the study of standards of right or wrong; that part of philosophy dealing with moral conduct, duty, and judgment." This definition leads the reader to believe that if managers are ethical or understand ethical concepts, they will always know right and wrong solutions to every problem. Unfortunately, this view is simplistic, because what is "right" in one situation may be totally wrong in the next situation. Human resource management presents many confounding variables that influence how a problem should be solved. Because there is no one best way to manage human resources, managers must select from among alternatives what is most appropriate at any given time for a particular unit. Often these problems have several equally desirable or undesirable alternatives.

For example, in the last ten years many changes have occurred in the health care industry in response to inadequate fiscal resources. As a result of inadequate federal fiscal resources, diagnostic-related groupings (DRGs) were implemented. Hospitals and other health care providers are now reimbursed for their services based on the Medicare patient's diagnosis and not on the acuity of their illness or length of stay. Although the implementation of DRGs may have eased or reduced the strain on governmental fiscal resources, it has created new ethical problems such as patient dumping, premature patient discharge, and inequality of care. There is cause to be concerned that this decision, as well as other major and sweeping health care decisions related to inadequate resources, have been made without adequate reflection about what new ethical concerns will be generated as a result.

The health care industry is now facing another crisis regarding inadequate resources, that of inadequate human resources — the nursing shortage. Already, organizations and managers have made quick, poorly thought out decisions to find short-term solutions to this long-term and severe problem. New workers have been recruited at a phenomenally high cost without development of solutions to the problems that caused high worker attrition in the first place. Managers must learn how to solve problems and make decisions about how to best utilize their limited resources. Because limited resources force choices, managers must expect to be confronted with many human resource management decisions that have an ethical component. Managers must be proactive in learning to use ethical frameworks and principles to assist them in this problem solving. These ethical frameworks and principles will assist managers in assessing the ethical impact of their decisions before they make them.

REFERENCES

World Book Dictionary, Volume One A–K, C. Barnhart and R. Barnhart (eds.), World-Book Childcraft International, Chicago, 1979.

24

Ethical Decision-Making in Human Resource Management

BECAUSE MANAGERS must make many difficult human resource management decisions, it is essential that they have good problem-solving and decision-making skills. When these decisions involve an ethical component, the decision-making process becomes even more complex, and the ramifications of making a "good" or a "bad" decision increase. Thus, managers must learn to use decision-making principles that result not only in high-quality decisions, but also in interpersonal satisfaction.

Learning how to make good decisions requires that individuals understand some basic principles regarding decision-making. One such principle is that the speed and ease of decision-making have no direct correlation with the quality of decision-making. Some individuals make decisions very quickly and easily, the resulting choices being of poor quality; others make good decisions seemingly effortlessly. Some persons agonize over each and every decision, yet still make poor choices. Lastly, some individuals delay making any decision and find that a positive outcome occurs anyway (i.e., problem resolves itself).

Much of the difficulty individuals have in making decisions can be attributed to a lack of formal education about decision-making principles and how to solve problems. Because many of the decisions that managers make have far-reaching implications, it is important that nurse managers not make decisions using trial and error. Trial-and-error decision-making does help some managers learn to make good decisions, but much is left to chance, and the cost to the decision-maker may be significant.

In addition to using trial and error, the inexperienced decision-maker frequently makes another decision-making error in utilizing the outcome of the decision as the sole basis for determining whether, in fact, the decision was a good one. Outcomes should never be used as the sole criteria in assessing the quality of the problem solving, as many variables affect outcome that have no reflection on whether the problem solving was appropriate.

Of all the far-reaching decisions nurse managers must make, perhaps the most important are human resource management decisions with ethical ramifications. These decisions must be made using a professional approach that eliminates trial and error and that focuses on proven decision-making models or problem-solving processes. Managers must be taught to use these models and processes in ethical problem solving. Using a systematic approach to problem solving allows managers to make better decisions and increases the probability that they will feel good about the decisions they have made.

There are many systematic approaches to ethical problem solving that are appropriate for the nurse manager. These approaches include the use of theoretical problem solving and decision-making models, ethical frameworks, and ethical principles. Human resource management case studies that involve ethical decisions will be presented in this chapter and analyzed according to these approaches. In addition, ethical concerns in human resource management, which have been suggested in various chapters of this book, will be summarized. Tools for implementation include two ethical human resource management case studies for managers to use for group and individual problem solving.

PROBLEM-SOLVING AND DECISION-MAKING MODELS

Although the terms *problem solving* and *decision-making* are frequently used interchangeably, they are distinctly different. Problem solving is an attempt to identify the root of a problem in situations and requires that time and energy be spent in eliminating the underlying problem. Decision-making in contrast, is triggered by a problem and results in a decision being made but may not involve examination of the underlying cause of the problem or any attempt to correct it (Marquis and Huston, 1987). If the manager feels that he or she can eliminate the problem itself, a problem-solving model is probably most appropriate. If the manager must take immediate action and make a decision regarding the consequences of some problem, or if the problem itself is unimportant or temporary, a decision-making model may be most appropriate.

The Traditional Problem-Solving Process

Although not recognized specifically as an "ethical" problem-solving model, one of the oldest and most frequently used tools for problem solving is the traditional problem-solving process. This process consists of seven steps, the actual decision being made at Step 5 (Table 24-1). Although many individuals use at least some of the steps in this model in their decision-making, they frequently fail to generate an adequate number of alternatives for analysis or to evaluate the results, two essential steps in the process.

Table 24-1.   Traditional Problem-Solving Process

1. Identify the problem
2. Gather data to analyze the causes and consequences of the problem
3. Explore alternative solutions
4. Evaluate the alternatives
5. Select the appropriate solution
6. Implement the solution
7. Evaluate the results

The following case study provides an example of how the traditional problem-solving process might be applied in reaching a human resource management decision with ethical ramifications.

THE CASE: THE MARGINAL EMPLOYEE

You are the oncology supervisor in a 400-bed hospital. There are 35 beds on your unit, which is generally full. It is an extremely busy unit, and your staff needs high-level assessment and communication skills in providing patient care. Because the nursing care needs on this floor are unique, and because you utilize primary nursing, it has been very difficult in the past to float staff from other units when additional staffing was required. Although you have been able to keep the unit adequately staffed on a day-to-day basis, there are two open positions for registered nurses on your unit that have been unfilled for almost 3 months. Historically, your staff have been excellent employees. They enjoy their work and are highly productive. Unit morale has been exceptionally good. However, in the last 3 months, the staff have begun complaining about "Judy," a full-time employee who has been working on the unit for about 4 months. Judy has been a registered nurse for about 15 years and has worked in oncology units at other facilities. References from former employers identified Judy's work as competent, although little other information was given. At Judy's 6-week and 3-month performance appraisals, you coached her regarding her barely adequate work habits, assessment and communication skills, and decision-making. Judy responded that she would attempt to work on improving her performance in these areas, as working on this unit was one of her highest career goals. Although Judy has been receptive to your coaching and has verbalized to you her efforts to improve her performance, there has been little observable difference in her behavior. You have slowly reached the conclusion that Judy is probably currently working at as high a level as she is capable and that she is a marginal employee at best. The other staff feel that Judy is not carrying her share of the workload and have asked that you remove her from the unit.

ANALYSIS

1. *Identify the problem.* The marginal performance of one employee is affecting the morale on the unit.

2. *Gather data to analyze the causes and consequences of the problem.* The following information should be gathered and considered by the nursing manager:

- Judy has been a registered nurse for 15 years and probably has always been a marginal employee.

- Judy states she is highly motivated to be an oncology nurse.

- Judy has been coached on several occasions regarding how she might improve her performance, and no improvement has been seen.

- It is difficult to recruit and retain staff nurses for this unit.

- The unit is already short two full-time RN positions.

- Judy's performance is not unsatisfactory; it is only marginal.

- Judy is the only marginal employee on the unit at this time.

- The other nurses on the floor considered Judy's performance to be disruptive enough to ask you to remove her from the floor.

3. *Explore alternative solutions.*

Alternative 1 – Terminate Judy's employment.

Alternative 2 – Transfer Judy to another floor.

Alternative 3 – Continue coaching Judy and help her identify specific and realistic goals about her performance.

Alternative 4 – Do nothing and hope that the problem resolves itself.

Alternative 5 – Work with the other staff nurses to create a work environment that will make Judy want to be transferred from the floor.

4. *Evaluate the alternatives.*

Alternative 1 – Although this would provide a rapid solution to the problem, there are many negative aspects to this alternative. Judy, although performing at a marginal level, has not done anything that warrants severe discipline or termination. Even though some staff have requested her removal from the unit, this action could be viewed as arbitrary and grossly unfair by a silent minority, decreasing employees' sense of security and unit morale even more. In addition, it would be difficult to fill Judy's position.

Alternative 2 — This alternative would immediately remove the problem and would probably please the staff. However, this alternative merely transfers the problem to a different unit, which is counterproductive to organizational goals. This might be an appropriate alternative if the supervisor could show that Judy could be expected to perform at a higher level on another unit. It is difficult to predict how Judy would feel about this alternative. Judy is probably aware of the other staff's frustration with her, and a transfer would provide at least temporary shelter from her colleagues' hostility. In addition, although Judy would be pleased at not being terminated, she would appropriately view the transfer as a negative reinforcement of her behavior. This recognition is demoralizing, and the opportunity for her to fulfill a long-term career goal would be denied.

Alternative 3 — This alternative requires a long-term and time-consuming commitment on the part of the manager. There is inadequate information given in the case to determine whether the supervisor can make this type of commitment, although it is significant that Judy would be the only marginal employee that the supervisor would have to work with. This would not be a realistic alternative if there were several marginal employees on a unit in terms of reduced unit productivity and supervisory time needed for coaching. In addition, there is no guarantee that setting short-term, specific, and realistic goals will improve Judy's work performance. It should, however, increase Judy's self-esteem and reinforce her supervisor's interests in her as a person. It also retains a registered nurse who is difficult to replace. This alternative does not address the staff's dissatisfaction.

Alternative 4 — There are few positive aspects to this alternative other than that the supervisor would not have to expend energy at this point. The problem, however, will probably snowball and unit morale will get worse.

Alternative 5 — Although most individuals would agree that this alternative is morally corrupt, there are some advantages. Judy would voluntarily leave the unit and the supervisor and staff would not have to deal with the problem. The disadvantages are similar to those cited in Alternative 1.

5. *Select the appropriate solution.* As in most decisions with an ethical component, there is no one right answer, and, in fact, all the alternatives have desirable and undesirable facets. Alternative 3 probably presents the least number of undesirable attributes. The cost to the supervisor is in time

and effort. She really has little to lose in attempting this plan to increase employee productivity, since there are no replacements to fill the position anyway. Losing Judy by termination or transfer merely increases the workload of the other employees due to short staffing. It also does not help the employee.

6. *Implement the solution.* In implementing Alternative 3, the supervisor should be very clear with Judy about her motives. She must also be sure that the goals they set are specific and realistic. Although the staff may continue to verbalize their unhappiness with Judy's performance, the supervisor should be careful not to discuss confidential information about Judy's coaching plan with them. She should, however, reassure the staff that she is aware of their concerns and that she will follow the situation closely.

7. *Evaluate the results.* The supervisor elected to review her problem solving 6 months after the plan was implemented. She found that although Judy was satisfied with her performance and appreciative of her supervisor's efforts, that performance had not improved appreciably. Judy continued to be a marginal employee but was meeting minimal competency levels. In this time, the supervisor did gain a better understanding of the cost to the unit of a marginal employee in terms of reduced productivity and supervisory time. The supervisor did find, however, that in time, the staff had become more accepting of Judy's level of ability and rarely verbalized their dissatisfaction with her anymore. In general, unit morale increased again.

It is important to recognize that even if the outcome of the selected alternative had negative consequences, the supervisor did make a "good" decision. It was a "good" decision because she utilized a structured approach to problem solving. This structured approach resulted in her gathering a great deal of important information about the problem, which she then utilized in thoroughly analyzing multiple alternatives. Regardless of the outcome, the supervisor could feel comfortable that she made the best possible decision at the time with the information and resources she had available.

The Nursing Process

Another problem-solving model not specifically designed for, but appropriate for, ethical analysis is the nursing process. Most nurses are aware of the nursing process and the cyclic nature of its components of assessment, planning, implementation, and evaluation (see Figure 24-1). However, most nurses do not recognize its use as a decision-making tool. The cyclic nature of the nursing process allows for feedback to occur in the decision-making at any step in the process. It also allows the cycle to repeat itself until adequate information is gathered to make a decision. It does not, however, require clear problem identification. The following case-study analysis shows how the nursing process might be used as an ethical decision-making tool.

THE CASE: ONE APPLICANT TOO MANY

The reorganization of the Public Health Agency has resulted in the creation of a new position of community health liaison. A job description has been written, and notice of the job opening has been posted. As the chief nursing executive of this agency, you will be responsible for selecting the best individual for the position. Because you are aware that all hiring decisions have some subjectivity, you want to eliminate as much personal bias as possible in making your decision. Two individuals have applied for the position, and one of these individuals is a close personal friend.

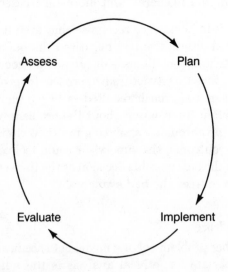

FIGURE 24-1. *The nursing process*

ANALYSIS

Assess. As the nursing executive, you have a responsibility to make personnel decisions as objectively as you can. This means that the hiring decision should be based solely upon which employee is best qualified for the position. You do recognize, however, that there may be a personal cost in terms of the friendship.

Plan. You must plan how you are going to collect this data. The tools you have selected are applications, résumés, references, and personal interviews.

Implement. Both applicants are contacted and asked to submit personal résumés and three letters of references from recent employers. In addition, both candidates are scheduled for structured format interviews with you and two of the board members of the agency. Although these board members will be asked to provide feedback regarding the applicant interviews, you have reserved the right to make the final hiring decision.

Evaluate. As a result of your plan, you have discovered that both candidates meet the minimal requirements posted for the job. One candidate clearly has higher level communication skills; the other candidate (your friend) has more experience in public health and is more knowledgeable regarding the resources of your community. Both employees have complied with the request to submit résumés and letters of reference, and these are of similar quality.

Assess. Your assessment of the situation is that you need more information to make the best possible decision. You must assess whether strong communication skills or public health experience and familiarity with the community would be most valuable in this position.

Plan. You plan how you can gather more information about what the employee will be doing in this newly created position.

Implement. If the job description is inadequate in providing this information, it may be necessary to backtrack and perform job analysis and job design. You may want to gather information from other public health agencies with a similar job classification.

Evaluate. Through job design and job analysis, you now feel that excellent communication skills are absolutely essential for the job. The candidate who has these skills also has an acceptable level of public health experience and seems motivated to learn more about the community and its resources. This means that your friend will not receive the job.

Assess. Now it is necessary for you to assess whether a good decision has been made.

Plan. You plan to evaluate your decision in 6 months using the established job description as a basis for your evaluation criteria.

Implement. You are unable to implement your plan, as this employee resigns unexpectedly 4 months after she has taken the position. Your friend is now working in a similar capacity in another state. Although you correspond on an infrequent basis, the relationship has changed as a result of your decision.

Evaluate. Did you make a good decision? This decision was based on a carefully thought out process, which included adequate data gathering and a weighting of alternatives. Variables beyond your control resulted in the employee's resignation, and there was no apparent reason for you to suspect that this would happen. The decision to exclude or minimize personal bias was a conscious one, and you were aware of the possible ramifications of this choice. The decision-making appears to have been appropriate.

Because the nursing process is so effective as a general decision-making tool, many authors have adapted the nursing process in some way to develop frameworks or tools that focus specifically on ethical decision-making. Two of these tools include the MORAL Decision-Making Model and Murphy and Murphy's Approach to Ethical Decision-Making.

The MORAL Decision-Making Model

The MORAL decision-making model, developed by Crisham (1985), is a model for ethical decision-making that incorporates the nursing process and principles of biomedical ethics. This model is especially useful in clarifying ethical problems that occur as a result of conflicting obligations. Managers frequently have conflicting obligations as a result of their differing responsibilities to patients, subordinates, self, and the organization. The MORAL model could appropriately have been used with the case study "One Applicant Too Many," as the manager experienced interpersonal conflict regarding her obligation to herself, her "friend and colleague," the other applicant, and the organization.

This model is represented by the mnemonic MORAL, representing:

M – Massage the dilemma; collect data about the ethical problem and who should be involved in the decision-making process.

O — Outline options; identify alternatives and analyze the causes and consequences of each.

R — Review criteria and resolve; weigh the options against the values of those involved in the decision. This may be done through a weighting or grid.

A — Affirm position and act; develop the strategy for implementation.

L — Look back; evaluate the decision-making.

The assessment phase of the nursing process is reflected in *M*assaging the dilemma. Planning occurs in the *O*utline of options and the *R*eview of criteria. The implementation phase of the nursing process is apparent in *A*ffirming one's position and acting; evaluation, the last step of the nursing process, corresponds with *L*ooking back. Another ethical problem-solving tool that is built upon the nursing process is Murphy and Murphy's approach to ethical decision-making.

The Murphy and Murphy Approach to Ethical Decision-Making

Murphy and Murphy (1976) developed the following systematic approach to ethical decision-making:

1. Identify the problem.
2. Identify why the problem is an ethical problem.
3. Identify the people involved in the ultimate decision.
4. Identify the role of the decision-maker.
5. Consider the short-term and long-term consequences of each alternative.
6. Make the decision.
7. Compare the decision with the decision-maker's philosophy of ethics.
8. Follow up on the results of the decision in order to establish a baseline for future decision-making.

This type of systematic decision-making approach differs from problem-solving models already discussed, as it does not attempt to solve the underlying problem. It is a decision-making model, as it requires that a decision be made. It is also specifically geared for ethical decision-making, as it helps the decision-maker clarify the basic beliefs and values of the individuals involved. The following case study analysis should help the reader understand how the Murphy and Murphy approach could be used in making a human resource management decision with ethical ramifications.

THE CASE: LITTLE WHITE LIES?

Sam is the nurse recruiter for a metropolitan hospital, which is experiencing an acute nursing shortage. He has been told to do whatever, or to say whatever, is necessary to recruit professional nurses so that the hospital will not have to close several units. He has also been told that his position will be eliminated if he does not produce a substantial number of applicants as a result of nursing career days that will be held the following week. Sam loves his job and is the sole provider for his family. Because many other organizations besides the one he is representing are experiencing severe shortages, the competition for employees is keen. After his third career day without a single prospective applicant, he begins to feel desperate. On the fourth and final day, Sam begins making many promises to potential applicants regarding shift preference, unit preference, salary, and advancement that he is not sure he can keep. At the end of the day, Sam has a lengthy list of interested applicants but also feels a great deal of interpersonal conflict.

ANALYSIS

1. *Identify the problem.* In a desperate effort to save his job, Sam finds he has taken action that has resulted in high interpersonal conflict regarding his values.

2. *Identify why the problem is an ethical problem.* This is an ethical problem because it involves personal values and beliefs, has far-reaching implications for all the individuals involved, and presents several alternatives for decision-making that are either equally desirable or undesirable.

3. *Identify the people involved in the ultimate decision.* Sam has the ultimate responsibility for knowing his values and acting in a manner that is congruent with his value system. The organization is, however, involved in the value conflict in that the organization's values and expectations are in conflict with Sam's. The potential applicants are also involved in this conflict, as there is some responsibility by Sam and the organization to these applicants, although this responsibility is one of the values in conflict.

4. *Identify the role of the decision-maker.* Because this is Sam's problem, and it is an interpersonal conflict, he must

decide the appropriate course of action. His primary role is to examine his values and act in accordance with those values.

5. *Consider the short-term and long-term consequences of each alternative.* Sam has several alternatives:

Alternative 1 — Quit his job immediately. This would prevent *future* interpersonal conflict provided that Sam became aware of his value system and behaved in a manner consistent with that value system in the future. It would not, however, solve the immediate conflict about the action Sam has already taken, and it would take away Sam's livelihood.

Alternative 2 — Do nothing. Sam could choose not to be accountable for his own actions. This would require that Sam rationalize that the philosophy of the organization is in fact acceptable or that he has no choice regarding his actions. The responsibility for meeting the needs and wants of the new employees would thus be shifted to the hospital, although Sam would have no credibility with the new employees. This alternative would have a negligible impact on his ability to recruit, at least on a short-term basis. Sam would continue to have a job and be able to support his family.

Alternative 3 — If, after value clarification, Sam has determined that his values are in conflict with the hospital's directive to do whatever, or say whatever, to recruit new employees, he could approach his superior and share these concerns. Sam should be very clear about what his values are and to what extent he is willing to compromise those values. He also should include in this meeting what, if any, action should be taken to meet the needs of the new applicant employees. It is important for Sam to be realistic about the time and effort usually required to change the values and beliefs of an organization. He also must be aware of his bottom line if the organization is not willing to provide a compromise resolution.

Alternative 4 — Sam could contact each of the applicants and tell them that it may not be possible to keep recruitment promises, but that he will do what he can to see that they are fulfilled. This alternative is risky. The applicants would probably become suspicious of both the recruiter and the organization, and Sam has little formal power at this point to fulfill their requests. This alternative also requires a time and energy commitment by Sam and does not prevent the problem from recurring.

6. *Make the decision.* Sam elected Alternative 3.

7. *Compare the decision with the decision-maker's philosophy of ethics.* In value clarification, Sam discovered that he valued truth telling. Alternative 3 allows Sam to present a recruiting plan to his superior that includes a bottom line that this value will not be violated.

8. *Follow up on the results of the decision in order to establish a baseline for future decision-making.* Sam approached his superior and was told that his beliefs were idealistic and inappropriate in an age of severe worker shortages. Sam was terminated. However, Sam felt that he had made an appropriate decision. He did become self-aware regarding his values and had attempted to communicate these values to the organization in an effort to work out a mutually agreeable plan. Although Sam was terminated, he knew that he could find some type of employment to meet immediate fiscal needs. Sam also utilized what he had learned in this decision-making process, in that he planned to more carefully evaluate the recruitment philosophy of the organization in relation to his own value system before accepting another job.

ETHICAL FRAMEWORKS FOR DECISION-MAKING

In addition to problem-solving and decision-making models, ethical frameworks for decision-making can assist managers in problem solving. These frameworks do not solve ethical problems, but they assist the individuals involved in problem solving to clarify their values and beliefs. Four of the most commonly used ethical frameworks are utilitarianism, duty-based reasoning, rights-based reasoning, and intuitionism (Marquis and Huston, 1987).

Using an ethical framework of *utilitarianism* encourages managers to make decisions based on what provides the greatest good for the greatest number of individuals. Managers using a utilitarian approach take action that stresses unit and organizational goals over individual goals. In the case study, "The Marginal Employee," the utilitarian manager might have appropriately dismissed Judy because of her low productivity and need for valuable supervisory time, which represented a significant cost at both the unit and organizational level. In "Little White Lies?", the organization might also have used utilitarianism to justify lying to employee applicants. This would be based on the fact that hiring new employees would benefit current employees, since it would help keep units in the hospital open.

According to *duty-based reasoning*, some decisions must be made because there is a duty to do what is right. There is a duty either to do something or to refrain from doing something. In the case "One Applicant Too Many," the supervisor felt a duty to hire the best qualified individual for the job, even if the personal cost was high. In "The Marginal Employee," the supervisor felt a duty to help Judy perform at the highest level possible through coaching. In doing so, she refrained from dismissing her as an employee.

Rights-based reasoning is based on the belief that some things are a person's just due; that is, that each individual has basic claims or entitlements that should not be interfered with. Rights are different from needs, wants, or desires. In "Little White Lies?" Sam felt that all individuals have the right to truth and, in fact, that he had the duty to be truthful. The supervisor in "One Applicant Too Many" felt that both applicants had the right to fair and impartial consideration of their applications.

The *intuitionist framework* allows the decision-maker to review each ethical problem or issue on a case-by-base basis, comparing the relative "weights" of goals, duties, and rights. This weighting is determined primarily by intuition, what the decision-maker feels is right for that particular situation. All of the cases solved in this chapter have involved some degree of decision-making by intuition.

PRINCIPLES OF ETHICAL DECISION-MAKING

Decision-makers may also use moral and ethical principles to assist them in systematically examining ethical issues. These principles of ethical reasoning, as they are called, further explore and define what beliefs or values form the basis for decision-making. Among the ethical principles identified by ethical theorists are the following:

1. *Autonomy.* This principle, a form of personal liberty, is also referred to as freedom of choice or accepting the responsibility for one's choice. The legal right of self-determination

supports this moral principle. The use of progressive discipline recognizes the autonomy of the employee. The employee, in essence, has the choice to meet organizational expectations or to be disciplined further. If the employee's continued behavior warrants termination, the principle of autonomy says that the employee made the choice to be terminated by virtue of his or her actions, not the manager's.

2. *Beneficence.* This principle states that the actions one takes should be done in an effort to promote good. The concept of nonmaleficence, which is associated with beneficence, says that if one cannot do good, then at least one should do no harm. Performance appraisals provide an example of how the manager might apply the concept of beneficence. The manager who uses this ethical principle in planning performance appraisals is much more likely to be focused on the performance appraisal as a means of promoting employee growth.

3. *Paternalism.* This principle is related to positive beneficence in that one individual assumes the authority to make a decision for another individual. Because paternalism limits freedom of choice, most ethical theorists feel paternalism is justified only to prevent an individual from coming to harm. Unfortunately, some managers use the principle of paternalism in subordinate career planning. In doing so, the manager may assume he or she has greater knowledge than the employee about what that employee's short- and long-term goals should be.

4. *Utility.* This principle reflects a belief in utilitarianism or the belief that what is best for the common good outweighs what is best for the individual. This principle justifies paternalism as a means of restricting the freedom of the individual. If the manager uses the principle of utility as a guiding belief in decision-making, the manager may become less humanistic and more focused on production.

5. *Justice.* This principle states that equals should be treated equally and unequals should be treated according to their differences. This principle is frequently applied when there are scarcities or competition for resources or benefits. The manager who uses the principle of justice will work to see that pay raises are reflective of performance and not just time of service.

6. *Truth telling and deception.* These principles are used to explain how the individual feels about the need for truth telling or the acceptability of deception. A manager who feels that deception is morally acceptable if it is done with

the objective of beneficence may tell all applicants rejected for a specific job that they were strongly considered, whether or not that is true.

ETHICAL DIMENSIONS IN HUMAN RESOURCE MANAGEMENT

In this book many aspects of human resource management have been discussed, and each chapter could appropriately have included a section on ethical issues or constraints affecting that particular topic. Ethical concerns that have been alluded to have included the following:

Unit I — Chapter 1 discussed the components of human resource management and the challenges faced by organizations in the future in dealing with an inadequate nurse applicant pool. In Chapter 2 individual values and organizational philosophy were identified as primary determinants of behavior, and the reader was strongly encouraged to work in an organization with congruent values and beliefs. Chapter 3 discussed the sometimes overlapping and conflicting responsibility for human resource management at each level of the organizational hierarchy. Examples of ethical concerns or questions generated in this unit included:

■ At what point do the needs of the organization become more important than those of the individual worker?

■ Is it necessary that each employee be assisted to achieve at optimal levels? Can the manager be selective in which employees are assisted to reach optimal productivity?

■ Should employees ever be coerced into changing their stated values to more closely align with those of the organization?

■ How can nursing managers allocate resources fairly in an environment in which virtually all resources are limited?

Unit II — The first chapter in this unit examined planning at the nursing service level and the importance of congruence between nursing service planning and planning at the organizational level. Chapter 5 discussed planning at the unit level in terms of patient care delivery mode, job design, and job analysis. Chapter 6 looked at staffing and scheduling as they affect worker satisfaction and productivity. Examples of ethical concerns or questions generated in this unit include:

■ At what point does short staffing become unsafe?

■ Should shift scheduling be used as a means of reward and punishment?

- Is it ever justified to develop a job or tailor a job description for a specific individual?

Unit III — This unit examined how external constraints, such as legal issues and unionization, affect nursing managers in managing human resources. Examples of ethical concerns or questions generated in this unit include:

- Is it ethical to promote union organizers to management, solely to reduce the possibility of union formation?
- Is affirmative action hiring as compensation for past discrimination ethically justifiable, or does it promote reverse discrimination?
- Should nurses be allowed to strike?

Unit IV — This unit addressed the personnel process of recruitment, interviewing, and selection. Of all the units, the personnel process is probably fraught with the greatest number of ethical concerns, primarily because there is currently an inadequacy of resources available. Examples of ethical concerns generated in this chapter were:

- Is "stealing" employees from other agencies ever ethical?
- How far can the truth be stretched in recruitment advertising before it becomes deceptive?
- Should pre-employment testing be required as a condition of employment?
- Is it ethical for an employee to take a position in an organization if he or she already plans to leave in a short time?
- When it is justified for an employee to lie in an interview?
- Are fringe benefits an employee's right, or are they a reward?

Unit V — This unit discussed the concepts of socialization/resocialization and the more traditional concepts of induction and orientation. Ethical concerns generated as a result of the content in these two chapters included:

- Who has the responsibility for socializing the new graduate into the professional nursing role? Academia, the hospital, or a joint process?
- What commitment does the organization have to the nurse who is reentering the profession after not practicing for many years?
- Should an employee's orientation be continued indefinitely until he or she feels ready to function autonomously?

Unit VI – Unit VI focused on the development of the employee through performance appraisal, coaching, career development, and education. Because the attitudes, values, and beliefs of the manager toward all of these practices has a tremendous impact on their implementation, many ethical concerns can be identified:

■ At what point does the power to evaluate the work of others become unhealthy?

■ Should the individual be allowed total self-determination in short- and long-term career planning?

■ Is it ethical to promote or transfer a less qualified individual in order to keep a valuable employee on a unit?

Unit VII – The three chapters in this unit examined how organizations can create a work environment that is focused on meeting employee needs and that results in high productivity and retention. This is done through the identification and formal education of leaders and managers, and through the provision of a climate that meets both motivator and hygiene needs. Examples of ethical concerns associated with this unit included:

■ To whom do managers owe their primary allegiance: the organization or their subordinates?

■ When is it appropriate to use money as the primary motivator?

■ Which is more important to the organization – good leaders or good managers?

■ If employees are producing at acceptable or higher levels, what new rewards and incentives should be introduced?

Unit VIII – This unit focused on troubled employees, including those who need discipline, those seeking grievance as a means of superior/subordinate conflict resolution, and those who are chemically impaired. Again, the values of the supervisor have a tremendous impact on how troubled employees are managed. For example:

■ Does the organization have an obligation to re-employ chemically impaired employees who seek rehabilitation?

■ Is it ever ethical to file a grievance against another individual for the purpose of harassment?

■ Can discipline administered in anger be fair?

■ When does the employee's right to privacy regarding the use of drugs or alcohol stop and the supervisor's right to that information begin?

- In pursuing beneficence, is it more appropriate to progressively discipline an employee who has made no effort to correct his or her behavior deficiencies or to terminate that employee?

Two case studies are included in Tools 24-1 and 24-2. The reader is encouraged to solve these case studies individually or in groups, using one of the systematic approaches to ethical problem solving that have been presented in this chapter. The reader is also encouraged to address several of the ethical concerns that have been highlighted in reviewing units of this book, as well as other ethical issues that were generated throughout this text. Managers new to structured or systematic ethical problem solving will need to examine many ethical issues or problems before they will be confident regarding their decision-making skills.

KEY CONCEPTS CHAPTER 24

1. Much of the difficulty some individuals have in making ethical decisions can be attributed to a lack of formal education in problem solving and decision-making.

2. There are many systematic approaches to ethical problem solving that are appropriate for the nurse manager. These approaches include the use of theoretical problem-solving and decision-making models, ethical frameworks, and ethical principles.

3. Outcomes should never be used as the sole criterion in assessing the quality of the problem solving, as many variables affect outcome that have no reflection on whether the problem solving was appropriate.

4. In problem solving, an attempt is made to identify the root of a problem, and time and energy are spent to eliminate the problem.

5. Decision-making is triggered by a problem and results in a decision being made, but it may not involve examination of the underlying cause of the problem or any attempt to correct it.

6. Four of the most commonly used ethical frameworks for decision-making are utilitarianism, duty-based reasoning, rights-based reasoning, and intuitionism. These frameworks do not solve ethical problems but assist the individuals involved in problem solving to clarify their values and beliefs.

Tool 24-1   Case Study: The Impaired Employee

You are a middle-level manager in a skilled nursing facility. Beverly is a 35-year-old, full-time nurse on the day shift and has been employed in your facility for ten years. There have been rumors for some time now that Beverly has been coming to work under the influence of alcohol. Staff have reported the smell of alcohol on her breath, unexcused absences from the unit, and an increase in the number of medication errors she has made. You have not directly observed any of these behaviors. When you arrive at work one day, you observe Beverly covertly drinking from a dark-colored flask in her locker. You immediately confront Beverly with your observation and ask her if she is drinking alcohol while on duty. Beverly tearfully admits that she is drinking alcohol but states that this is an isolated incident and begs you to forget it. She promises not to ever consume alcohol at work again.

In an effort to reduce the emotionalism of the event and give yourself time to think, you send Beverly home and schedule a conference with her for later in the day. At this conference, Beverly is defensive and states that she does not have a drinking problem and that you are overreacting. You share the data you have gathered during the day, which supports that Beverly is probably chemically impaired. Beverly offers no explanation for these behaviors. Your plan for Beverly is to suspend her for 2 weeks without pay and to require her to attend three alcohol support group meetings before she can return to work. She is also informed that failure to do so and any further evidence of intoxication while on duty will result in immediate termination. Beverly again becomes very tearful and begs you to reconsider. She states that she is the sole provider for her four small children and that her frequent sick days have taken up all available vacation and sick pay she might have coming. You feel your decision is fair and again encourage Beverly to seek guidance regarding her drinking. Four days later in the newspaper, you read that Beverly committed suicide the day after the meeting.

Questions for analysis:

Evaluate the problem solving of the manager. Would your actions have differed if you were the manager? Are there conflicting legal and ethical obligations? To whom does the manager have the greatest obligation — patients, staff, or the organization? Was there a helping relationship between the manager and Beverly? Could the outcome have been prevented?

Tool 24-2   Case Study: The Valuable Employee

Gina is the supervisor of a 16-bed ICU/CCU in a 200-bed urban hospital. She has been the supervisor for eight years and is respected and well liked by her staff. Her staff retention level and productivity are higher than that of any other unit in the hospital. Gina relies heavily on Mark, her permanent charge nurse on the day shift for the last six years. He is bright, motivated, and has excellent clinical and management skills. Mark seems satisfied and challenged in his current position, although Gina has not had any formal career-planning meetings with Mark to discuss his long-term career goals. It would not be unfair to say that Mark's work has greatly increased Gina's scope of power and enhanced the reputation of the unit.

Recently, one of the physicians approached Gina regarding wanting to open an outpatient cardiac rehabilitation program. The program will require a strong leader and manager who is self-motivated. It will be a lot of work but also provides many opportunities for advancement. He suggests that Mark would be an excellent choice for the job, although he has given Gina full authority to make the final decision.

Gina is aware that Lynn, a bright and dynamic staff nurse from the Open Heart Surgery Floor would also be very interested in the job. Lynn has only been employed at the hospital for 1 year but has a proven track record and would be very successful in the job. In addition, there is a staffing surplus right now on the Open Heart Surgery Floor, as two of the surgeons have recently retired. It would be difficult and time consuming to replace Mark as charge nurse in the CCU/ICU.

Questions for Analysis:

What process should this supervisor pursue to determine who should be hired for the position? Should the position be posted? Is paternalism justified in this case? When does the benefit of using transfers/promotions as a means of reward outweigh the cost of reduced productivity? Could autocratically selecting Lynn be justified by utilitarianism?

---

7. Principles of ethical reasoning explore and define what beliefs or values form the basis of our decision-making. These principles include autonomy, beneficence, paternalism, utility, justice, truth telling, and deception.

REFERENCES

Chrisham, P., "MORAL: How Can I Do What is Right?", cited in Sullivan, E., and Decker, P., *Effective Management in Nursing*, Second Edition, Addison Wesley, Menlo Park, CA, 1988.

Marquis, B. and Huston C., *Management Decision Making for Nurses: 101 Case Studies*, J.B. Lippincott, Philadelphia, 1987.

Murphy, M., and Murphy, J., "Making Ethical Decisions Systematically," *Nursing 76*, 6:13, 1976.

ADDITIONAL READINGS

Aroskar, M., "Anatomy of an Ethical Dilemma: The Theory and Practice," *AJN*, 80(4): 634–658, 1980.

Beauchamp, T., and Childress, J.F., *Principles of Biomedical Ethics*, Oxford University Press, New York, 1983.

Benjamin, M., and Curtis, J., *Ethics in Nursing*, Oxford University Press, New York, 1981.

Corey, G., Corey, M.S., and Callahan, P. *Issues and Ethics in the Helping Professions*, Third Edition, Brooks/Cole, Pacific Grove, CA, 1988.

Curtin, L., "Ethics in Nursing Administration," in Marriner, A. (ed.), *Contemporary Nursing Management*, C.V. Mosby, St. Louis, 1982.

Curtin, L. Flaherty, M., *Nursing Ethics: Theories and Pragmatics*, Prentice-Hall, Bowie, MD, 1982.

Mappes, T.A., and Zembatty, J. S., *Biomedical Ethics*, Second Edition, McGraw-Hill, New York, 1986.

Quinn, C.A., and Smith, M.D., *The Professional Commitment: Issues and Ethics in Nursing*, W. B. Saunders, Philadelphia, 1987.

Veatch, R.M., and Fry, S.T., *Case Studies in Nursing Ethics*, J. B. Lippincott, Philadelphia, 1987.

Yarling, R.R., and McElmurry, B.J., "The Moral Foundation of Nursing," *Advances in Nursing Science*, 8(2):63–73, 1986.

management development, 314–317,
318–319
needs assessment and, 312–313
staff development, 313–314
theories of learning and, 306–310
education department, responsibilities of,
305–306
education differential, 365
Edwards Personal Preference Schedule,
197
effectiveness report, 241. *See also*
performance appraisal
emotional stress, 10–11
employee assistance programs, 374, 375
employee handbook, 210, 211, 212–213
employee indoctrination, 207–236
defined, 207
induction, 207, 209–211, 213–214
orientation, 207, 209–210, 211–220
purposes of, 208
socialization/resocialization, 207,
223–235
employee releases, 294
employer policy violations, 410
employment process, 149–204
interviewing, 150, 171–184
recruitment, 149–150, 153–168
selection and placement, 150, 185–204
encouraging manager, 351–353, 355–356
entrepreneur role of manager, 336
environment, organizational, 27–28
external, 61–65
fairness of, 412, 414
internal, 60–61, 62–63
motivation and, 349–357
positive, 371–372
Equal Employment Opportunity
Commission (EEOC), 141
equal employment opportunity (EEO)
laws, 136, 139–144
Equal Pay Act of 1963, 138
essay performance appraisal, 249–251
ethical decision-making, 439–462. *See*
also values
case studies in, 461–462
ethical frameworks for, 454–455
in human resource management,
457–460
MORAL model for, 450–451
Murphy and Murphy approach to,
451–454
principles of, 455–457
in recruitment, 165, 168
ETSA, 194
Executive Orders
10988 (Kennedy), 121
11246 (Johnson), 140
11375 (Johnson), 140
expectancy model (Vroom), 344–346

external environment, 61–65
extrinsic motivation, 348–349

facilitator, 405
fact finding, 131
fair employment legislation, 141
Fair Labor Standards Act (FLSA),
137–138
falsehoods, 389, 456–457
featherbedding, 139
Federal Mediation and Conciliation
Service, 402, 406
feedback, 263, 348, 350. *See also*
performance appraisal
Fielder, F., 328–329
fighting, 389
figurehead role of manager, 332
first-level managers, 38, 39–40, 41
fiscal accountability, for middle-level
managers, 107–113
forced distribution ranking, 246–247
forecasting, 94
formal grievance process, 404–406
free-form review, 249–251
free speech, law on, 130
fringe benefits, 167, 364–369
FTE (full-time equivalent), 110
functional nursing, 76–77

Gellerman, S. W., 346–347
George Washington University Series
Nursing Tests, 195
goals and objectives
examples of, 66, 67
planning and, 54, 57–59
writing, 65
grievance process, 126–127, 394, 395,
401–415
arbitration in, 130, 400, 402–403,
406–407
formal, 404–406
informal, 401–404
rights and responsibilities in, 411–415
rules for positive outcome of, 413–414
unions and, 401, 404–405, 406,
409–411
grievances, 130, 394, 395, 399–415
common, 408–409, 410
defined, 407–408
gripes, 407–408. *See also* grievances
Guilford-Zimmerman Temperament
Survey, 196

"halo" effect, 243
handbook, employee, 210, 211, 212–213
handicapped, legislation protecting, 140,
141–142
Hawthorne effect, 4
health and safety legislation, 144–145

ISBN 0-397-54739-0

9 780397 547395